Surgical Management of Low Back Pain

Second Edition

American Association of Neurological Surgeons

and the American Association of Neurosurgeons

American Association of Neurosurgeons • Rolling Meadows, Illinois

Thieme

Surgical Management of Low Back Pain

Second Edition

Daniel K. Resnick, MD
Associate Professor
Vice Chairman
Department of Neurological Surgery
University of Wisconsin School of Medicine and Public Health
University of Wisconsin Hospital and Clinics
Madison, Wisconsin

Regis W. Haid Jr., MD
Neurosurgeon and Founding Partner
Atlanta Brain and Spine Care
Atlanta, Georgia

Jeffrey C. Wang, MD
Professor
Departments of Orthopaedic Surgery and Neurosurgery
David Geffen School of Medicine
University of California–Los Angeles
Chief, Orthopaedic Spine Service
University of California–Los Angeles Comprehensive Spine Center
Los Angeles, California

Thieme
New York • Stuttgart

American Association of Neurosurgeons
Rolling Meadows, Illinois

Thieme Medical Publishers, Inc.
333 Seventh Ave.
New York, NY 10001

American Association of Neurosurgeons (AANS)*
5550 Meadowbrook Drive
Rolling Meadows, Illinois 60008-3852

The abbreviation AANS refers to both the American Association of Neurological Surgeons and the American Association of Neurosurgeons.

Executive Editor: Kalen Conerly
Associate Editor: Ivy Ip
Vice President, Production and Electronic Publishing: Anne T. Vinnicombe
Production Editor: Print Matters, Inc.
Vice President, International Marketing and Sales and Marketing: Cornelia Schulze
Chief Financial Officer: Peter van Woerden
President: Brian D. Scanlan
Compositor: Aptara
Printer: Maple-Vail Book Manufacturing Group

Library of Congress Cataloging-in-Publication Data

Surgical management of low back pain / [edited by] Daniel K. Resnick, Regis W. Haid, Jeffrey C. Wang.—2nd ed.
p. ; cm.
Includes bibliographical references and index.
ISBN 978-1-60406-035-5 (alk. paper)
1. Backache–Surgery. I. Resnick, Daniel K. II. Haid, Regis W. III. Wang, Jeffrey C.
[DNLM: 1. Low Back Pain—surgery. WE 755 S961 2008]
RD771.B217S874 2008
617.5′64059–dc22

2008018145

Important note: Medical knowledge is ever-changing. As new research and clinical experience broaden our knowledge, changes in treatment and drug therapy may be required. The authors and editors of the material herein have consulted sources believed to be reliable in their efforts to provide information that is complete and in accord with the standards accepted at the time of publication. However, in view of the possibility of human error by the authors, editors, or publisher of the work herein or changes in medical knowledge, neither the authors, editors, or publisher, nor any other party who has been involved in the preparation of this work, warrants that the information contained herein is in every respect accurate or complete, and they are not responsible for any errors or omissions or for the results obtained from use of such information. Readers are encouraged to confirm the information contained herein with other sources. For example, readers are advised to check the product information sheet included in the package of each drug they plan to administer to be certain that the information contained in this publication is accurate and that changes have not been made in the recommended dose or in the contraindications for administration. This recommendation is of particular importance in connection with new or infrequently used drugs.

Some of the product names, patents, and registered designs referred to in this book are in fact registered trademarks or proprietary names even though specific reference to this fact is not always made in the text. Therefore, the appearance of a name without designation as proprietary is not to be construed as a representation by the publisher that it is in the public domain.

The material presented in this publication by the AANS is for educational purposes only. The material is not intended to represent the only, nor necessarily the best, method or procedure appropriate for the medical or socioeconomic situations discussed, but rather it is intended to present an approach, view, statement, or opinion of the faculty, which may be helpful to others who face similar situations.

Neither the content, the use of a specific product in conjunction therewith, nor the exhibition of any materials by any parties coincident with this publication, should be construed as indicating endorsement or approval of the views presented, the products used, or the materials exhibited by the AANS, or its Committees, Commissions, or Affiliates.

Printed in the United States

5 4 3 2 1

ISBN 978-1-60406-035-5

To our wives—Nicole, Betsy, and Christina—for their unwavering support

Contents

Continuing Medical Education Credit Information and Objectives

■ Objectives

Upon completion of this activity, the learner should be able to:

1. Discuss the indications for the performance of common surgical approaches for painful disorders of the lumbar spine.
2. Describe techniques used for the performance of common surgical approaches for painful disorders of the lumbar spine.
3. Describe common complication avoidance maneuvers as well as the management of commonly encountered complications affecting patients treated for disorders of the lumbar spine.

■ Accreditation

This activity has been planned and implemented in accordance with the Essentials and Standards of the Accreditation Council for Continuing Medical Education through the AANS*. The AANS is accredited by the Accreditation Council for Continuing Medical Education to provide continuing medical education for physicians

■ Credit

The AANS designates this educational activity for a maximum of 15 *AMA PRA Category 1 credits*™. Physicians should only claim those hours of credit commensurate with the extent of their participation in the activity.

The Home Study Examination is online on the AANS Web site at:
www.aans.org/education/books/surgicalmgmt.asp

Estimated time to complete this activity varies by learner, and activity equaled up to 15 Category 1 credits of CME.

■ Release/Termination Dates

Original Release Date: **10/15/2008**
The CME termination date is: **10/15/2011**

**The abbreviation AANS refers to both the American Association of Neurological Surgeons and the American Association of Neurosurgeons.*

Continuing Medical Education Disclosure

Disclosure Information

The AANS controls the content and production of this CME activity and attempts to ensure the presentation of balanced, objective information. In accordance with the Standards for Commercial Support established by the Accreditation Council for Continuing Medical Education, authors (and the significant others of those mentioned) are asked to disclose any relationship they or their co-authors have with commercial companies that may be related to the content of their chapter.

Authors (and the significant others of those mentioned) who have disclosed a relationship* with commercial companies whose products may have a relevance to their chapter are listed below.

Author Name	Disclosure	Type of Relationship
Howard S. An	NIH, Rush University Medical Center	University Grant
	Stryker Inc.	Industry Grant Support
	Medtronics	Industry Grant Support
	Depuy Spine	Industry Grant Support
	N Spine Inc.	Stockholder
	ULI Inc.	Stockholder
Paul A. Anderson	Medtronic	Industry Grant Support
	Medtronic	Consultant Fee
	Stryker	Consultant Fee
	Pioneer	Consultant Fee
Ray M. Baker	DePuy	Industry Grant Support, Consultant Fee
	Kyphon	Industry Grant Support, Consultant Fee
	Relievant Medical	Stockholder
	Smith and Nephew	Honorarium
	Baylis Medical	Speaker's Bureau
	BOD NASS and ISIS	Fiduciary Position
Edward C. Benzel	Orthomena	Research Support
	Zimmer	Industry Grant Support
	Mazor	Consultant Fee
	Axiomed	Consultant Fee
	Axiomed	Stockholder

Author Name	Disclosure	Type of Relationship
Richard Guyer	Depuy	Consultant Fee
Regis W. Haid Jr.	Medtronic	Other Financial/Material Support
Robert Heary	Depuy Spine	Industry Grant Support
	Depuy Spine	Consultant Fee
James D. Kang	Sofamor	University Grant
	Medtronics	University Grant
	Danek	University Grant
Mark McLaughlin	Medtronics	Consultant Fee
	Integra Life Sciences	Consultant Fee
	Spine Wave	Consultant Fee
Paul Matz	Synthes Spine	Honorarium
Praveen V. Mummaneni	Medtronic	Honorarium Speaking
	Depuy Spine	Consultant Fee
Steven L. Ondra	Medtronic	Industry Grant Support
	Medtronic	Consultant Fee
	Medtronic	University of Wisconsin
David W. Polly	Medtronic	Consultant Fee
	Medtronic	Speakerís Bureau
	Scoliosis Research Society	Fiduciary Position
	Broadwater	Honorarium
Daniel Resnick	Medtronic	Consultant Fee
Rick Sasso	Medtronic	Research Support
	Stryker	Research Support
	Synthes	Research Support
	Medtronic	Consultant Fee
Michael Steinmetz	Kyphon	Consultant Fee
	Stryker	Honorarium
Jeffrey C. Wang	Synthes	Speaker's Bureau
	Stryker	Speaker's Bureau
Michael Y. Wang	Depuy Spine	University Grant
	Depuy Spine	Consultant Fee
	Aesculap Spine	Consultant Fee

*Relationship refers to receipt of royalties, consultantship, funding by research grant, receiving honoraria for educational services elsewhere, or any other relationship to a commercial company that provides sufficient reason for disclosure.

Authors (and the significant others of those mentioned) who have reported they do not have any relationships with commercial companies:

Author Name:

Dani Bidros
John H. Chi
Richard Derby
Victor Haughton
Jason M. Highsmith
Daniel Hoh
Langston Holly
Alex Hughes
Wellington K. Hsu
David H. Kim
Sanjeev Kumar
Thomas E. Mroz
Prithvi Narayan
Brian A. O'Shaughnessy
Corey A. Pacek
Sharad Rajpal
Alexander Kirk Reichard
Raphael R. Roybal
Edward R. G. Santos
Nirav Shah
Shenil Shah
Gwendolyn Sowa
Eve Tsai
Gregory Trost
Kene Ugokwe

Foreword

Low back pain is one of the most frequent physical ailments suffered by mankind now and in the past. Surgical management of this entity is certainly a last resort. This volume contains chapters not only on surgical techniques, but also, and even more importantly, on patient selection for surgical treatment (Chapter 7), on which fusion techniques are supported by the literature (Chapter 1), and on the pathophysiology of low back pain and its treatment (Chapter 2), which is important to understanding how to treat this entity surgically or nonsurgically.

Other chapters are also valuable but not necessarily directly related to the surgical treatment of low back pain. For example, Chapters 17 and 18 discuss gene therapy and tissue engineering for spinal fusion as well as tissue engineering and strategies for disk regeneration. Controversial treatments, such as interdiskal electrothermal therapy (Chapter 20) and radiofrequency nuclear decompression nucleoplasty (Chapter 21) for low back pain, are also discussed. Chapters 22 and 23 deal with lumbar disk arthroplasty. In both chapters, the authors rightly emphasize that early clinical success with this technique is good (equivalent to spinal fusion) but that good-quality long-term outcome data are unavailable. The remaining chapters nicely describe the different surgical techniques used to fuse the lumbar spine and the importance of maintaining or restoring sagittal balance.

Although low back pain is still difficult to treat, this book makes it easier to understand. It also clearly describes the surgical options that should be considered and which techniques should be in the surgeon's armamentarium. Consequently, this volume should be in the library of every surgeon who considers surgical intervention for the treatment of patients with low back pain.

Volker K. H. Sonntag, MD, FACS
Vice Chairman, Division of Neurological Surgery
Barrow Neurological Institute
Director, Residency Program
Chairman, BNI Spine Section
Clinical Professor of Surgery (Neurosurgery)
University of Arizona
Phoenix, Arizona

Foreword

Over the past decade there have been major advances in the diagnosis and treatment of low back pain and degenerative lumbar disk disease. This text, *Surgical Management of Low Back Pain*, second edition, by Drs. Resnick, Haid, and Wang, is a comprehensive and timely treatise, as it discusses the scientific basis for various treatments and provides a detailed review of the pathophysiology, biomechanics, and various imaging modalities. Of importance to the spine surgeon are the detailed reviews of various operative techniques for treating low back pain.

The scientific analysis of the biology of bone healing that is provided in this book furthers our understanding of the techniques of arthrodesis. A major advance in the performance of fusions has been the introduction of growth factors and bone morphogenic protein.

The importance of the economics of lumbar fusion is also reviewed here, as well as the controversial disk arthroplasty.

I believe this text furthers our understanding of low back pain and will greatly enhance the treatment of this common and disabling disorder.

Henry H. Bohlman, MD
Professor of Orthopaedic Surgery
Case Western Reserve University School of Medicine
Director
The University Hospitals Spine Institute
Cleveland, Ohio

Preface

This text is intended to be used primarily by practicing spinal surgeons as well as residents and fellows who are training to become spinal surgeons. Those interested in the thought processes behind the development of current and evolving technologies, such as corporate representatives and venture capitalists may also benefit from the discussions of evolving technologies and the emphasis on evidence-based review of technologies contained herein. Spinal surgery is an evolving field, and while this text can only capture a snapshot of the current technology and thought, it illustrates the processes used by leading practicing surgeons in choosing the correct procedure for the correct patient. While our ideas and tools will evolve over time, these basic processes will not.

Chapters are organized using a "basic principles to advanced concepts" approach. The initial chapters focus on anatomy, biomechanics, and physiology of back pain and the use of the literature to provide information regarding the effectiveness of our various interventions. A discussion of the latest imaging techniques follows, with updates on magnetic resonance imaging sequences and dynamic imaging. A discussion of the use of diskography immediately follows the imaging chapter, allowing the reader to compare the utility of the various imaging techniques. Individual techniques for the management of back pain are then presented. Traditional, percutaneous, and minimally incisional techniques are discussed with a focus on patient selection, technical pearls, and complication avoidance. The final chapters deal with evolving technologies that may not be familiar to many readers.

The first version of this text was very popular but limited in scope. When it came time to revise the text, we made a concerted effort to include evolving technologies such as arthroplasty, tissue engineering, and gene therapy as well as discussions of cost effectiveness of existing and emerging technologies. The use of minimally incisional techniques and the application of techniques traditionally used for simple degenerative problems to more complex deformities are also new additions. The chapter authors include recognized innovators as well as recognized critics of new technologies in order to provide some balance and perspective.

Daniel K. Resnick, MD
Regis W. Haid Jr, MD
Jeffrey C. Wang, MD

Contributors

Howard S. An, MD
Director and Chair
Department of Orthopedic Surgery
Rush University Medical Center
Chicago, Illinois

Paul A. Anderson, MD
Professor
Department of Orthopaedic Surgery and Rehabilitation
University of Wisconsin School of Medicine and Public Health
Madison, Wisconsin

Ray M. Baker, MD
Clinical Associate Professor
Department of Anesthesiology
University of Washington School of Medicine
Seattle, Washington

Edward C. Benzel, MD
Chair
Department of Neurological Surgery
Director
Center for Spine Health
Neurological Institute
Cleveland Clinic
Cleveland, Ohio

Dani S. Bidros, MD
Resident
Department of Neurological Surgery
Cleveland Clinic
Cleveland, Ohio

John H. Chi, MD, MPH
Instructor
Department of Neurosurgery
Johns Hopkins University School of Medicine
Baltimore, Maryland

Richard Derby, MD
Medical Director
Spinal Diagnostics and Treatment Center
Daly City, California

Richard D. Guyer, MD
Associate Clinical Professor
Department of Orthopaedic Surgery
University of Texas Southwestern Medical School
Dallas, Texas
Texas Back Institute
Plano, Texas

Regis W. Haid Jr., MD
Neurosurgeon and Founding Partner
Atlanta Brain and Spine Care
Atlanta, Georgia

Victor Haughton, MD
Professor
Department of Radiology
University of Wisconsin School of Medicine and Public Health
Madison, Wisconsin

Robert F. Heary, MD
Professor and Program Director
Department of Neurological Surgery
University of Medicine and Dentistry of New Jersey
Newark, New Jersey

Jason M. Highsmith, MD
Charleston Brain and Spine
Charleston, South Carolina

Daniel J. Hoh, MD
Clinical Instructor
Department of Neurological Surgery
Keck School of Medicine
University of Southern California
Los Angeles, California

Langston T. Holly, MD
Assistant Professor
Division of Neurosurgery
David Geffen School of Medicine
University of California–Los Angeles
University of California–Los Angeles Health System
Los Angeles, California

Wellington K. Hsu, MD
Clinical Instructor
Department of Orthopaedic Surgery and Rehabilitation
University of Wisconsin School of Medicine and Public Health
Madison, Wisconsin

Alex Hughes, MD
Department of Orthopaedic Surgery
David Geffen School of Medicine
University of California–Los Angeles
University of California–Los Angeles Health System
Los Angeles, California

James D. Kang, MD
Professor
Departments of Orthopaedic Surgery and Neurological Surgery
University of Pittsburgh School of Medicine
Department of Orthopaedic Surgery
University of Pittsburgh Medical Center
Pittsburgh, Pennsylvania

David H. Kim, MD
Assistant Clinical Professor
Department of Orthopaedic Surgery
Tufts University School of Medicine
New England Baptist Hospital
Boston, Massachusetts

Sanjeev Kumar, MD
Department of Neurological Surgery
University of Medicine and Dentistry of New Jersey
Newark, New Jersey

Daniel C. Lu, MD, PhD
Chief Resident
Department of Neurological Surgery
University of California–San Francisco School of Medicine
San Francisco, California

Paul G. Matz, MD
Associate Professor
Department of Surgery, Division of Neurosurgery
University of Alabama–Birmingham
Division of Neurosurgery
University of Alabama–Birmingham Health System
Birmingham, Alabama

Mark R. McLaughlin, MD
Princeton Brain and Spine Care
Langhorne, Pennsylvania

Thomas E. Mroz, MD
Staff
Departments of Orthopaedic and Neurological Surgery
Cleveland Clinic Lerner College of Medicine
Case Western Reserve University
Center for Spine Health
Neurological Institute
Cleveland Clinic
Cleveland, Ohio

Praveen V. Mummaneni, MD
Associate Professor
Department of Neurological Surgery
University of California–San Francisco School of Medicine
Codirector
UCSF Spine Center
San Francisco, California

Prithvi Narayan, MD
Princeton Brain and Spine Care
Langhorne, Pennsylvania

Stephen L. Ondra, MD
Professor
Department of Neurological Surgery
Feinberg School of Medicine
Northwestern University
Northwestern Memorial Hospital
Chicago, Illinois

Brian A. O'Shaughnessy, MD
Chief Resident
Department of Neurological Surgery
Feinberg School of Medicine
Northwestern University
Chicago, Illinois

Corey A. Pacek, MD
Department of Orthopaedic Surgery
University of Pittsburgh Medical Center
Pittsburgh, Pennsylvania

David W. Polly Jr, MD
Professor and Chief
Departments of Orthopaedic Surgery and Neurosurgery
University of Minnesota Medical School
University of Minnesota Medical Center
Minneapolis, Minnesota

Sharad Rajpal, MD
Chief Resident
Department of Neurological Surgery
University of Wisconsin School of Medicine and Public Health
Department of Neurosurgery
University of Wisconsin Hospitals and Clinics
Madison, Wisconsin

A. Kirk Reichard, MD
Resident
Department of Orthopaedic Surgery
Indiana University School of Medicine
Indianapolis, Indiana

Daniel K. Resnick, MD
Associate Professor
Vice Chairman
Department of Neurological Surgery
University of Wisconsin School of Medicine and Public Health
University of Wisconsin Hospital and Clinics
Madison, Wisconsin

Gerald Rodts Jr, MD
Professor
Department of Neurosurgery
Emory University School of Medicine
Chief
Neurosurgery Service
Crawford W. Long Hospital
Atlanta, Georgia

Raphael R. Roybal, MD, MBA
Chatham Orthopaedic Associates
Savannah, Georgia

Edward Rainier G. Santos, MD
Assistant Professor
Department of Orthopaedic Surgery
University of Minnesota Medical School
University of Minnesota Medical Center
Minneapolis, Minnesota

Rick C. Sasso, MD, FACS
Indiana Spine Group
Indianapolis, Indiana

Nirav K. Shah, MD
Princeton Brain and Spine Care
Langhorne, Pennsylvania

Shenil Shah, BA
Wabash College
Crawfordsville, Indiana

Gwendolyn A. Sowa, MD, PhD
Assistant Professor
Department of Physical Medicine and Rehabilitation
University of Pittsburgh School of Medicine
University of Pittsburgh Medical Center
Pittsburgh, Pennsylvania

Michael P. Steinmetz, MD
Associate Staff
Center for Spine Health
Neurological Institute
Cleveland Clinic
Cleveland, Ohio

Gregory R. Trost, MD
Professor
Department of Neurological Surgery
University of Wisconsin School of Medicine and Public Health
Department of Neurosurgery
University of Wisconsin Hospitals and Clinics
Madison, Wisconsin

Eve Tsai, MD, PhD, CIP, FRCS
Division of Neurosurgery
Ottawa Hospital
Ottawa, Ontario, Canada

Kene T. Ugokwe, MD
Resident
Department of Neurological Surgery
Neurological Institute
Cleveland Clinic
Cleveland, Ohio

Jeffrey C. Wang, MD
Professor
Departments of Orthopaedic Surgery and Neurosurgery
David Geffen School of Medicine
University of California–Los Angeles
Chief, Orthopaedic Spine Service
University of California–Los Angeles Comprehensive Spine Center
Los Angeles, California

Michael Y. Wang, MD
Department of Neurological Surgery
University of Miami Leonard M. Miller School of Medicine
Miami, Florida

1 Lumbar Fusion for Degenerative Disease of the Spine: What the Literature Supports

Daniel K. Resnick

The number of lumbar fusions procedures performed in the United States has increased substantially over the last several years and exhibited an upswing in the late 1990s. There are distinct regional differences in the rate of fusions performed per 1000 patients, a fact that has been interpreted in support of the hypothesis that fusion is overused.[1] Recent editorials in the popular press and general medical literature have strongly condemned a perceived overutilization of lumbar fusion and have suggested that the increase in the frequency of fusion surgery noted over the last decade is a result of financial incentives to surgeons and instrumentation companies.[2–4] This condemnation is largely based on an apparent lack of evidence to support the role of fusion for the treatment of low back pain. Indeed, Gibson et al,[5] in the 1999 Cochrane review, stated, "There is no scientific evidence on the effectiveness of any form of surgical decompression or fusion for degenerative lumbar spondylosis compared with natural history, placebo, or conservative management." This opinion was essentially reiterated in a 2005 update.[6] The Center for Medicare Services (CMS), the body that determines whether or not various procedures are paid for has called spine surgeons to task.

In November 2006, representatives of the various societies of spinal surgeons (the American Association of Neurosurgeons [AANS], the American Association of Orthopedic Surgeons, the Congress of Neurological Surgeons, the North American Spine Society, and the Scoliosis Research Society) were asked to testify before the Medical Care and Advisory Panel of the CMS to justify the performance of lumbar fusion. An extensive literature review was performed as part of our preparation for this session. This chapter reviews the literature support for the performance of lumbar fusion using an evidence-based medicine paradigm similar to that employed by the AANS/CNS in past publications.[7,8] In terms of disclosure, it is important to realize that not all of the reviews described here have been vetted through an official committee structure, and that many of the statements made are my opinion. Furthermore, I am a practicing spine surgeon, and thus may be considered biased. But I do not apologize for this potential bias, and I will point out instances where alternative interpretations of data may be supported.

What Is Evidence-Based Medicine?

Evidence-based medicine is a process by which the literature may be evaluated in a comprehensive and systematic fashion to answer clinical questions with varying levels of certainty. In short, evidence-based medicine combines a critical evaluation of the literature with physician judgment and patient values to arrive at a "best-guess" solution for a particular problem. When there is high-quality medical evidence to support a particular treatment strategy, then the best guess is likely to be the best treatment strategy for that particular patient with that particular disorder. If the medical evidence is questionable, then the best guess may simply be a treatment strategy that truly represents a well-intentioned and informed guess.

The main strength of the evidence-based medicine process is the ability to combine a comprehensive literature review with a disciplined and transparent process of evaluation to make treatment recommendations in accordance with the strength of the medical evidence. If a treatment strategy is supported by incontrovertible evidence, it should be offered to almost all relevant patients. If a treatment strategy is supported only by poor-quality evidence, then the application of that strategy to a given patient should be substantially guided by physician judgment and patient preference.

There are limits to what evidence-based medicine can address. The literature cannot be interpreted in the absence of common sense and clinical experience. A frequently cited example of the inappropriate application of evidence-based medicine techniques is the assertion that there is no scientific evidence on the effectiveness of parachute use for life preservation following falls from aircraft.[9] Indeed, no randomized controlled trial or even a well-designed cohort comparison has ever been performed to provide such evidence. There are case reports of survival following falls without parachutes and reports of deaths in skydivers using parachutes. Therefore, just because a treatment is not supported by high-quality medical evidence does not mean that a treatment has no value. Failure to appreciate this conundrum led to the Cochrane review conclusions cited above. The Cochrane group considers only randomized

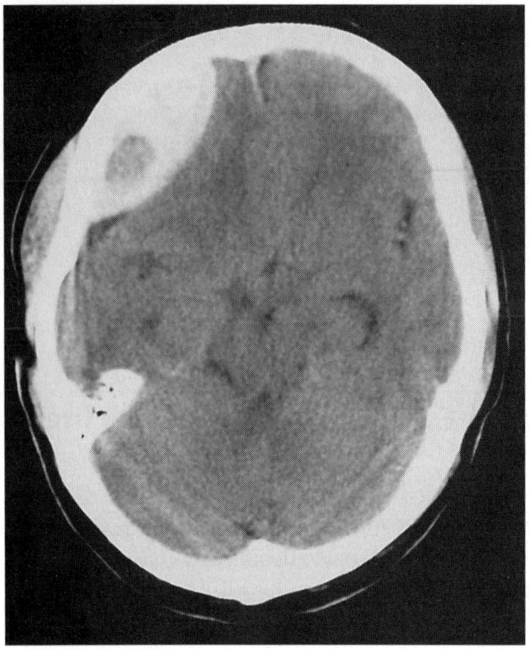

Fig. 1.1 This computed tomography (CT) scan demonstrates a large intracranial epidural hematoma. The patient is suffering from a transtentorial herniation syndrome and will almost certainly die without prompt surgical treatment. If the Cochrane parameters are applied to the literature regarding operative head trauma, the reviewers would have to conclude that there is no evidence supporting the evacuation of such intracranial mass lesions in trauma victims. The fact that no such trial could ever be performed is not recognized. Randomized controlled trials are only appropriate where there is genuine therapeutic equipoise. This illustrates why most medical societies have resorted to using graded recommendation schemes as described in the text. In the absence of randomized controlled trials, physicians must rely on what evidence is available, clinical judgment, patient desires, and common sense.

controlled studies as valid sources of medical evidence. The absence of such studies, in their opinion, equates with the absence of evidence[5,6] **(Fig. 1.1)**.

■ Evidence-Based Medicine and Lumbar Fusion

To identify high-quality evidence, it is important to establish some ground rules. The highest quality evidence comes from well-designed and properly executed randomized controlled studies. In order for a study to be considered properly designed, it needs to be appropriately powered to answer the clinical question asked, and the treatment groups and control groups need to be comparable and representative of the population of patients normally treated for a particular disorder. Appropriate outcome measures should be applied prospectively, follow-up must be relatively complete, and the statistical analysis should be appropriate for the question asked. If a study fails to meet any of these criteria, evidence derived from that study may be considered of lower quality.[8]

In order for a study to provide high-quality evidence, in addition to reasonable timing of assessment, the outcome measure used must be valid, reliable, and responsive. For example, when considering patients with low back pain, it is probably reasonable to use an outcome measure that reflects patient pain complaints regarding the back and legs. It is also reasonable to use a measure of functional outcome to determine if patients have derived improved ability to function within society, take care of themselves, continue their employment, and enjoy their pastimes. Such measures would be considered *valid*, as they seem to reflect the goals of treatment for surgical intervention.

Reliability refers to the ability of the outcome measure to be consistently applied and to provide consistent results when employed by the same individual or different individuals to a similar patient population. For example, patient satisfaction scores are notoriously unreliable because patients give different answers depending on the interviewer and the situation. Reliability can be measured, and is generally reported as a kappa value. The higher the value, the more reliable the measure. *Responsiveness* describes the ability of a measure to reflect change that is clinically relevant. In theory, if treatment A works better than treatment B, then the outcomes achieved with treatment A should be measurably better than those achieved with treatment B.[10]

Finally, outcome measures appropriate for one population undergoing lumbar fusion may not be appropriate for other populations undergoing fusion. For example, the return to work rate may be a valid, reliable, and responsive outcome measure for patients undergoing anterior lumbar interbody fusion. But is this outcome measure appropriate when we are studying the results of fusion versus no fusion in patients undergoing decompression for degenerative spondylolisthesis associated with lumbar stenosis?

Several commonly used, responsive, validated, and reliable outcome measures are available for the assessment of outcomes following lumbar fusion.[10] The choice of the appropriate outcome measure is based on the particular characteristics of the population to be studied and the anticipated beneficial effect.

Once we have established a valid, reliable, and responsive outcome measure, we then need to determine how much of a change is really important. For example, the National Acute Spinal Cord Injury Study (NASCIS) is frequently cited as a justification for the use of steroids following spinal cord injury.[11] In fact, for many years steroids were considered a treatment standard for patients with spinal cord injury. This conclusion has been criticized by many authors due to the relatively small treatment effect noted and due to deleterious effects of steroids that occurred with similar or even greater frequency than the beneficial effects.[7,12] The issue appears to be that although the improvement noted was statistically significant, it was clinically irrelevant and the risk of complications appeared to be just as likely.[7,12]

Study design may also influence the significance of results. The most common problems relate to sample size.

Fritzell et al,[13,14] in a randomized series comparing fusion techniques for low back pain, found that there was significant functional improvement in 70% of patients treated with posterolateral fusion (PLF) with pedicle screws compared with 60% of those patients treated with PLF alone. The study was not designed to detect this level of improvement, and therefore this difference in outcomes was not found to be significant.

Study design also includes the development of inclusion and exclusion criteria for patients entered into the study. It is important to recognize that the population entered into a randomized clinical trial performed at high-volume academic centers may not reflect the overall population of patients treated with a particular strategy. Consider the inclusion criteria and control groups employed in the Charite disk arthroplasty study.[15] The authors of this study excluded patients with spondylolisthesis, disk space collapse, facet arthropathy, or spondylosis from their study. The comparison procedure was a stand-alone anterior lumbar interbody fusion (ALIF). Do these patients represent the population of patients who are treated with lumbar fusion? Several authors have applied the Charite inclusion criteria to their own fusion populations and found that between 0% and 6% of patients treated with single-level interbody fusion in their practices would have been eligible for the Charite study.[16] Furthermore, the appropriateness of the comparison group may be questioned because few spinal surgeons would recommend a stand alone ALIF without evidence of disc space collapse.[17,18]

There have been five randomized controlled clinical trials performed evaluating the efficacy of lumbar fusion for degenerative disease of the spine. The remainder of this chapter is devoted to an analysis of these papers and a comment on the quality of evidence that exists supporting or refuting the efficacy of lumbar fusion as a treatment for low back pain due to degenerative disease of the lumbar spine.

Randomized Controlled Studies

Fritzell and colleagues[13] published the results of a multicenter randomized controlled trial from the Swedish Lumbar Spine Study Group in 2001. The authors assumed that very few patients would improve with conservative care and that a modest proportion of patients treated surgically would improve. They performed a power analysis based on this premise to have an 80% power to detect a significant difference in the effect of surgery versus the effect of nonsurgical treatment (in other words, they determined how much of an improvement they thought would be clinically relevant, and calculated how many patients they needed to include to be able to detect that degree of improvement 80% of the time). In this study, 294 patients with disabling back pain who were thought to be surgical candidates were randomized to conservative care (physical therapy supplemented with education and other pain relieving technologies at the discretion of the treating physician), or one of three surgical treatment arms. Patients were required to have suffered from back pain for at least 2 years and to have radiographic and clinical evidence of spondylosis at L4-L5, L5-S1, or both levels. The groups were comparable in all demographic variables measured with the exception of a higher incidence of medical comorbidity in the surgical group. Patients were followed for 2 years with intermediate evaluations at 6 months and at 1 year following onset of treatment. Outcomes were assessed using multiple well-validated outcome measures including pain visual analogue scales, the Oswestry Low Back Pain Questionnaire, the Million Visual Analogue Scale, the General Function Scale (GFS), return to work status, a patient satisfaction survey, and an independent functional assessment by a second spinal surgeon.

Follow-up was achieved in 98% of patients. Appropriate statistical analysis was performed based on the type of data derived from the different outcome measures. The surgical group did significantly better in terms of pain relief, degree of disability as measured by the Oswestry, Million, and GFS, return to work status, and degree of satisfaction reported by the patients and by the independent observer. Statistical analysis was rigorous, employing both "intention to treat" as well as a "worst-case" scenario. In short, all primary outcome measures evaluated in the study were significantly improved in the surgical group compared with the nonsurgical group.

In 2003, Brox et al[19] conducted a randomized study evaluating the relative efficacy of instrumented posterolateral fusion versus a specific protocol of cognitive intervention and physical therapy in a group of 64 patients (27 fusion, 37 nonfusion). The primary outcome measure used was a modified Oswestry Disability Index (ODI; modified for the Norwegian population). Secondary outcome measures included pain visual analogue scales, daily use of medication, the GFS, Waddel's Fear Avoidance Belief Questionnaire, and a patient satisfaction score. Outcomes were assessed by physical therapists or rehabilitation physicians at 1 year following initiation of treatment.

Patients enrolled in the surgical arm were treated with instrumented posterolateral fusion. The patients enrolled in the physiotherapy arm underwent a specifically designed program for patients with low back pain that had been previously demonstrated to be more effective than standard conservative care.[19] This program included cognitive therapy designed to address patient fear behavior as well as supervised physiotherapy averaging 25 hours per week for 8 weeks. Because of the intensity of the program, most patients stayed at the treatment center in patient hotels. This intensive course was followed by a home exercise program, physician and therapist consultations, various lessons, group therapy sessions, and participation in peer-led discussion groups.

Ninety-seven percent of patients were followed for 1 year. Patients in both arms of the study improved significantly from baseline on all outcome measures. The improvement in the primary outcome measure, the modified ODI, in the surgical group was 15.6 and the improvement in the physiotherapy group was 13.3. There were very large confidence intervals noted in this as well as other outcome measures assessed, almost certainly due to sample size. This difference in the degree of improvement between the surgical and physiotherapy group was not found to be significant. The surgical group did do significantly better in terms of relief of lower limb pain and tended to do better than the physiotherapy group in terms of improvement in back pain, emotional distress, and overall success ratings by both the patient and the independent observer. The physiotherapy group scored better fear avoidance activity and work as well as in fingertip-floor distance. Nonsignificant trends were also seen in favor of the physiotherapy group in terms of the GFS, and life satisfaction score.

The authors interpret their findings as demonstrating equivalence between their program of physiotherapy and lumbar fusion. The fact that both groups improved significantly supports the efficacy of both strategies as superior to the natural history of chronic low back pain treated in a conservative fashion. Given the small size of the study groups and the very large confidence intervals reported in the paper, the study was underpowered to detect a difference between two relatively effective treatment modalities. The use of psychological outcome measures to support nonoperative therapy may also be questioned, particularly as only one of the groups (nonoperative) had been treated with any psychological counseling. The outcomes from this study were also reported at 1 year as opposed to the usual 2-year time point. Because of concerns regarding methodologic flaws related to study size, outcome measures, and follow-up interval, this paper may be considered to provide lower quality evidence regarding the relative efficacy of fusion compared with the authors' aggressive nonoperative treatments.

Fairbank et al[20] published the results of a larger randomized controlled trial comparing lumbar fusion to aggressive conservative therapy (a regimen somewhat similar to that described by Brox). These authors enrolled 349 patients, of whom 176 were assigned to surgery and 173 were assigned to aggressive nonoperative management. These patients were selected based on the physician's opinion regarding whether or not they were surgical candidates. This eliminated patients with medical contraindications to surgery, but also eliminated patients with clear surgical indications such as instability, deformity, or neurologic deficits. The actual pathologic diagnoses were not well described, although the majority of patients in both groups suffered from degenerative disk disease. The surgical procedures were not standardized, and it appears that a mixture of anterior, posterior, rigid, and dynamic fixation procedures were performed. The primary outcome measures were the ODI and a shuttle walking test. Methodologic flaws included a 20% lost to follow-up rate for the Oswestry outcome measure, and a 30 to 40% lost to follow-up rate for the shuttle walking test and other secondary outcome measures. The authors performed an intent-to-treat analysis, meaning that patient outcomes were grouped in accordance with the initial assignment as opposed to the ultimate treatment received.

An intent-to-treat analysis is problematic in surgical trials, because although it is generally possible to cross over from nonsurgery to surgery, there is no way to cross over in the opposite direction (except very early on, after assignment and before surgery is performed). In this particular study, 48 patients (28% of the nonoperative group) crossed over from nonoperative treatment to surgery. The final results from these patients were considered with the nonoperative therapy group, significantly biasing the study against surgical intervention. (In effect, the authors are comparing the overall results of surgery in one group of patients with the results of nonoperative treatment in the best responders in the nonoperative group because nonresponders or poor responders went on to have surgery. Furthermore, any benefit derived from surgery in the worst 29% was ascribed to nonoperative therapy.) In any case, despite these biases, the authors found that the surgical group did significantly better in terms of improvement on the ODI both with the primary analysis ($p < .045$) and then with a secondary analysis intended to account for some of the crossover effect and loss to follow-up rate ($p < .02$). The surgical group also tended to do better on the Short Form–36 (SF-36) and shuttle walking outcome measures but these improvements were not statistically significant (not surprising with a 30 to 40% lost to follow-up rate). These results provide strong support for the role of surgery in the treatment of chronic low back pain due to degenerative disk disease, especially considering the lack of a standardized surgical approach, requirement for therapeutic equipoise, and inherent bias against surgery due to the intent-to-treat analysis.

The authors of the Fairbank study were less impressed by the advantages of surgery and concluded that surgery had, if anything, a very minor benefit compared with nonoperative techniques.[20] This conclusion differs from my conclusion, despite an analysis of the same outcomes data. This nicely illustrates how bias can color the interpretation of data, and the reader is encouraged to review the primary reference and come up with his or her own conclusions.

Ekman et al[21] published a randomized controlled study involving 111 patients with adult isthmic spondylolisthesis. These patients were randomized to one of three groups; group one was assigned to a 1-year exercise program, group two underwent a noninstrumented posterolateral fusion, and group three underwent an instrumented lumbar interbody fusion. The primary outcome measures were the ODI, the SF-36, and several global subjective outcome measures. In addition to 2-year outcomes in 106 of 111 patients, this group was able to obtain long-term (approximately 9-year) outcomes in 101 of the 111 patients. There was a significant crossover; nine of the 34 patients (26%) randomized to nonoperative treatment crossed over to surgery, and an intent-to-treat analysis was performed. In this study, the statistical analysis was repeated without inclusion of these patients, and attempts were again made to account for the crossover. At both the 1- and 2-year time points, the surgical group enjoyed significant benefits in all outcome measures. At last follow-up, the surgical group continued to enjoy benefits compared with baseline; however, the differences between the surgical and nonsurgical groups diminished. At final follow-up, the only significant difference between the groups was a greater degree of global improvement in the surgical group. The authors concluded that surgery resulted in modest but long-lasting benefits for this particular patient population. It is important to consider that a decade of pain relief is probably valuable even if the surgical procedure does not prevent the normal aging process.

In 2006, Brox et al[22] described the results of a small randomized controlled study limited to patients with low back pain following lumbar diskectomy for radiculopathy. This study was designed to detect a 10-point difference in the ODI and compared 1-year outcomes between patients treated with the aggressive conservative protocol described previously and an instrumented posterolateral fusion. The inclusion criteria were quite strict and excluded patients with neurologic deficits or radiographic evidence of nerve root compression. These authors found that both groups enjoyed significant improvement compared with baseline; however, there were no significant differences between the groups in terms of the primary outcome measures. This paper again provides evidence that fusion and aggressive conservative therapy are both effective treatments for chronic low back pain. In this particular patient population, either strategy appears to be equally effective.

■ Conclusion

Based on the randomized controlled trials described above, it can be stated unequivocally that lumbar fusion is an effective treatment for properly selected patients with chronic low back pain whose symptoms have not responded to nonoperative measures. The issue of patient selection is critical, as each of the studies reviewed had specific inclusion and exclusion criteria. The Fritzell study had the most liberal inclusion criteria, whereas the Ekman study was limited to patients with adult isthmic spondylolisthesis and the 2006 Brox study was limited to postdiskectomy patients. The data presented do not exclude the fact that other treatments are also effective for the management of low back pain in properly selected patients. The reader should also note that the inclusion criteria for each of these studies may not correlate well with the selection criteria generally used to select patients for surgery in a modern practice.

One point that should be emphasized when interpreting any of the studies described is that patients considered for surgery should have already failed nonoperative measures prior to consideration for surgery. Therefore, an upfront comparison between surgical and nonsurgical treatments is probably not realistic in terms of how these patients are generally treated. A treatment continuum is a more realistic and appropriate concept, with nonoperative measures employed first and surgery reserved for patients who fail these measures. Although the use of such a continuum will result in poorer apparent results for patients treated surgically (these patients are the more recalcitrant group and will have had a longer duration of symptoms), the overall treatment results are improved as patients who can improve with nonsurgical means are saved the potential complications of surgery.

Further research is necessary to help define the selection criteria for various fusion techniques. There is currently no data from randomized trials that supports the use of any specific instrumentation technique over any other or over the nonuse of instrumentation for the performance of lumbar fusion. In fact, the Fritzell and Ekman studies indicate that the use of instrumentation may not in fact be associated with improved outcomes. It is likely true that the universal application of one particular technique is not appropriate as different patients have different requirements. An elderly woman with a fixed grade one spondylolisthesis in association with central stenosis probably does not require the same fixation construct as a 38-year-old laborer with a mobile spondylolisthesis, associated foraminal stenosis, and retained disk space height. The Fritzell study lumped these patients together, potentially hiding a beneficial effect of instrumentation on the latter patient.

It is important that we continue to refine our techniques, refine our patient selection criteria, and objectively study our results. The information gleaned from these studies must be combined with an intimate knowledge of anatomy, pathophysiology, and natural history of patients with back pain, as well as with the particular history, desires, and needs of the individual patient to make appropriate decisions regarding the treatment of patients with intractable lower back pain.

References

1. Weinstein JN, Lurie JD, Olson PR, et al. United States' trends and regional variations in lumbar spine surgery: 1992–2003. Spine 2006;31:2707–2714
2. Abelson R, Peterson M. An operation to ease back pain bolsters the bottom line, too. New York Times, 2003 (December 31):A1
3. Deyo RA, Nachemson A, Mirza S. Spinal-fusion surgery—the case for restraint. N Engl J Med 2004;350:722–726
4. Deyo RA, Gray DT, Kreuter W, et al. United States trends in lumbar fusion surgery for degenerative conditions. Spine 2005;30:1441–1445

5. Gibson JN, Grant IC, Waddell G. The Cochrane review of surgery for lumbar disc prolapse and degenerative lumbar spondylosis. Spine 1999;24:1820–1832
6. Gibson JN, Waddell G. Surgery for degenerative lumbar spondylosis: updated Cochrane Review. Spine 2005;30:2312–2320
7. Hadley MN, Walters BC, Grabb PA, et al. Guidelines for the management of acute cervical spine and spinal cord injuries. Clin Neurosurg 2002;49:407–498
8. Resnick DK, Choudhri TF, Dailey AT, et al. Guidelines for the performance of fusion procedures for degenerative disease of the lumbar spine. Part 1: introduction and methodology. J Neurosurg Spine 2005;2:637–638
9. Smith GC, Pell J. Parachute use to prevent death and major trauma related to gravitational challenge: systematic review of randomised controlled trials. BMJ 2003;327:1459–1461
10. Resnick DK, Choudhri T, Dailey A, et al. Guidelines for the performance of lumbar fusion for degenerative disease of the lumbar spine. Part 2: assessment of functional outcome. J Neurosurg Spine 2005;2:637–644
11. Bracken MB, Holford T. Neurological and functional status 1 year after acute spinal cord injury: estimates of functional recovery in National Acute Spinal Cord Injury Study II from results modeled in National Acute Spinal Cord Injury Study III. J Neurosurg 2002;96:259–266
12. Hurlbert RJ. The role of steroids in acute spinal cord injury: an evidence-based analysis. Spine 2001;26:S39–S46
13. Fritzell P, Hagg O, Wessberg P, et al. 2001 Volvo Award Winner in Clinical Studies: Lumbar fusion versus nonsurgical treatment for chronic low back pain: a multicenter randomized controlled trial from the Swedish Lumbar Spine Study Group. Spine 2001;26:2521–2532
14. Fritzell P, Hagg O, Wessberg P, et al. Chronic low back pain and fusion: a comparison of three surgical techniques: a prospective multicenter randomized study from the Swedish lumbar spine study group. Spine 2002;27:1131–1141
15. Blumenthal S, McAfee PC, Guyer RD, et al. A prospective, randomized, multicenter Food and Drug Administration investigational device exemptions study of lumbar total disc replacement with the CHARITE artificial disc versus lumbar fusion: part I: evaluation of clinical outcomes. Spine 2005;30:1565–1575
16. Simmons JW. Inclusion Criteria for Disc Arthroplasty. Philadelphia: North American Spine Society, 2005
17. Zindrick MR,Lorenz MA,Bunch WH. Editorial response to the Charite LumbarDisc Arthroplasty Study parts 1 and 2. Spine2005;30:E388–E390
18. McAfee PC, Cunningham BW, Lee GA, et al. Revision strategies for salvaging or improving failed cylindrical cages. Spine 1999;24:2147–2153
19. Brox JI, Sorensen R, Friis A, et al. Randomized clinical trial of lumbar instrumented fusion and cognitive intervention and exercises in patients with chronic low back pain and disc degeneration. Spine 2003;28:1913–1921
20. Fairbank J, Frost H, Wilson-MacDonald J, et al. Randomised controlled trial to compare surgical stabilisation of the lumbar spine with an intensive rehabilitation programme for patients with chronic low back pain: the MRC spine stabilisation trial. BMJ 2005;330:1233
21. Ekman P, Moller H, Hedlund R. The long-term effect of posterolateral fusion in adult isthmic spondylolisthesis: a randomized controlled study. Spine J 2005;5:36–44
22. Brox JI, Reikeras O, Nygaard O, et al. Lumbar instrumented fusion compared with cognitive intervention and exercises in patients with chronic back pain after previous surgery for disc herniation: a prospective randomized controlled study. Pain 2006;122:145–155

2 Pathophysiology and Treatment of Low Back Pain

Dani S. Bidros, Michael P. Steinmetz, and Daniel K. Resnick

Low back pain (LBP) is the most expensive benign medical condition in industrialized countries and the most common cause of activity limitation in persons younger than 45 years. It is estimated that 50 to 80% of the adult population suffers from at least one memorable episode of low back pain per year.[1] Around 15 to 20% develop protracted pain, and 2 to 8% have chronic pain. Every year, 3 to 4% of the population is temporarily disabled, and 1% of the working-age population is disabled permanently because of LBP.[2] LBP is second only to the common cold as a cause of lost work time; it is the fifth most frequent cause of hospitalization and the third most common reason to undergo a surgical procedure.[3] LBP accounts for 19% of all Workers' Compensation claims in the United States. Productivity losses from chronic LBP approach $28 billion annually in the United States.[4]

Differentiation of acute low back pain from chronic is essential because the management differs. LBP is defined as chronic after 3 months of symptoms. Acute pain is most often due to disruption of normal connective tissues, which usually heal within 6 to 12 weeks. Traumatic or degenerative conditions of the spine are the most common causes of chronic LBP. The evolution of chronic LBP is complex and can include physiologic, psychological, and psychosocial influences.[5] Although acute LBP has a favorable prognosis, the effect of chronic LBP and its related disability on society is tremendous.

A significant number of individuals suffering from low back pain improve with conservative treatments. The scope of conservative treatments has evolved over time. Whereas most surgeons would probably define conservative treatment as a several-month trial of physical therapy and nonsteroidal antiinflammatory medications, there has been recent expansion in the nonoperative treatment of LBP. Several new products and procedures and many different philosophies have been formulated as a result of the significant number of people suffering from LBP. Whereas many of these treatments are safe (magneto-therapy, acupuncture, herbal medications), most are costly, and some are certainly invasive (facet rhizotomy, epidural steroid injections) with unproven benefit.

In addition to the advent of many new nonoperative treatment modalities, nonfusion procedures for LBP, including intradiskal electrothermy and dorsal column stimulation, have been developed and are playing an increasing role in the management of patients with LBP. New fusion techniques have led to a significant increase in the spine surgeon's ability to treat LBP. Minimally invasive spine surgery has grown over the last decade, and with the premise of faster postoperative recovery and shorter hospital course, patients are now given more surgical options. Moreover, lumbar spine arthroplasty has provided nonfusion strategies, which have only recently become available. Better understanding of the biomechanics of the spine, the natural history of degenerative disk disease, improved localization of source of back pain, and extensive use of diagnostic imaging techniques have all contributed to the rapid evolution of spine surgery techniques.

The emergence of competing new technologies for the operative and nonoperative treatment of LBP is both exciting and frustrating. The majority of these new techniques have not been subject to randomized, controlled clinical trials. Patient selection criteria as well as outcome measures vary between various surgical and nonsurgical series. Finally, as soon as relatively concrete clinical data are gathered regarding one methodology, another "new and improved" methodology is aggressively marketed. This situation has reemphasized the need for the physician treating patients with LBP to have a clear understanding of the anatomy, pathophysiology, and natural history of LBP. The only way that a physician can make an informed judgment regarding the need for and appropriateness of a given treatment modality (be it magnetism or instrumented fusion) is with a firm grasp of these basic principles. This chapter reviews the anatomic substrate and basic pathophysiology of LBP.

■ Nociception in the Lumbar Spine

Nociception is the neurochemical process whereby specific nociceptors convey information regarding potentially harmful stimuli through peripheral neural pathways to the central nervous system (CNS). Nociceptors are present in the outer annular fibrosis, facet capsule, posterior longitudinal ligament, associated muscles, and other structures of the spinal motion segment. Noxious mechanical, thermal, and chemical stimuli activate peripheral nociceptors that transmit the pain message through thinly myelinated A (fast) fibers and unmyelinated C (slow) fibers. The quality of pain sensation depends on the nociceptor being stimulated; stimulation of A fibers leads to pricking pain, whereas stimulation of cutaneous C nociceptors results in a burning, dull sensation.[6]

Peripheral transmission of pain stimuli through A fibers and C fibers leads to the release of excitatory amino acids, such as glutamine and asparagine, which then act on *N*-methyl-D-aspartic acid (NMDA) receptors, causing the release of the neuropeptide substance P (SP).[7] Neuropeptides, such as SP, calcitonin gene–related protein (CGRP), and vasoactive intestinal polypeptide (VIP) are transported to the endings of nociceptive afferents, which inflammation and other algogenic mechanisms sensitize.[8] These neurochemical changes sensitize nociceptors so that they respond to mild or normal sensory stimuli, such as light touch or temperature change, which may result in the pain syndrome allodynia.

Sensory pain impulses arising from the lumbar spine are projected to the bipolar nerve cell body located within the dorsal root ganglion (DRG). The DRG is mechanically sensitive and capable of independent pain transduction, transmission, and modulation. Lindblum and Rexed[9] implicated the DRG as a modulator of LBP. Howe et al[10] demonstrated that chronic injury to the dorsal root produces a marked increase in sensitivity to mechanical stimulation. Several of the aforementioned peptides, including CGRP and SP, have been localized to the small dorsal root ganglion cells. CGRP has been shown to be the most abundant peptide in the DRG.[11] Several studies have shown increases in the concentrations of SP and VIP following stimulation of the DRG.[12,13] Sensory afferent information is processed by the dorsal root ganglion and then transmitted to the CNS.

The cells in the DRG are divided into different classes according to their diameters, large unmyelinated fibers, small unmyelinated (C) fibers, and finely myelinated (A) fibers. The central terminations of the primary afferent fibers, derived from the small cells, end mainly in Rexed lamina II (the substantia gelatinosa) of the spinal cord. Small interneurons within Rexed lamina I and II produce both excitatory and inhibitory neurotransmitters and project to the dendrites of multiple dorsal horn cells within several adjacent levels of the spinal cord.[14] These interneurons are responsible for modulation of the stimulus that is ultimately projected centrally.

In the setting of peripheral nerve injury, acute tissue damage can cause the upregulation of certain neuropeptides including galanin and VIP, as well as the downregulation of others such as SP, somatostatin, and CGRP. When the peripheral source of pain persists, intrinsic mechanisms that reinforce nociception influence the pain. In addition to this change in the neurotransmitter milieu, damage to the supporting structures of the nerve can lead to alterations in the anatomy of the pain system. Damage to Schwann cells can result in the upregulation of neurotrophins responsible for nerve regeneration.[15] It has been postulated that these growth factors may promote aberrant forms of regeneration and abnormal pain states. Woolf et al[16] showed that large myelinated afferents, supplying mechanoreceptors, grew into lamina II after a peripheral nerve injury. Abnormal connections of these large afferents to nociceptive processing circuits of the dorsal horn may contribute to allodynia, a sensation of pain that is provoked in pathologic circumstances by innocuous stimuli.

Transduction is the process whereby noxious afferent stimuli are converted from chemical to electrical neural messages in the spinal cord that communicate cephalad to numerous regions of the brainstem and diencephalons, including the thalamus, periaqueductal gray, parabrachial region, reticular formation, and limbic structures. There is a high level of redundancy in nociceptive projections to higher processing centers (**Fig. 2.1**). The spinothalamic tract mediates the sensations of pain, cold, warmth, and touch. These neuron cell bodies are located primarily in lamina I and lamina IV to lamina VI. These axons decussate via the anterior white commissure and ascend in the contralateral lateral spinothalamic tract and anterior spinothalamic tract to terminate on the posterior part of the ventral medial nucleus, ventral posterior lateral nucleus, and medial dorsal nucleus. Nociceptive information is also transmitted to the multiple spinal cord relay nuclei via the spinomesencephalic and spinoreticular tracts. A multisynaptic pathway carries information about noxious inputs to the medial thalamus, where it is relayed to the nucleus accumbens, septal nuclei, and amygdala of the limbic system. This pathway is relevant to the motivational aspects of pain.[17]

Multiple higher centers can directly modulate nociception at the spinal level through descending projections (**Fig. 2.2**). Reynolds[18] demonstrated that stimulation of the midbrain periaqueductal gray (PAG) inhibits the perception of noxious stimuli during surgical manipulations on rats. The PAG neurons project to the nucleus raphe magnus (NRM) and adjacent reticular formations and to the spinal cord.[19] These pathways utilize several different neurotransmitters, including opioids, serotonin, and catecholamines. These descending inputs, largely from the cortex and thalamus, alter the perception of pain.[20] Cortical areas most prominently involved in this process include the S1 and S2 somatosensory cortex, the anterior insula, and the cingulate gyrus.[21,22] The lentiform nucleus and cerebellum also provide descending input to the pain pathway. This activity is thought to allow for processing of reflexive motor responses to painful stimuli. Ventrally directed tactile processing from S1 to the temporal lobe limbic structures via relays in S2 and the insula may subserve tactile learning and memory.[23] These descending pathways may be manipulated surgically to alter pain transmission and used to treat pain syndromes.

■ Pain Generators in the Spine

The low back contains several potential anatomic sources of pain. The paraspinal musculature, facet joints, and

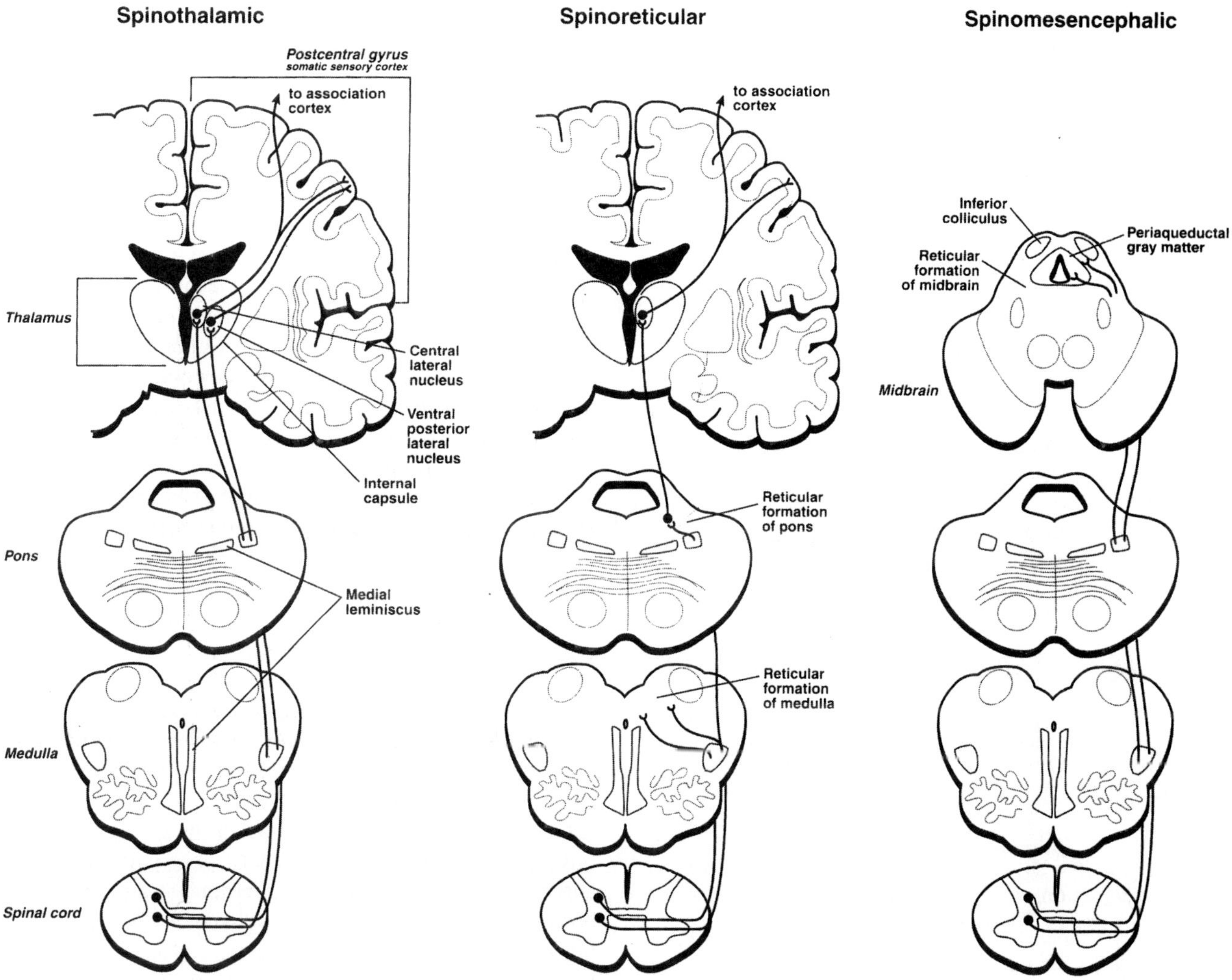

Fig. 2.1 The three major ascending pain pathways (spinothalamic, spinoreticular, spinomesencephalic) are illustrated in a schematic format. In addition to the well-described thalamic projections, these tracts project to other brainstem nuclei. These include the nucleus raphe magnus (NRM), nucleus magnocellularis (NMC), nucleus reticularis gigantocellularis (NRC), and periaqueductal gray (PAG). Other fibers simultaneously project to the reticular formation of the medulla and pons, as well as to the nucleus raphe dorsalis (NRD). At each relay point, information can be modified by descending pathways from the cortex.

ligaments of the intervertebral disk complex are innervated by nociceptive fibers and can all play a role in the pathogenesis of LBP. Various authors have tried to characterize the pain patterns that are thought to be produced by abnormalities of these structures. Persistent pain from a primarily muscular origin is often referred to as a *myofascial pain syndrome.* Pain syndromes thought to occur as the result of facet arthropathy have been referred to as *facet syndromes.* Finally, there has been much written about the nature and cause of *discogenic* LBP. Each of these pain syndromes is felt to respond to therapy directed toward the presumed source of pain.

There is significant controversy regarding the existence of a "facet syndrome," and differentiating pain derived from facet arthropathy versus degenerative changes in the intervertebral disk may be impossible and, in the case of fusion, irrelevant. Muscle-derived pain may present as a distinct syndrome, the myofascial pain syndrome, which is distinct from pain derived from the axial spine. This discussion focuses on axial back pain, or pain derived from the axial spine. Because persistent LBP of muscular origin is relatively common, a brief discussion of its nature, pathophysiology, and treatment follows.

Myofascial Pain Syndrome

Pain in this syndrome occurs when the muscles and tendons as one contractile unit are exposed to single or recurrent episodes of biomechanical overloading. Pain receptors in this unit are sensitive to a variety of mechanical stimuli, including pressure, pinching, cutting, and stretching. Injured muscles are usually abnormally shortened, with increased tone and tension due to spasm or overcontraction. Injured muscles often meet the diagnostic criteria for myofascial pain syndrome.

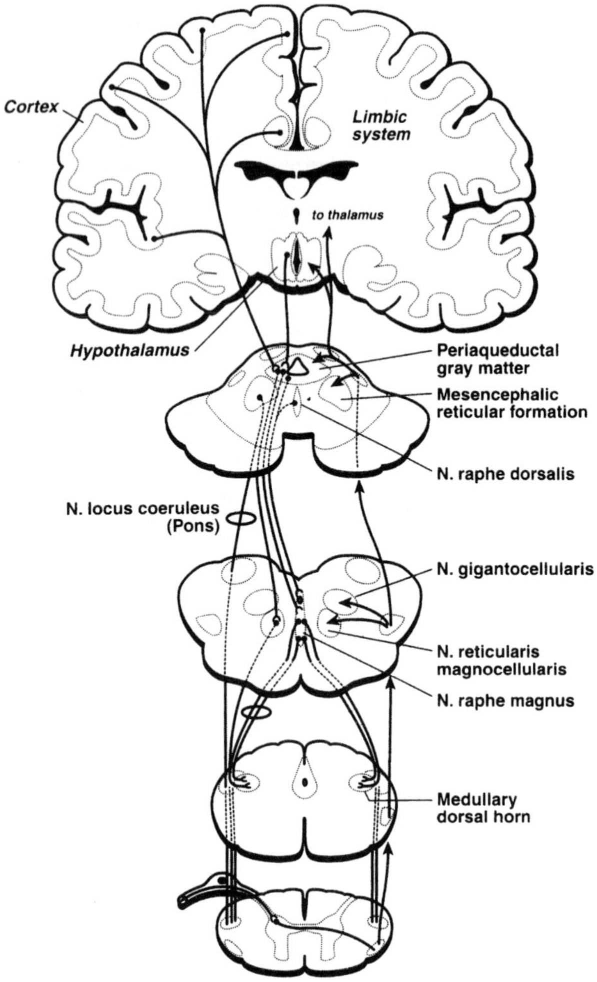

Fig. 2.2 The diagram depicts the endogenous descending pain inhibitory systems. Cortical projections, as well as projections from the hypothalamus, terminate in the periaqueductal gray and then project to the dorsal horn of the spinal cord. Some mesencephalic neurons (containing the neurotransmitters enkephalin, dynorphin, serotonin, and neurotensin) project directly to the dorsal lateral funiculus of the spinal cord.

Myofascial pain syndrome, a condition originally described by Simons and Travell, is characterized by muscles that are in a shortened or contracted state, with increased tone and stiffness, and that contain trigger points. Trigger points are tender, firm, 3- to 6-mm nodules that are identified on palpation of the muscles.[24] Palpation of the trigger points provokes radiating, aching pain into localized reference zones. These trigger points are characterized by local tenderness, an associated taut contracted muscle band (often palpable in the spine), a local twitch response, referred pain, and autonomic phenomena. Trigger point palpation can elicit a jump sign, an involuntary reflex disproportionate to the palpatory pressure applied.[25] The pain is usually caused by factors such as direct or indirect trauma, exposure to cumulative and repetitive strain, postural dysfunction, and physical deconditioning.[26] Myofascial pain can occur at the site of tissue damage or due to radicular and other neuropathic disorders at sites where pain is referred. Muscles affected by neuropathic pain may be injured due to prolonged spasm, mechanical overload, or metabolic and nutritional deficiency.

Some research suggests that myofascial dysfunction with characteristic trigger points is a spinal segmental reflex disorder. Animal studies showed that trigger points can be abolished by transecting efferent motor nerves or infusing of lidocaine; however, spinal transection above the level of segmental innervation of a trigger point-containing muscle does not alter the response. Simons et al[24] postulate that abnormal or excessive acetylcholine release at the neuromuscular junction generates sustained muscle contraction and a continuous reverberating cycle resulting in painful and dysfunctional muscle contraction. There are currently no diagnostic tests for myofascial pain syndrome. Treatment options include spray and stretch, trigger point injection with local anesthetics, and various manipulation techniques.[27,28]

Facet-Joint Pain

Chronic LBP secondary to involvement of the facet joints is a common problem. Facet joints have been recognized as potential sources of back pain when they were first recognized by Goldthwait[29] in 1911. In 1933, Ghormley[30] first used the term *facet syndrome,* which he defined as lumbosacral pain with or without sciatic pain, particularly occurring suddenly after a twisting or rotary strain of the lumbosacral region. The syndrome is characterized by hip and buttock pain, cramping leg pain (primarily above the knee), low back stiffness, and the absence of paresthesias. Patients usually exhibit local paraspinal tenderness; pain on spine hyperextension; hip, buttock, or back pain with straight leg raising; and no neurologic deficit.[30,31]

The facet joints are paired diarthrodial synovial articulations between the posterior elements of the adjacent vertebrae that share compressive loads and other biomechanical forces with the intervertebral disk.[32] Lumbar facet joints are innervated by medial branches of the dorsal rami of the spinal nerves from the L1 to L4 levels. At L5, the dorsal ramus travels between the ala of the sacrum and its superior articular process and divides into medial and lateral branches at the caudal edge of the process.[33–37] Each segmental medial branch of the dorsal ramus supplies at least two facet joints[38,39] **(Fig. 2.3).** In one study, Ashton and colleagues[40] found nociceptive fibers within the capsule of the facet and were unable to locate similar fibers in the annulus. Injections into the facets caused back, hip, and buttock pain in six normal human volunteers, providing further evidence of the presence of nociceptive fibers with overlapping fields in the facet capsules.[41]

Like other synovial joints, the facets react to trauma and inflammation by manifesting pain, stiffness, and dysfunction with secondary muscle spasm, leading to joint stiffness

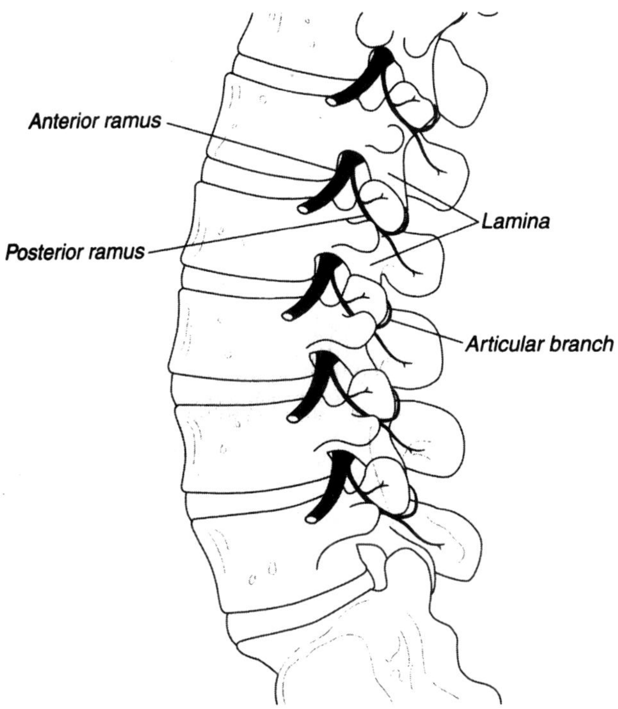

Fig. 2.3 Facet joint innervation. A lateral view of the lumbar vertebral column demonstrating lumbar spinal nerves exiting from the neural foramina. The dorsal ramus of the lumbar spinal nerve divides into several branches that innervate the superior facet of one joint and the inferior facet of the adjacent joint.

and degeneration. Numerous radiologic and histologic studies have shown that diskal and facet degeneration are linked and with time, degeneration of the segment leads to osteoarthritis of the facets.[42] Neuroanatomic and immunohistochemical studies have demonstrated free and encapsulated nerve endings in facet joints as well as nerve fibers containing the neuropeptides SP and CGRP that mediate and modulate nociception.[43,44] Substance P nerve fibers have been found in degenerative lumbar facets subjected to aging and cumulative biomechanical loading, and its levels are correlated with the severity of joint arthritis. Studies have shown that infusion of SP into joints with mild disease reportedly accelerated the degenerative process. Furthermore, these chemicals and inflammatory mediators have been linked to proteolytic and collagenolytic enzymes that cause degradation of the cartilaginous matrix and osteoarthritis. Therefore, evidence of nociceptive afferents and the presence of algogenic neuropeptides, such as SP and CGRP, in facets and periarticular tissues support a role for these structures as spinal pain generators.

Multiple studies utilizing controlled diagnostic blocks have established the relevance of lumbar facet joint involvement in patients with chronic LBP, ranging from 15 to 52%, based on the type of population and setting studied.[33–37] Long-term therapeutic benefit has been reported from three types of interventions in managing lumbar facet joint pain, including intraarticular injections, medial branch blocks, and neurolysis of medial branches.

Discogenic Pain

Axial back pain is usually thought to arise from abnormalities involving the vertebral bodies and intervertebral disks. It is generally described as deep, midline, aching pain. There may be some radiation of pain into the buttocks or upper thighs, and the pain is often positional in nature, worse when upright as opposed to supine. This type of pain is thought to be produced by the visceral afferents that innervate the intervertebral disk. The innervation of the intervertebral disk is via the sinuvertebral nerves, which were first described by Luschka[45] in the mid-1800s. He showed that this nerve was derived mainly from the spinal nerve, with contribution from the sympathetic system **(Fig. 2.4)**. Malinsky, in 1959, demonstrated multiple types of nerve endings in the outer portion of the annulus fibrosis, and this finding has been repeatedly corroborated and further defined by others.[38,46–48]

The sinuvertebral nerves (SVNs) arise from two roots, one from the ventral primary ramus and the other from the ramus communicans. The SVN enters the neural canal

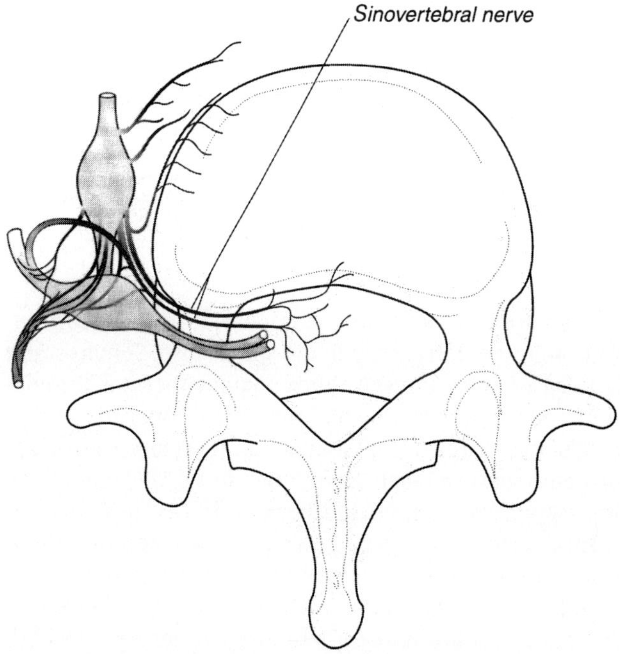

Fig. 2.4 Innervation of the spinal canal. The sinuvertebral nerve (SVN) is composed of two primary inputs. The diagram depicts the SVN contributions from the ventral primary ramus and the ramus communicans. The nerve enters the spinal canal through the neural foramina crossing the vertebral body caudal to the pedicle. The SVN then ramifies rostrally and caudally along the posterior longitudinal ligament. The nerve innervates the intervertebral disk at the level of the parent nerve and one level rostrally.

through the intervertebral foramen. Within the canal the nerve ramifies into two branches. The major branch ascends rostrally along the lateral border of the posterior longitudinal ligament. A second division passes medially and dorsally to innervate the intervertebral disk at the level of origin of the parent nerve. Bogduk et al[46] demonstrated through anatomic studies that an SVN, through its two primary branches, innervates two separate intervertebral levels. The inferior branch innervates the superior aspect of the disk at the level of entry, and the rostral branch provides innervation to the disk one level above. The SVN, therefore, provides the majority of innervation to the spinal canal. This network of nerve endings provides innervation of the dura matter, ligaments, and blood vessels, including the posterior longitudinal ligament and posterior aspect of the annulus fibrosis.

The nucleus pulposus of the intervertebral disk is composed of collagen, mucopolysaccharides, and water. During adulthood, the large proteoglycan molecules break into small molecules that bind less water than the original molecule. Repair by means of proteoglycan synthesis is slow. The degeneration of proteoglycans results in changes in the local pH and the accumulation of prostaglandins and other inflammatory mediators.[49] Recent elucidation of biochemical behaviors and neurophysiologic factors affecting the disk and other regional pain-sensitive tissues may account for this discrepancy. In humans, painful disks have a lower pH than that of nonpainful disks.[49] Also, experimental lowering of the pH in animal models induced pain-related behaviors and hyperalgesia. Diskography of canine disks that were normally or experimentally deformed seemed to show increased concentrations of neuropeptides, such as SP, CGRP, and VIP in the DRG, implicating their possible role in the transmission or the modulation of pain. SP probably modulates initial nociceptive signals received in the gray matter of the dorsal spinal cord.

Somatostatin is another neuropeptide in dense concentration in the dorsal gray of the spinal cord. Somatostatin is released from the DRG after noxious thermal stimulation and likely plays a role in pain transmission and in producing neurogenic inflammation. Therefore, the release of neuropeptides such as SP, VIP, and CGRP may occur in response to noxious biochemical forces and environmental factors (biomechanical stress, microtrauma, vibration), stimulating the synthesis of inflammatory agents (cytokines, prostaglandin E_2) and degradative enzymes (proteases, collagenase). These factors cause progressive deterioration of the motion segment structures, especially the intervertebral disk.

The annulus fibrosis also undergoes changes over time. Fissuring and disruption of annular lamellae further exacerbate molecular breakdown and dehydration of the disk and causing annular tears.[50,51] Radial lesions are macroscopic deformities that extend radially from the nucleus to the periphery.[52] They are seen in increasing frequency after age 30.[53] These tears extend into the outer portion of the annulus that has a vascular supply, thus allowing for the ingrowth of vascular granulation tissue along the edges of the radial rupture.[50] Small tears may bridge the defect by forming fibrotic scar tissue. Large tears, subject to continuous movement, may be prevented from healing. Studies of experimental injuries to the annulus fibrosis of dogs demonstrate the limited healing potential of the annular fibers to radial tears.[54]

The nucleus pulposus and inner two thirds of the annulus are void of nerve endings. A rich network of nerve fibers innervates the supporting structures of the intervertebral disk. The latter aspect of the vertebral column and the posterior longitudinal ligament are invested with a rich plexus of nerves derived from the SVN and the gray rami of the lumbar sympathetic trunks.[55] Nerve fibers extend beyond the longitudinal ligament deep into the outer third of the annulus fibrosis.[56] It is postulated that the intervertebral disk may become a pain producer when the outer third of the annulus is exposed to a painful stimulus.

The normal intact lumbar intervertebral disk does not produce pain. This is supported by diskography studies that were unable to elicit a painful stimulus upon injection of the normal disk space.[57] This is explained by the fact that injection into the nucleus pulposus of a healthy disk does not aggravate the outer portion of the disk, which is protected by a healthy annulus. The annulus is designed to withstand high pressures within the nucleus pulposus. Disk degeneration produces injuries in the form of radial tears to the inner third of the annulus. Provocation diskography of a diseased disk space produces a painful response when increased intradisk pressure is communicated via the injured annular channels to the nerve endings in the outer third of the annulus.[58,59]

Several authors have provided direct in vivo studies that provide substantial evidence pointing toward the intervertebral disk as the source of pain for the majority of patients with LBP. As discussed previously, numerous authors have identified nociceptive fibers within the outer annulus, posterior longitudinal ligament, and in granulation tissue associated with radial tears. Wiberg[60] reported selective reproduction of back pain with stimulation of the intervertebral disk (posterior annulus) in a series of patients undergoing awake lumbar diskectomy. Kuslich et al[61,62] also noted the pain-generating potential of the annulus fibrosis by using local anesthesia to perform lumbar diskectomies in awake patients. They stimulated various structures, including the facet capsule, ligamentum flavum, and annulus fibrosis. Patients reliably reported the occurrence of axial back pain with stimulation of the annulus fibrosis. Stimulation of the other structures did not reliably result in the reproduction of LBP. Information derived from these studies, as well as the evidence presented previously, provides strong evidence for the hypothesis that the intervertebral disk is an important generator of pain in a substantial number of patients with LBP.

Inflammatory factors may be responsible for axial back pain in which epidural steroid injections provide relief. Levels of phospholipase A_2 (PLA_2), which plays a role in inflammation, are elevated in surgically extracted samples of human herniated disks. Furthermore, PLA_2 may play a dual role, inciting disk degeneration and sensitizing annular nerve fibers. Afferent nociceptors in nerve roots may be sensitive to various proinflammatory mediators, which are inhibited by corticosteroids.[63]

Research suggests that proinflammatory cytokines may also contribute to discogenic pain by sensitizing nociceptors and their effect on disk degeneration by suppressing proteoglycan synthesis and increased diskal matrix degradation. Cytokines are produced in response to neural injury in the CNS and may play a role in spinal neural hypersensitization and chronic neuropathic pain. Cytokines known to play a role in nociception include nerve growth factor, interleukin-1 (IL-1), IL-6, IL-10, and tumor necrosis factor-α (TNF-α).[64,65]

Corticosteroids can inhibit activity of TNF-α, which induces IL-1 and prostaglandin E_2 production. Once released, these substances contribute to early and late effects of the inflammatory process and stimulate nociception.[66] A nociceptive role for nitric oxide (NO) in discogenic pain syndromes is under investigation. NO levels are elevated in hu man disk herniations, and when the hydrostatic pressure of the disk is increased due to biomechanical stressors, NO inhibits proteoglycan synthesis in cells in the nucleus pulposus, leading to proteoglycan loss, reduced water content, and disk degeneration.[67]

Neurotransmitters and biochemical factors may sensitize neural elements in the motion segment so that the normal biomechanical stresses induced by previously asymptomatic movements or lifting tasks cause pain. Furthermore, injury and the consequential neurochemical cascade may initiate the degenerative and inflammatory changes described above, which mediate additional biochemical and morphologic changes and which modify or prolong the pain stimulus. Whether the biochemical changes that occur with disk degeneration are the consequence or cause of these painful conditions is unclear. However, chemical and inflammatory factors may create the environmental substrata through which biochemical stress and forces cause axial or limb pain with various characteristics and degrees.

■ Surgery for Low Back Pain

In cases of neurologic deficit or structural instability of the spine, decompression of neural elements and reconstruction to the spine may result in restoration of function and elimination of severe pain. In a recent animal study, disk distraction alone demonstrated evidence of regenerative potential in degenerated intervertebral disks.[68] The vast majority of patients who present with LBP have no neurologic deficit and no evidence of acute instability of the spine. Most have some evidence of degenerative disk disease, and many display evidence of chronic or glacial instability (modic changes, disk space collapse, low-grade spondylolisthesis). The major purpose of medical or surgical intervention in these patients is to relieve their LBP. Theoretically, any interruption of the pain pathway, from the low back to the cerebral cortex, has the potential to relieve LBP.[69]

Spinal fusion is designed to eliminate the lumbar pain generator. It is hypothesized that stimuli for pain-generating afferents within the annulus (or facet joint) are eliminated with the removal of the disk and the elimination of motion at the fusion site. Conflicting reports in the literature exist concerning the efficacy of fusion for LBP. Different diagnostic tests, surgical approaches, the use or nonuse for rigid, semirigid, or interbody instrumentation, and varying patient selection criteria and outcome measures make global statements difficult. It does appear certain, however, that there are patients with degenerative disk disease and LBP who respond very well to surgical fusion. Description of this patient population as it relates to several different fusion techniques follows in ensuing chapters. Nonfusion strategies such as disk arthroplasty and dynamic fixation have been promoted to treat LBP. They avoid the elimination of segmental motion and theoretically decrease the incidence of adjacent segment spondylosis following surgery.

Intradiskal electrothermy is a recently developed method used to denature the collagen of the annulus fibrosus.[70] Exposure of the collagen to temperatures of 60°C leads to shortening of the collagen strands, which apparently leads to a "sealing" of annular tears. Passive heat spread leads to exposure of the outer annulus to temperatures in the range of 42°C, hot enough to coagulate local nociceptors. This technology would therefore (at least temporarily) destroy pain-generating structures in the annulus fibrosis but would not affect the facet capsule. Although still employed in some centers, this technique has fallen out of favor with many spine physicians. Its efficacy has been called into question. See Chapter 20 for a discussion of this technique to eliminate back pain.

Another means by which pain generated at the level of the low back can be alleviated is interruption of the pain signal. Dorsal column stimulation employs an electrical current to create a localized electromagnetic field around the spinal cord. This electromagnetic field causes tonic stimulation of large fibers in the dorsal column, causing a sensation of buzzing or tingling in the region of the body served by the particular group of fibers stimulated. This stimulation overrides the transmittal of information to higher centers from smaller diameter nociceptive tracts, thus eliminating the sensation of pain. Other options such as deep brain stimulation of the periaqueductal gray matter or other CNS regions have also been employed for the management of LBP. Intrathecal pumps to deliver analgesics such as opioids may also be used to treat pain.

■ Conclusion

Low back pain is very common. The vast majority of patients with LBP improve spontaneously. The rationale for nonoperative treatment has been based on findings from clinical and autopsy studies, which demonstrate that protruding or extruded disk material can be resorbed over time.[71] There exists a population of patients, however, whose pain does not improve over time and with noninvasive therapy. Clearly, the capsule of the facet joint and the annulus of the intervertebral disk are potential pain generators. Regardless of the pain generator, once a painful stimulus is generated, several pathways exist for the transmittance of painful sensation to the CNS. The source of LBP may be difficult to identify in an individual patient. There are a large number of diagnostic tests and therapeutic modalities that are designed to identify or eliminate specific pain generators in the lumbar spine (e.g., anterior lumbar interbody fusion [ALIF], facet rhizotomy, intradiskal electrotherapy [IDET]). The patient selection criteria and the technical aspects of, and success rates of, many of these procedures are discussed in ensuing chapters. Other methodologies nonselectively eliminate several potential pain generators (consider the effect of posterior lumbar interbody fusion on the facet joint and the intervertebral disk) or interrupt the pathways responsible for the perception of pain (dorsal column stimulation). This text reviews these various tests and therapies to clarify the rationale, the patient selection criteria, the technical aspects, and the expected outcomes of each of these therapies.

References

1. Loeser JD, Volinn E. Epidemiology of low back pain. Neurosurg Clin North Am 1991;2:713–718
2. Anderssen GBJ. The epidemiology of spinal disorders. In: Frymoyer JW, ed. The Adult Spine: Principles and Practice. New York: Raven Press, 1997:93–141
3. Cavanaugh JM, Weinstein JN. Low back pain: epidemiology, anatomy and neurophysiology. In: Wall PD, Melzack R, eds. Textbook of Pain, 3rd ed. London: Churchill Livingstone, 1994:441–455
4. Bats-Baril WL, Frymoyer JW. The economics of spinal disorders. In: Frymoyer JW, ed. The Adult Spine: Principles and Practice. New York: Raven Press, 1991:85–105
5. Chaturvedi SK. Prevalence of chronic pain in psychiatric patients. Pain 1987;29:231–237
6. Ochoa J, Torebjork E. Sensations evoked by intraneural microstimulation of C nociceptor fibers in human skin nerves. J Physiol 1989;415:583–599
7. De Biasi S, Rustioni A. Glutamate and substance P coexist in primary afferent terminal in the superficial laminae of spinal cord. Proc Natl Acad Sci U S A 1988;85:7820–7824
8. Schaible HG, Schmidt RF. Time course of mechanosensitivity changes in articular afferents during a developing experimental arthritis. J Neurophysiol 1988;60:2180–2195
9. Lindblum K, Rexed B. Spinal nerve injury in dorsolateral protrusions of lumbar disks. J Neurosurg 1948;5:413–432
10. Howe JF, Loeser JD, Calvin WH. Mechanosensitivity of dorsal root ganglia and chronically injured axons: a physiological basis for the radicular pain of nerve root compression. Pain 1977;3:25–41
11. Gibson SJ, Polak JM, Bloom SR, et al. The distribution of nine peptides in rat spinal cord with special emphasis on the substantia gelatinosa and on the area around the central canal (lamina X). J Comp Neurol 1981;201:65–79
12. Weinstein J, Pope M, Schmidt R, et al. Neuropharmacologic effects of vibration on the dorsal root ganglion. An animal model. Spine 1988;13:521–525
13. Yaksh TL, Jessell TM, Gamse R, et al. Intrathecal morphine inhibits substance P release from mammalian spinal cord in vivo. Nature 1980;286:155–157
14. Cruz F, Lima D, Zieglgansberger W, et al. Fine structure and synaptic architecture of HRP-labeled primary afferent terminations in lamina Ili of the rat dorsal horn. J Comp Neurol 1991;305:3–16
15. Ernfors P, Rosario CM, Merlio JP, et al. Expression of mRNAs for neurotrophin receptors in the dorsal root ganglion and spinal cord during development and following peripheral or central axotomy. Brain Res Mol Brain Res 1993;17:217–226
16. Woolf CJ, Shortland P, Reynolds M, et al. Reorganization of central terminals of myelinated primary afferents in the rat dorsal horn following peripheral axotomy. J Comp Neurol 1995;360:121–134
17. Burstein R, Giesler GJ. Retrograde labeling of neurons in spinal cord that project directly to nucleus accumbens or the septal nuclei in the rat. Brain Res 1989;497:149–154
18. Reynolds DV. Surgery in the rat during electrical analgesia induced by focal brain stimulation. Science 1969;164:444–445
19. Besson JM, Chaouch A. Peripheral and spinal mechanisms of nociception. Physiol Rev 1987;67:67–186
20. Chudler EH, Anton F, Dubner R, et al. Responses of nociceptive SI neurons in monkeys and pain sensation in humans elicited by noxious thermal stimulation: Effect of interstimulus interval. J Neurophysiol 1990;63:559–569
21. Casey KL, Minoshima S, Berger KL, et al. Positron emission tomographic analysis of cerebral structures activated specifically by repetitive noxious heat stimuli. J Neurophysiol 1994;71:802–807
22. Rainville P, Duncan GH, Price DD, et al. Pain affect encoded in human anterior cingulated but not somatosensory cortex. Science 1997;277:968–971
23. Friedman DP, Murray EA, O'Neill JB, et al. Cortical connections of the somatosensory fields of the lateral sulcus of macaques: evidence for a corticolimbic pathway for touch. J Comp Neurol 1986;252:323–347
24. Simons DG, Travell JG, Simons LS. Myofascial Pain and Dysfunction. The Trigger Point Manual, 2nd ed. Baltimore: Williams & Wilkins, 1999
25. Rivner MH. The neurophysiology of myofascial pain syndrome. In: Fields HP, ed. Current Pain Headache Report: Pain. New York: McGraw-Hill, 2000:432–440
26. Panjabi MM. A hypothesis of chronic back pain: ligament subfailure injuries lead to muscle control dysfunction. Eur Spine J 2006;15:668–676
27. Gerwin RD. Myofascial aspects of low back pain. Neurosurg Clin N Am 1991;2:761–784
28. Goldby LJ, Moore AP, Doust J, Trew ME. A randomized controlled

trial investigating the efficiency of musculoskeletal physiotherapy on chronic low back disorder. Spine 2006;31:1083–1093
29. Goldthwait JE. The lumbosacral articulation: An explanation of many cases of lumbago, sciatica, and paraplegia. Boston Med Surg J 1911;164:365–372
30. Ghormley R. Low back pain with special reference to the articular facets with presentation of an operative procedure. JAMA 1933;101:1773–1777
31. Lippitt AB. The facet joint and its role in spine pain. Management with facet joint injections. Spine 1984;9:746–750
32. Fujiwara A, Tamai K, An HS, et al. The relationship between disc degeneration, facet joint osteoarthritis, and stability of the degenerative lumbar spine. J Spinal Disord 2000;13:444–450
33. Manchikanti L, Singh V, Pampati V, et al. Evaluation of the relative contributions of various structures in chronic low back pain. Pain Physician 2001;4:308–316
34. Manchikanti L, Pampati V, Singh V, et al. Evaluation of role of facet joints in persistent low back pain in obesity: A controlled, perspective, comparative evaluation. Pain Physician 2001;4:266–272
35. Manchikanti L, Pampati V, Baha A, et al. Contribution of facet joints to chronic low back pain in postlumbar laminectomy syndrome: a controlled comparative prevalence evaluation. Pain Physician 2001;4:175–180
36. Manchikanti L, Pampati V, Rivera J, et al. Role of facet joints in chronic low back pain in the elderly: a controlled comparative prevalence study. Pain Pract 2001;1:332–337
37. Manchikanti L, Pampati V, Fellows B, et al. Influence of psychological factors on the ability to diagnose chronic low back pain of facet joint origin. Pain Physician 2001;4:349–357
38. Pedersen HE, Blunck CF, Gardner E. Anatomy of lumbosacral posterior rami and meningeal branches of spinal nerve (sinu-vertebral nerves); with an experimental study of their functions. J Bone Joint Surg Am 1956;38-A:377–391
39. Yamashita T, Cavanaugh JM, el-Bohy AA, et al. Mechanosensitive afferent units in the lumbar facet joints. J Bone Joint Surg Am 1990;72:865–870
40. Ashton IK, Ashton BA, Gibson SJ, et al. Morphological basis for back pain: the demonstration of nerve fibers and neuropeptides in the lumbar facet joint capsule but not in the ligamentum flavum. J Orthop Res 1992;10:72–78
41. McCall IW, Park WM, O'Brien JP. Induced pain referral from posterior elements in normal subjects. Spine 1979;4:441–446
42. Fujiwara A, Lim TH, An HS, et al. The effect of disc degeneration and facet joint osteoarthritis on the segmental flexibility of the lumbar spine. Spine 2000;25:3036–3044
43. Cavanaugh JM, Lu Y, Chen C, et al. Pain generation in lumbar and cervical facet joints. J Bone Joint Surg Am 2006;88(suppl 2):63–67
44. Giles LG, Harvey AR. Immunohistochemical demonstration of nociceptors in the capsule and synovial folds of human zygapophyseal joints. Br J Rheumatol 1987;26:362–364
45. Luschka HV. Die Nerven des menshlichen Wirbelkanales. Tubingen: Laub, 1850
46. Bogduk N, Tynan W, Wilson AS. The nerve supply to the human lumbar intervertebral discs. J Anat 1981;132:39–56
47. Malinsky J. The ontogenetic development of nerve terminations in the intervertebral discs of man. Acta Anat (Basel) 1959;38:96–113
48. Yoshizawa H, O'Brien J, Thomas-Smith W, et al. The neuropathology of intervertebral discs removed for low back pain. J Pathol 1980;132:95–104
49. Nachemson A. Intradiscal measurements of pH in patients with lumbar rhizopathies. Acta Orthop Scand 1969;40:23–42
50. Vernon-Roberts B, Pirie CJ. Degenerative changes in the intervertebral discs of the lumbar spine and their sequelae. Rheumatol Rehabil 1977;16:13–21
51. Vernon-Roberts B, Pirie CJ. Healing trabecular microfractures in the bodies of lumbar vertebrae. Ann Rheum Dis 1973;32:406–412
52. Kirkaldy-Willis WH, Wedge JH, Yong-Hing K, et al. Pathology and pathogenesis of lumbar spondylosis and stenosis. Spine 1978;3:319–328
53. Hilton RC, Ball J. Vertebral rim lesions in the dorsolumbar spine. Ann Rheum Dis 1984;43:302–307
54. Hampton D, Laros G, McCarron R, et al. Healing potential of the annulus fibrosus. Spine 1989;14:398–401
55. Groen GJ, Baljet B, Drukker J. Nerves and nerve plexuses of the human vertebral column. Am J Anat 1990;188:282–296
56. Hirsch C, Ingelmark B, Miller M. The anatomical basis for low back pain. Acta Orthop Scand 1963;33:1–17
57. Walsh TR, Weinstein JN, Spratt KF, et al. Lumbar discography in normal subjects. A controlled, prospective study. J Bone Joint Surg [A] 1990;72:1081–1088
58. Mooney V. Where is the lumbar pain coming from? Ann Med 1989;21:373–379
59. Vanharanta H, Sachs BL, Spivey MA, et al. The relationship of pain provocation to lumbar disc deterioration as seen by CT/discography. Spine 1987;12:295–298
60. Wiberg G. Back pain in relation to the nerve supply of the intervertebral disc. Acta Orthop Scand 1949;19:211–221
61. Kuslich S, Ahern J, Garner M. An in-vivo, prospective analysis of tissue sensitivity of lumbar spinal tissues. New York: 12th Annual Meeting of the North American Spine Society, 1997.
62. Kuslich SD, Ulstrom CL, Michael CJ. The tissue of origin of low back pain and sciatica. Orthop Clin North Am 1991;22:181–187
63. Saal JS, Franson RC, Dobrow R, et al. High levels of inflammatory phospholipase A2 activity in lumbar disc herniations. Spine 1990;15:674–678
64. Sorkin LS, Xiao WH, Wagner R, et al. TNF-alpha applied to the sciatic nerve trunk elicits background firing in nociceptive primary afferents fibers. 8th world congress for pain, IASP abstracts, Vancouver, IASP Press, August 1996:354
65. Wagner R, Myers RR. Endoneurial injection of TNF-alpha produces neuropathic pain behaviors. Neuroreport 1996;7:2897–2901
66. Carette S, Marcoux S, Truchon R, et al. A controlled trial of corticosteroid injections into facet joints for chronic low back pain. N Engl J Med 1991;325:1002–1007
67. Liu GZ, Ishihara H, Osada R, et al. Nitric oxide mediates the change of proteoglycan synthesis in the human lumbar intervertebral disc in response to hydrostatic pressure. Spine 2001;26:134–141
68. Guehring T, Omlor GW, Lorez H, et al. Disc distraction shows evidence of regenerative potential in degenerated intervertebral discs as evaluated by protein expression, magnetic resonance imaging, and messenger ribonucleic acid expression analysis. Spine 2006;31:1658–1665
69. Arnau JM, Vallano A, Lopez A, Pellise F, Delgado MJ, Prat N. A critical review of guidelines for low back pain treatment. Eur Spine J 2006;15:543–553
70. Andersson GB, Mekhail NA, Block JE. A randomized, double-blind, controlled trial: intradiscal electrothermal therapy versus placebo for the treatment of chronic discogenic low back pain. Spine 2006;31:1637–1638
71. Weber H. Lumbar disc herniation. A controlled, prospective study with ten years of observation. Spine 1983;8:131–140

3 Imaging Modalities for Low Back Pain: Magnetic Resonance Imaging

Victor Haughton

Imaging patients with low back pain, once oriented to anatomic changes in the spine, now includes the evaluation of functional integrity of the spine. When computed tomography (CT) and magnetic resonance (MR) were developed, they were used primarily as alternatives to myelography, for the detection of herniated disks and nerve root compression. With the high resolution available now, cross-sectional imaging achieves nearly perfect accuracy for disk herniations.[1] Despite this accuracy, MR fails in the majority of cases to distinguish the degenerative changes that cause a patient's back pain. Changes in the intervertebral disk and facet joints characterized as degeneration are found in patients with back pain but also in subjects without back pain.[2] The poor specificity of MR for the anatomic changes that cause back pain has been a popular topic.[3] MR has now been adapted to the evaluation of changes in the spine produced by an applied load or force. The study of the spine under various load conditions is generally referred to as dynamic imaging. Dynamic imaging is relatively new and incompletely evaluated, but offers additional possibilities for diagnosis.

This chapter describes the applications of magnetic resonance imaging (MRI) to the diagnosis of back pain. Gross anatomic changes in the intervertebral disk, facet joint, and osseous spine associated with aging and degeneration that result in specific MR changes are described. The MR sequences used in spine imaging are reviewed. The major imaging findings in spine disorders are noted briefly.

■ Magnetic Resonance Imaging Techniques

To minimize artifact and maximize spatial and contrast resolution, specialized MR techniques are required in spine imaging. Localized or surface coils are used in place of body coils to improve the signal from spine tissues. The coil's sensitive volume is matched to the structures to be imaged, improving the resolution in the region of interest by eliminating the signal from tissues anterior and lateral to the spine. Technical parameters such as time to repetition (TR), time to echo (TE), field of view, matrix, and number of excitations are chosen to achieve optimal spatial and contrast resolution. Other techniques may be used to improve images, such as cardiac gating, which reduces artifacts from pulsations in the cerebrospinal fluid (CSF). Multiple planes are used for imaging the spine. Sagittal images are acquired usually with T1 and T2 weighting and with 3- to 5-mm slice thickness. Axial images are acquired, preferably with the plane of sectioning parallel to the adjacent vertebral end plate to minimize geometric distortion. Three-dimensional (3D) volume acquisitions can be obtained to permit reconstruction in any selected plane or presentation as a pseudo-3D image.

Magnetic Resonance Pulse Sequences for Spine Imaging

The most frequently used MR spine imaging techniques can be classified as spin echo (SE) or gradient echo (GE). Images obtained with short TR and short TE provide T1 weighting and a high signal-to-noise ratio (SNR). These images are characterized by high signal intensity from lipid-containing tissues such as epidural fat and bone marrow, intermediate signal intensity from spinal cord, low signal intensity from CSF, and no signal from cortical bone. These images depict the vertebrae, neural foramina, facet joints, and epidural space effectively. T1-weighted images effectively demonstrate herniations of the intervertebral disk that displace epidural fat, or spinal stenosis and facet joint degeneration that cause bony sclerosis and neural foraminal narrowing. T2-weighted images, acquired with a long TR and a long TE, display high signal intensity from CSF and from intramedullary lesions, intermediate signal intensity from spinal cord, and low signal intensity from bone and fat. With a longer TR and TE, the T2-weighted images take longer to acquire and have lower SNR. T2-weighted images are especially useful for demonstrating intramedullary lesions, like demyelination, edema, and tumor infiltration because of the high signal intensity of these processes. T2-weighted images demonstrate reduction in signal intensity from the intervertebral disk during the process of degeneration, due to the loss of water and glycosaminoglycans. T2-weighted images also detect the "high-intensity zone" (HIZ) in the annulus fibrosus, which is found in disk degeneration.

Spin Echo

Spin echo sequences use two radiofrequency pulses, one applied to excite the tissues and another to reverse the

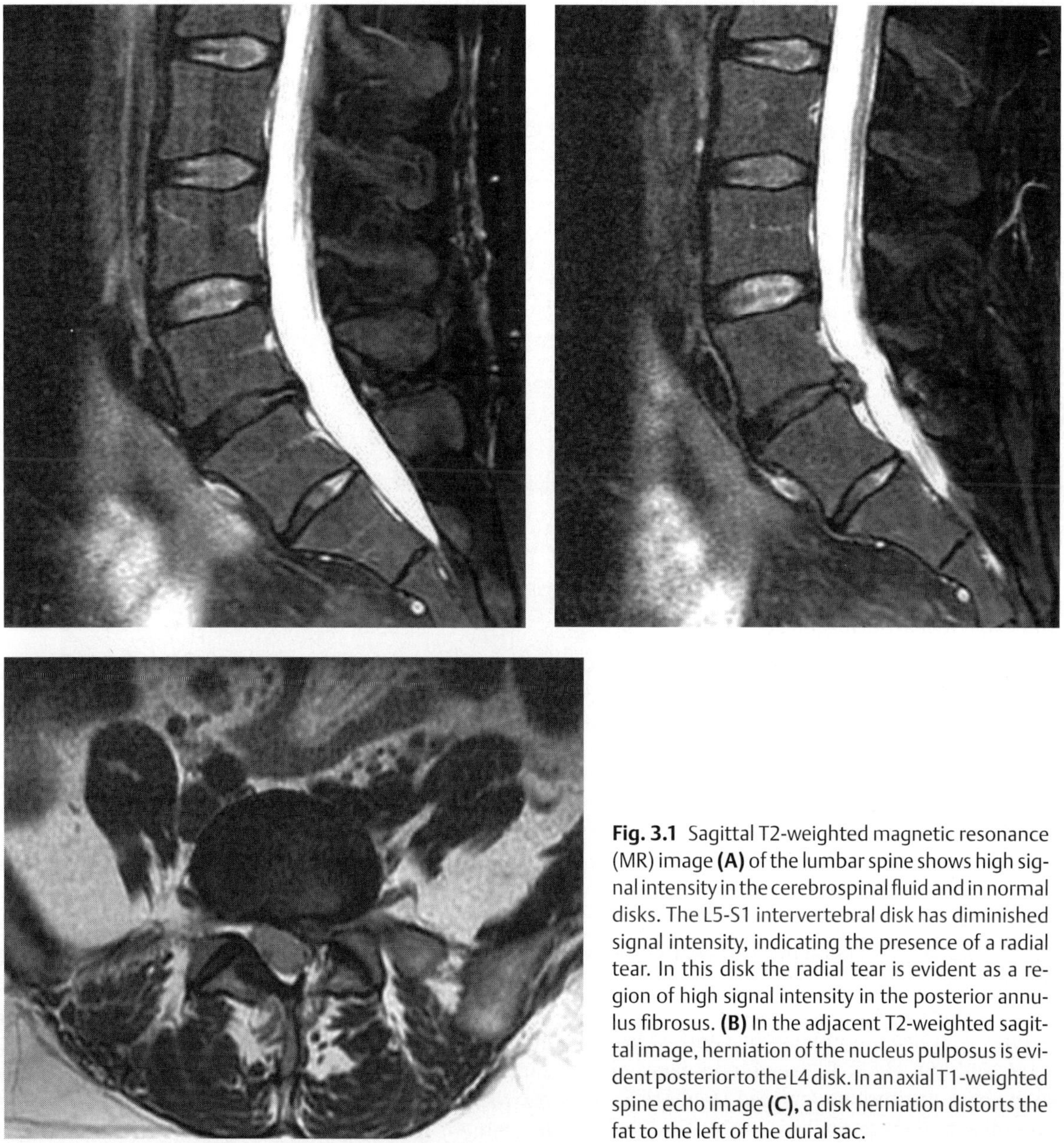

A B C

Fig. 3.1 Sagittal T2-weighted magnetic resonance (MR) image **(A)** of the lumbar spine shows high signal intensity in the cerebrospinal fluid and in normal disks. The L5-S1 intervertebral disk has diminished signal intensity, indicating the presence of a radial tear. In this disk the radial tear is evident as a region of high signal intensity in the posterior annulus fibrosus. **(B)** In the adjacent T2-weighted sagittal image, herniation of the nucleus pulposus is evident posterior to the L4 disk. In an axial T1-weighted spine echo image **(C),** a disk herniation distorts the fat to the left of the dural sac.

precession of the excited protons and create a signal that can be detected with the MR receiver coil. The time between consecutive excitation pulses (TR) and the time between the excitation and refocusing pulse (TE) determine whether a sequence is T1 weighted (short TE, short TR) or T2 weighted (long TR, long TE). Producing good resolution in disks and spinal cord, spin echo has been a standard sequence for spine imaging **(Fig. 3.1).** A fast spin echo (FSE) technique is used now to acquire T2-weighted images because it shortens the acquisition time compared with the conventional SE. FSE T2-weighted images may have less edge sharpness and less signal intensity from the intervertebral disk compared with SE. They also produce higher signal intensity in fat compared with conventional SE. A technique to reduce the signal intensity of fat (fat saturation) may be used in conjunction with FSE.

Gradient Echo

In another method of signal detection, gradient echo, reversing the direction of the applied magnetic field produces the coherent signal that the MR imager detects. Inhomogeneity in the local magnetic field cases a more rapid loss of signal (referred to as T2*) than in SE images **(Fig. 3.2).** Hemorrhage is easily detected with GE sequences. At the interface between bone and soft tissue or air or screws or metallic devices, signal is diminished more severely than in spin echo techniques. Radiofrequency (RF)

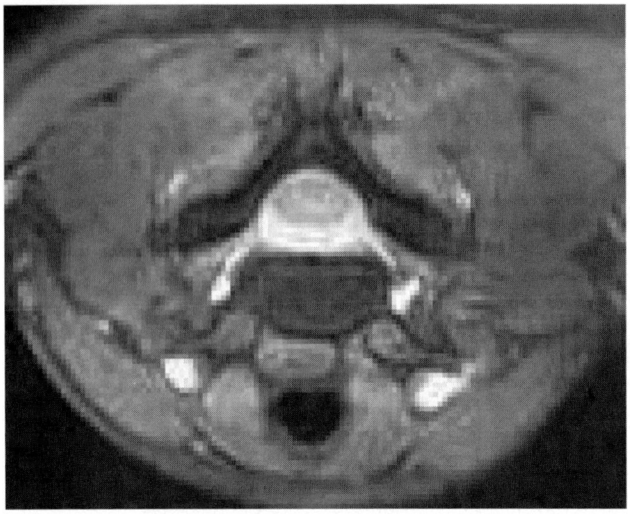

Fig. 3.2 Axial gradient echo (GE) image through the cervical spine demonstrates the spinal cord, subarachnoid space, and spinal column with little distortion and motion artifact.

"spoiler" pulses (un sequences such as SPGR) are used to reduce T2 contrast and reveal the proton density or T1 contrast between tissues. GE images have generally shorter acquisition times than SE images. GE images, having less sensitivity to CSF motion, are typically used in place of axial SE images for imaging the cervical spine.

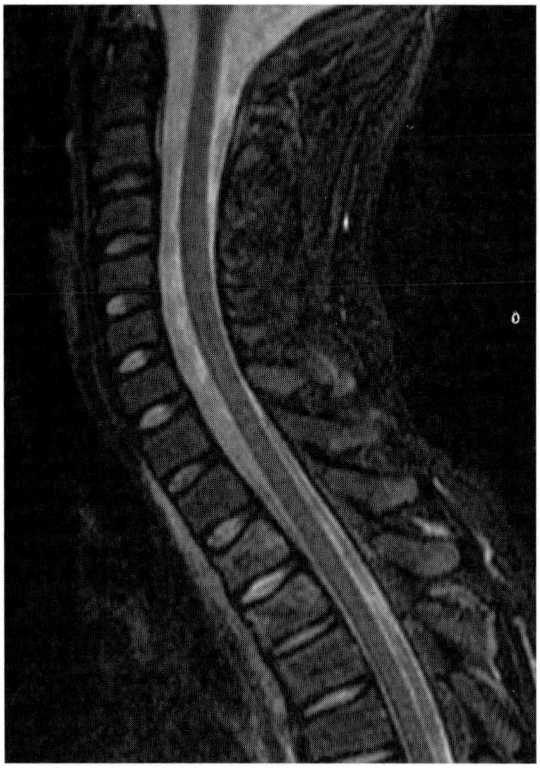

Fig. 3.3 Sagittal short tau inversion recovery (STIR) image of the spine showing increased signal intensity in the T2 and T3 vertebrae and slight wedging secondary to acute injury.

Inversion Recovery

Inversion recovery techniques use an RF pulse to invert the magnetization vector prior to the application of the excitation pulse. Contrast in the image can be substantially altered with the preliminary inversion pulse. One application of inversion recovery is the fluid-attenuated inversion recovery (FLAIR) sequence. With this technique, the signal from pure fluids is nulled, improving the contrast between soft tissues and CSF. FLAIR T1-weighted images of the spine have in some institutions replaced standard SE images. With an inversion pulse applied a short time interval (tau) before the excitation and refocusing pulse, the short tau inversion recovery (STIR) images are created. The STIR images have reduced signal intensity from fat, enhancing contrast between tissues with differing water content **(Fig. 3.3).** One important application of STIR images in general is to demonstrate lesions in bone marrow effectively **(Fig. 3.3).** Inversion recovery techniques include fast spine echo inversion recovery (FSEIR) and fast STIR.

Contrast Enhancement

Paramagnetic contrast media are used in MR to increase the signal intensity of specific structures and processes in T1-weighted images. Tissues that have a blood supply, a fenestrated capillary endothelium, and an extravascular space demonstrate an increase in signal intensity in T1-weighted images acquired after the administration of intravenous paramagnetic contrast media. Within the central nervous system, normally protected by tight capillary junctions in the endothelium, enhancement does not occur. With a breakdown of the blood–brain barrier, contrast enhancement may be detected in the brain or spinal cord. Contrast enhancement characterizes most tissues outside of the central nervous system. Therefore, muscle, fat, meninges, marrow, and epidural veins all demonstrate contrast enhancement to some degree **(Fig. 3.4).** The intervertebral disk, lacking a blood supply, enhances little immediately after the injection of contrast medium. Because contrast medium diffuses slowly into the intervertebral disk after intravenous administration, enhancement can be detected in the normal disk if larger amounts of contrast medium are administered and longer delays are used between contrast medium administration and acquisition of the image.[4,5]

Radial tears in the intervertebral disk may demonstrate contrast enhancement, probably due to the presence of granulation tissue. In experimentally created tears of the annulus fibrosus[6] and in excised degenerated intervertebral disk tissues,[7] granulation tissue is evident in the radial tear **(Fig. 3.4).** The use of contrast medium increases the detection of radial tears;[8] however, a suspected radial tear is not usually considered a sufficient indication for the use of contrast medium in the scan.

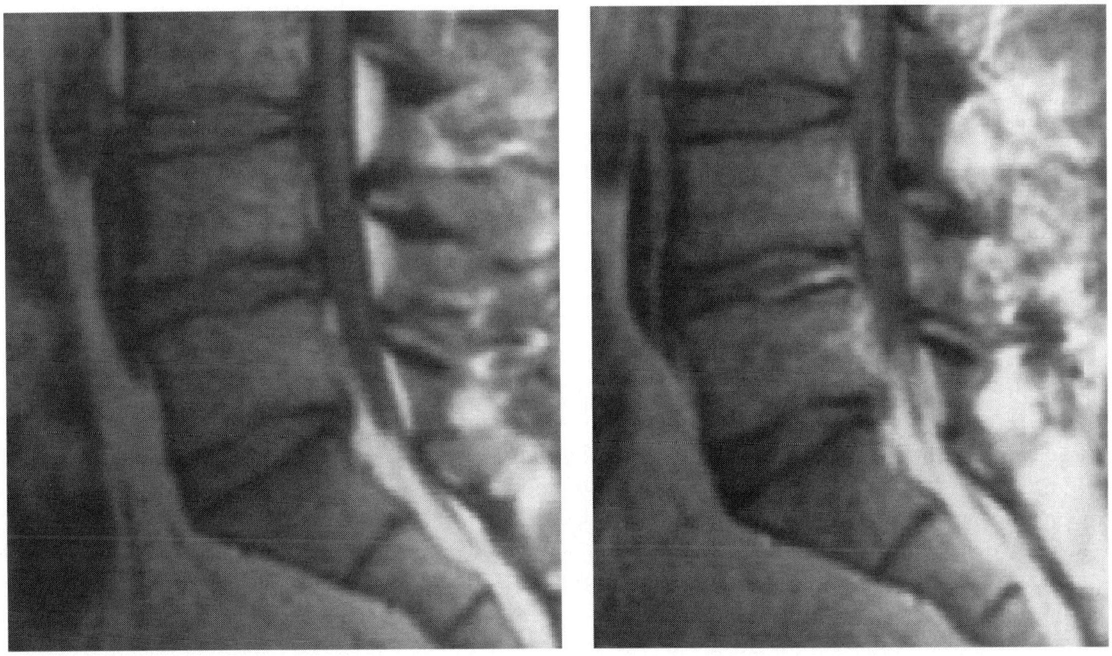

A B

Fig. 3.4 Sagittal T1-weighted images of the lumbar spine before the administration of contrast medium **(A)** and after **(B)**. Contrast enhancement in the L4-L5 intervertebral disk indicates the presence of granulation tissue in a radial tear of the annulus fibrosus.

One of the indications for contrast medium is to differentiate a recurrent herniated disk and an epidural scar. In patients who have had a previous laminectomy and diskectomy, scar usually shows contrast enhancement and disk fragments do not. Often in patients with failed back surgery, heterogeneous enhancement is present in the epidural space, suggesting the presence of both scar tissue and disk fragments. MR distinguishes scar and disk with an accuracy of 90%; CT does so with less accuracy.[9] In the immediate postoperative period, detection of a recurrent herniated disk is complicated by the presence (in approximately 70% of cases) of a hematoma or an epidural mass of poorly organized connective tissue resembling a herniated disk on MR images.[10]

Contrast medium may also be used to measure diffusion into the intervertebral disk. Normally diffusion into the disk is slowed by the presence of fixed negative charges attached to glycosaminoglycans in the disk. The rate of diffusion into the disk depends on the nature and amount of the glycosaminoglycans.[11] Disk degeneration increases the rate of diffusion into the disk. The substitution of the nonionic media gadoteridol (ProHance) and gadodiamide (Omniscan) for the ionic medium gadopentetate (Magnevist) increases the rate of diffusion in both normal and degenerating intervertebral disks.[12] In the detection of recurrent herniated disk, the ionic medium is also preferred because it produces greater contrast between the disk fragment and the adjacent scar.

Contrast enhancement in nerve roots of the cauda equina is reported in patients with herniated disks.[13] The enhanced nerve usually correlates with the nerve that is suspected clinically to be involved. However, prominent radicular veins may simulate nerve root enhancement in some cases. Following laminectomy, nonspecific nerve root enhancement is often seen. The clinical significance of nerve root enhancement at this time is uncertain.

Dynamic Magnetic Resonance Imaging of the Spine

With MR, changes in the anatomic relationships in the spine secondary to physiologic loading can be measured. Several strategies have been described. One method uses one of several devices that compress the body axially while it is in the MR scanner.[14] Images are acquired of the spine with and without the compression applied, and anatomic changes are detected. In another method, the patient is placed in an "upright" MR scanner and can assume a variety of sitting or standing positions while MR images are taken to determine the effect of the position on anatomic relationships in the spine.[15] In another technique, the spine is imaged with varying degrees of spinal rotation to measure the mobility of one spinal segment in relation to the adjacent one.[16] Motion segments with a normal-appearing disk allow rotations of up to 1 degree. Disks having degenerative changes allow more rotation. Rotation is significantly greater in disks that evoke "concordant pain" at diskography than in disks that do not.[17] More research is needed to determine the value of these techniques in clinical practice.[18]

Clinical instability has been defined as the failure of the spine to maintain normal patterns of deformation and to resist painful deformity under physiologic loading.[19] The criteria for selecting patients for spinal fusion may be heavily weighted to the clinical findings.[20] Physical examination and history may be sufficient to detect instability; however, spinal fusion should be reserved for patients with supporting functional imaging evidence of instability, according to some spine surgeons. A functional imaging study that accurately distinguishes stable and unstable segments would be helpful in selecting patients for fusion.

The primary imaging modality at present for diagnosing instability is flexion-extension radiography, despite its poor accuracy rate. False positives and false negatives are found with all methods for calculating instability from flexion/extension radiographs.[21] The rotations and translations of normal and degenerating motion segments have been extensively studies in biomechanical experiments. Disk degeneration has a greater effect on the resistance of the disk to axial rotational torques than to flexion, extension, or lateral bending torques.[22] Normal intervertebral disks resist axial rotational because of the radial orientation of collagen fibers in the annulus fibrosus. Although not effectively measured with radiographs, axial rotations can be measured with CT or MRI.[16,17] Axial rotatory motions of segments with normal and abnormal disks differ more significantly than do the motions secondary to extension, flexion, and lateral bending motions. Functional imaging with applied axial rotatory torques may be useful in future studies to determine the effect of disk degeneration of the motions of spinal segments.

Dynamic imaging of the spine is in the initial stages of evaluation. Applications may include the assessment of spinal canal dimensions, ligamentous injury, spinal instability, and union versus non-union. Where roentgenographic stereophotogrammetry (RSA) is used, noninvasive dynamic imaging is likely to replace it. With dynamic imaging, motions of the spinal column can be measured with the same accuracy as with RSA.[23] The relative mobility of spinal motion segments can be measured and hypermobility can be detected with dynamic imaging. The study of degenerative spinal instability should benefit from the use of dynamic imaging.

Other Techniques for Magnetic Resonance Imaging of the Spine

Magnetic resonance provides several useful techniques that will in the future contribute to the diagnosis of back pain. One is the measurement of the T2 relation time of the intervertebral disk.[24,25] This technique reports the T2 relaxation times throughout the nucleus and annulus of the disk. Because T2 relaxation time is closely related to the free water content, T2 relaxation measurements provide a useful continuous and reproducible measure of disk aging and degenerations. It may provide a more sensitive technique to detect early intervertebral disk degeneration. Studies have shown an increase in T2 and presumably in water content in the disk in the second decade of life.[26] Further studies are indicated to validate its role in spine research and in the clinical evaluation of disk degeneration.

Another technique is MR spectroscopy (MRS). With this technique, metabolites within the disk, such as lactate, may be measured. It has been applied to the evaluation of water and fat in the spine in storage diseases.[27] MRS may have applications in differentiation of tumor from nonneoplastic disease, spinal cord injury, and metabolic disorders.

Diffusion weighted imaging (DWI) and diffusion tensor imaging (DTI) have been applied effectively to spine imaging. Contrast in DWI is produced by the effect of body tissues and pathologic processes on the diffusion of protons. DWI, used effectively for detection of cerebral infarction, has been reported to be effective in distinguishing pathologic fractures from benign compression fractures.[28] In the former, diffusion is restricted, producing a high signal in DWI, whereas in the latter diffusion is unrestricted, producing relatively low signal intensity in DWI. The effects of pulsation in the CSF and susceptibility effects complicate measuring diffusion in the spinal cord. In the detection and characterization of an epidural abscess, DWI has an important application because restricted diffusion in a cavity is relatively specific for abscess.

The DTI technique provides a more complete assessment of diffusion than the DWI. It demonstrates the magnitude of diffusion and the direction of diffusion. It is a noninvasive technique that demonstrates the orientation of fibers in the annulus fibrosus.[29] Used to measure diffusion in the more amorphous disk regions, DTI has been shown to detect early degeneration in the disk, which is characterized by a change in water content and the structure of the disk matrix. DTI has applications in research and potentially in clinical evaluations of disk disease.

Ultrashort TE imaging (UTE) provides a means of imaging the osseous tissues in the spine. Unlike most MR techniques, this one allows the detection of the MR signal within bone.[30] Contrast enhancement in bone can be detected with the technique. It is likely to be useful in orthopedic research and probably clinical evaluations.

With pulse sequences sensitive to motion, MR angiography (MRA) is possible. In the spine, MRA may be used to identify the artery of Adamkiewicz or abnormal vessels associated with an arteriovenous fistula or arteriovenous malformation (AVM).

Spine Anatomy, Aging, and Degeneration

This section describes the tissues that determine the MR appearance of the spine. Other texts should be consulted for a thorough discussion of the anatomy of the spine.

Intervertebral Disk

Normal Anatomy

The normal intervertebral disk is a highly complex structure of specialized living connective tissue. The disk is composed of fibrocartilage, hyaline cartilage, and dense collagen tissue. It has anatomic relationships to the anterior longitudinal, posterior longitudinal and transforaminal ligaments. The disk confers flexibility to the spine by allowing flexion, extension, and lateral bending. It provides limited rotation between vertebral segments because of the oblique orientation of fibers in the annulus fibrosus. It changes dynamically in volume, releasing water when the spine is under additional load and absorbing water when it is under reduced loads. The changes in disk volume result in a diurnal variation of approximately 1 to 2 inches of stature and in a change in the T2 relaxation time of the disk that can be measured with quantitative MRI.[31] Cells in the disk respond to changes in pressure with changes in the metabolism of glycosaminoglycans.[32] This effect is related to the frequency of the pressure application.

Disregarding the anterior longitudinal ligament and the osseous and cartilaginous end plates, the remaining tissue in the intervertebral disk can be divided into three parts for the purpose of description: outer annulus fibrosus, inner annulus fibrosus, and nucleus pulposus. The outer annulus fibrosus has thick lamellae of dense connective tissue. The dense fibers in the outer annulus originate and insert in the bone contained within the adjacent ring apophysis. Each layer has fibers that run parallel at approximately 60 degrees with respect to the end plate. Fibers in adjacent layers run in different directions, although making the same angle with respect to the end plate. The major chemical constituent of the outer annulus is collagen, and the predominant cell type is the fibroblast. Histologically it resembles a tendon such as the Achilles tendon. It contains 10 to 15% type VI collagen, which probably contributes to the stiffness of the intervertebral disk. In T2-weighted MR images, it has a low signal intensity, like tendons. The inner annulus, containing collagenous lamellae that are interspersed with a gel containing glycosaminoglycans, has greater signal intensity. Like the lamellae in the outer annulus, those in the inner annulus run obliquely. They insert and originate not in bone but in the hyaline cartilage that forms the cartilaginous end plate. The predominant cell type is the chondrocyte. The nucleus pulposus is fibrocartilage like the inner

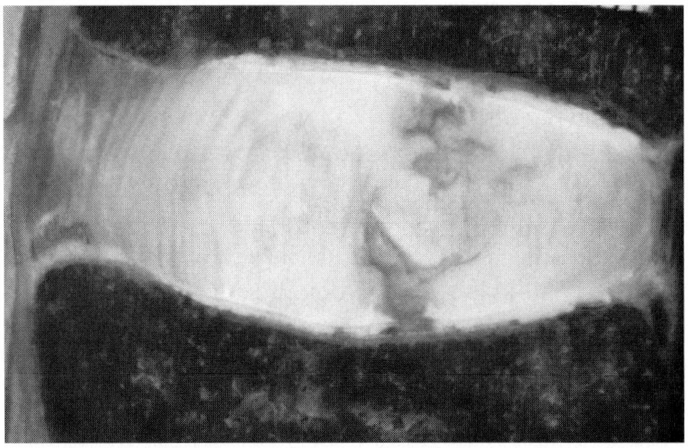

Fig. 3.5 Sagittal anatomic section through a normal adult lumbar intervertebral disk. The section shows a thin layer of hyaline cartilage covering a portion of the upper and lower margins of the disk. It shows brownish collagenous fibers in the peripheral annulus fibrosus in the anterior and posterior disk. Centrally, the lamellae in the annulus become less and less distinct until they are indistinguishable from the amorphous-appearing nucleus pulposus.

annulus but with less organized fibrous structure. It also contains glycosaminoglycans, collagen, and chondrocytes. The inner annulus fibrosus and the nucleus fibrosus have high signal intensity on T2-weighted images, reflecting the glycosaminoglycans and water content.

The anterior and posterior longitudinal ligaments blend with the anterior and lateral margin of the intervertebral disk. The anterior longitudinal ligament, which contains predominantly collagen and contacts the anterior and lateral surfaces of the disk, cannot be distinguished from the outer annulus fibrosus on MR images **(Fig. 3.5).** The posterior longitudinal ligament where it attaches to the posterior intervertebral disk margin cannot be distinguished from the posterior disk margin in MR images. Where the ligament passes posterior to the epidural venous plexus behind the vertebral body, it may be distinguished on MR.

Another morphologic feature of the intervertebral disk that may be distinguished on MR images is the low signal intensity in the central portion of the disk. This is a region in the equator of the intervertebral disk that is not characterized by increased density of collagen, elastic, and reticulin fibers. The lower signal intensity of the cleft represents the lower concentration of glycosaminoglycans due to the higher fiber content. Although not a cleft, it is sometimes referred to as the "intranuclear cleft."

The intervertebral disk has several thousand cells (chondrocytes or fibroblasts) in each cubic milliliter. These cells produce precursors of collagen and glycosaminoglycans that are released into the disk matrix. The production of these precursors is necessary to replace the collagen and glycosaminoglycans in the disk that is degraded by collagenases and proteinases in the disk. The glycosaminoglycans and collagen in the disk turn over approximately every 180 days. Reduction in the diffusion processes in the intervertebral disk may contribute to disk degeneration by interrupting the normal synthetic processes in the cell population in the disk.

The cells in the intervertebral disk receive their nutrition via diffusion because the intervertebral disk has no perfusion from arteries or capillaries. Oxygen, glucose, sulfates, and other nutrients diffuse into the disk through the vertebral end plates, and carbon dioxide and other waste products diffuse out. Diffusion into the intervertebral disk can be imaged with MR as an increase in signal intensity in the disk after the intravenous administration of a paramagnetic contrast medium.

Aging and Degeneration

Aging and degeneration of the disk are sometimes considered indistinguishable. Both are associated with a decrease of water and glycosaminoglycans in the disk and an increase in collagen. Degeneration differs from aging in the rate of biochemical change. Aging is associated with slow changes in chemical constituents and degeneration with much more rapid change. From the perspective of biochemistry, degeneration seems like accelerated aging.

The biomechanical changes associated with degeneration differ from those associated with aging. Disks with an intact annulus fibrosus retain resistance to axial rotatory torque throughout life, whereas disks that have radial tears of the annulus fibrosus do not. A characteristic of degenerating disks is that they allow the motion segment to rotate more in response to an axial rotatory torque than disks with an intact annulus. In biomechanical testing, an axial rotatory torque produces two to three times as much rotation in degenerating disks as in normal disks. In biomechanical terms, disk degeneration represents a mechanical failure of the intervertebral disk.

Aging Changes In the neonate, the disk appears as a colorless, translucent structure between the partially ossified vertebral bodies. In the periphery of the neonatal disk, an outer annulus with conspicuous lamellae and low signal intensity on MR images is evident. In the center of the disk are some streaks, which represent syncytial cells that are remnants of the primitive notochord. Adjacent to the disk, the unossified cartilage of the intervertebral disk has a similar color in anatomic sections and similar signal intensity on MR images. The vertebral cartilage contains large blood vessels. On MR images, the peripheral annulus fibrosus and the central disk are sharply differentiated from each other **(Fig. 3.6)**.

From birth to adolescence the intervertebral disk changes rapidly in height, diameter, and structure, as the skeleton matures. The lamellae in the outer annulus fibrosus become better defined in the first two decades of life. The collagen content of the inner annulus and the nucleus pulposus increases rapidly in the first two decades of life,

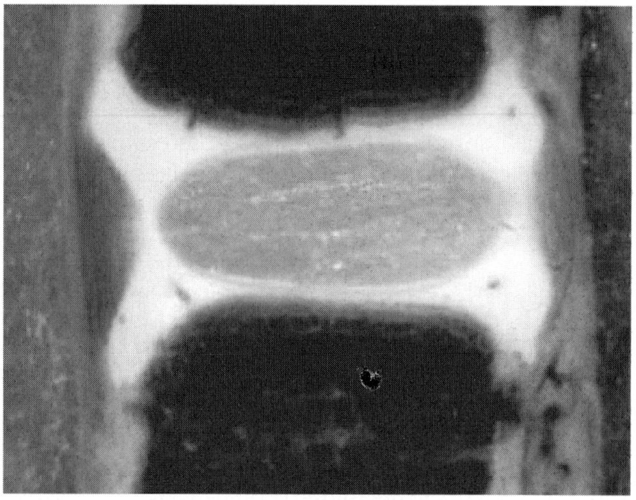

Fig. 3.6 Sagittal anatomic section through a lumbar intervertebral disk in a neonate. The nucleus pulposus is translucent and nearly colorless. Surrounding it is an opaque, ivory colored tissue, the inner annulus fibrosus. The collagenous fibers in the peripheral annulus fibrosus are evident in the anterior and posterior parts of the disk. A few small blood vessels are present in the inner annulus fibrosus.

with an increase in the stiffness of the disk. The disk in the second decade of life has a longer T2 relaxation time, likely due to greater water content.[26] Ossification of the vertebral body concludes in this time period. All blood vessels in the cartilage around the disk and the notochordal cells in the center of the disk disappear. In histologic sections, the intervertebral disk has a white, opaque appearance. A central region of lower signal intensity develops in the second decade of life because of increasing fiber content at the same time that the disk increases generally in water content. Compared with the juvenile disk, the adult disk has a less distinct transition between the peripheral annulus and the inner annulus and nucleus pulposus. Because of the different MR appearance of the normal juvenile and the mature intervertebral disk, the former is graded as a stage I on the Pfirrmann scale for grading intervertebral disk degeneration[33] and the latter as a stage II.

After the second decade of life, change continues in the intervertebral disk at a slower rate. In all regions of the disk, especially in the central region, the concentration of viable cells declines. The proportion of aggregating proteoglycans and the size of the aggregants in the disk diminish. In the nucleus pulposus and inner annulus fibrosus, collagen and noncollagen proteins increase in concentration. These changes result in a gradual decrease in T2 relaxation times and in signal intensity in T2-weighted images.

With aging, fissures and cracks develop in the annulus fibrosus **(Fig. 3.7)**. In the majority of intervertebral disks in people over the age of 50, transverse and concentric tears are present in the annulus fibrosus. Transverse tears are disruptions of the peripheral annular fibers near their attachment to the ring apophysis. They are found in disks

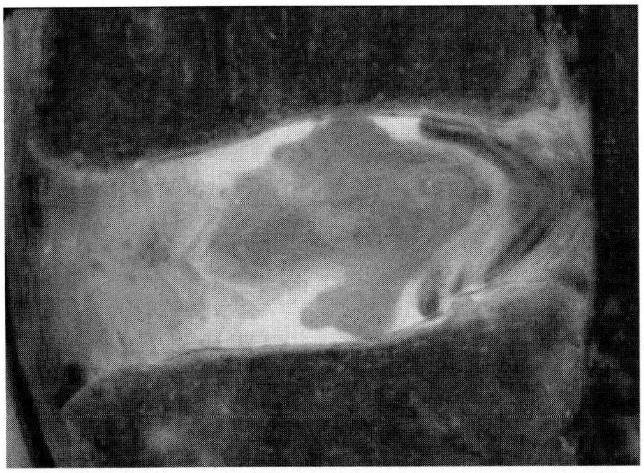

Fig. 3.7 Sagittal anatomic section through an adult intervertebral disk that has posteriorly a concentric tear, appearing as delamination of lamellae in the annulus fibrosus, and, anteriorly adjacent to the superior and inferior end plates, transverse tears of the annulus fibrosus, which appear as small cystic cavities in the peripheral annulus fibrosus.

that have no bulging of the annulus fibrosus, no loss of height or signal intensity or other signs of degeneration.[34] They are therefore most accurately characterized as age-related changes. The transverse tears that contain mucoid material appear on T2-weighted MR images as regions of increased signal intensity in the annulus fibrosus. If the transverse tears contain gas, they may appear as regions of low density on radiographs or of low signal intensity on MR images.[35] Concentric tears are small crescent-shaped gaps between lamellae of the annulus fibrosus. They may occur in disks without other signs of degeneration. They occasionally have sufficient mucoid material to permit their detection on MR. Neither concentric nor transverse tears demonstrate contrast enhancement. They do not likely cause pain because the peripheral portion of the intervertebral disk is not innervated.

Degenerative Changes The feature common to all degenerating intervertebral disks is a radial tear of the annulus fibrosus. Disks with reduced height, reduced signal intensity, or bulging of the annulus have a radial tear that is not found in aging disks with normal height and signal intensity[36,37] (**Fig. 3.8**). The definition of a radial tear is one that involves all layers of the annulus fibrosus; therefore, it differs from transverse and concentric tears that involve only a portion of the annulus. The radial tear, a fatigue failure of the disk, may be produced in the biomechanical laboratory by the application of repetitive loading or axial torsion. The radial tear may affect the anterior disk only, the posterior disk only, or extend across the full equator of the disk with disruption of both the anterior and the posterior lamellae of the annulus fibrosus. Radial tears are most prevalent at the L4-L5 and L5-S1 disk levels.

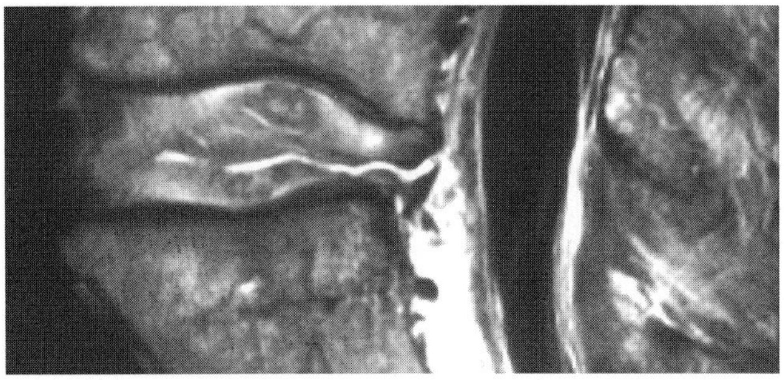

Fig. 3.8 Sagittal T2-weighted MR image of a cadaver L5-S1 intervertebral disk with a radial tear of the annulus fibrosus. This disk has a defect through the posterior annulus, which has high signal intensity due to the presence of mucoid material in it. The disk has lost some signal intensity compared with more normal disks in the same cadaver.

Magnetic resonance demonstration of a radial tear in an intervertebral disk is an excellent predictor of "concordant pain" at diskography. Intradiskal injection of contrast medium or saline exactly reproduces the patient's pain in most disks with annular disruption and causes pain in few normal intervertebral disks.[38–41]

Radial tear of the annulus fibrosus may produce pain that is essentially indistinguishable from that of a herniated disk,[42] even though a nerve root is not compressed. The radial tear of the annulus fibrosus may produce pain by one or more of several mechanisms. The presence of nociceptors within the disk is one possibility. Granulation tissue in the intervertebral disk, with nerve endings from the spinal nerves adjacent to the disk, may be the source of pain, which is experienced as referred pain in a lower extremity.[43] The leakage of substances from the degenerating disk into the epidural space where it irritates a spinal nerve is another mechanism.[44] Glycosaminoglycans, lactic acid, and immunogenic substances have been implicated as potential causes of pain after escape from a degenerating intervertebral disk.[45] Another possibility is increased motions of the spine at the level of a disk with a radial tear.[22] The loss of stiffness in the disk results in greater stresses in other spinal ligaments when physiologic loads and torques are applied. In the presence of a radial tear, a torque applied to the motion segment produces greater rotation than in a motion segment with a normal disk, especially in the case of an axial rotatory torque. The hypermobility of a motion segment that contains a radial tear hypothetically may cause pain. The hypothesis has not been adequately tested. Correlation has been demonstrated between larger rotations in a motion segment and "concordant pain" at diskography.[17] Changes in posture and physiologic loading of the spine may produce intermittent nerve root compression, in the presence of a degenerated disk that reduces the stiffness of the motion segment. Critical changes in the anatomic relationships within the neural foramina adjacent to a radial tear have been observed secondary to physiologic forces that would not significantly affect a normal disk level.[22] The foramen narrowing resulting from a radial tear, however, is unlikely to be visualized in routine clinical imagining in which the patient is placed supine in a position of comfort with minimal loading of the spine.

The radial tear permits herniation of nuclear material, which is implicated in the pathogenesis of sciatic pain. The pathogenesis of pain from a herniated nucleus pulposus cannot be explained simply in terms of compression or displacement of a spinal nerve or nerve root. Pressure on a normal spinal nerve does not cause pain. Smyth and Wright's[46] classic study in patients operated on for herniated disks showed that traction on a normal spinal nerve caused little symptomatology, whereas traction on a spinal nerve that had recently undergone decompression caused exquisite pain. The study suggests that spinal nerves chronically traumatized by a herniated disk fragment behave differently than normal nerves when compressed. Chronic or intermittent compression of a spinal nerve or roots leads to demyelination.[47] Demyelination changes the electrical conduction properties, resulting in repetitive depolarization of pain fibers that does not occur in normal nerves. In a demyelinated nerve root, weak mechanical stimuli, hypoxia, chemical mediators, inflammation, and sympathetic efferent activity may elicit nerve impulses ("ectopic hyperexcitability").

With loss of disk height the ligamentum flavum shortens, due to the shortening of elastic fibers within it, and thickens. Cysts and fissures may develop in the ligamentum flavum as part of the degenerative process.[48] The thickened ligament may contain fissures or foci of calcification. The thickened ligament decreases the size of the central spinal canal and of the neural foramen. Spinal nerves in the neural foramen or the dural sac within the central spinal canal may be affected by the thickening of the ligamentum flavum. Ligamentum flavum thickening contributes to spinal stenosis.

Spinal Zygapophyseal (Facet) Joints

The zygapophyseal (facet) joint is the articulation between the superior and inferior articular processes at each spinal intervertebral level between C2 and S1. The anatomy of the facet joints varies from level to level. The flat or gently curving articular surfaces of the facet joint vary in inclination from one level to another. In the cervical region the plane is typically oblique to the vertical and the axial plane. In the lumbar region the plane is typically vertical and varying from a plane nearly parallel with a sagittal plane (at L1) to one nearly perpendicular to the sagittal plane (at L4 and L5).

The zygapophyseal joint consists of the superior and inferior articular processes, which each have a thin uniform layer of dense cortical bone and thin layers of cartilage. The posterior surface of the zygapophyseal joint has a tough, thick fibrous capsule, which covers the joint space and portions of the adjacent articular processes. Anteriorly the zygapophyseal joint has no capsule or barrier between it and the spinal canal except the ligamentum flavum. Within the periphery of the facet joint, a thin synovial lining is found. The synovium may extend a variable distance from the joint between the ligamentum flavum and the lamina. Within the joint is a small fibrous meniscus, which varies in appearance with spinal level and age.[49] It probably facilitates motion and weight bearing.

Aging Changes Facet joint architecture changes with age. Uniform layers of cartilage and subarticular cortical bone characterize the cervical facet joints in cadavers less than 20 years of age. Most adult cervical facet joints have only a discolored or microscopically thin layer of cartilage and have irregularly thickened subarticular cortical bone.[50] The meniscus that characterizes zygapophyseal joints in children under the age of 10 disappears in most adults over age 40.[49] This change in the facet joints, which is essentially universal, can be characterized as an age-related change. In adults, zygapophyseal joints retain a thin relatively smooth rim of subchondral bone.[51]

Degenerative Changes Facet joint degeneration includes the loss of articular cartilage, sclerosis in the subcortical bone, erosions of subcortical bone, and hypertrophy of the facet articulating processes.[52] CT or MR demonstrates these changes effectively. Degeneration of the facet joint is initially characterized by loss of cartilage from the articular surface. Initially the degeneration has superficial crevasses described as "crabmeat degeneration." With additional destruction of cartilage, the articular bone is exposed. At this stage, subarticular erosions, bony sclerosis, and hypertrophy occur in the articular processes. MR and, to a greater extent, CT demonstrate the osseous and cartilaginous changes in the joint.[53]

Facet joint degeneration may contribute to back pain in a variety of ways. The process of sclerosis and subarticular erosions may be associated with painful arthropathy, which in the facet joints may results in pain referred to the lower extremities in the distribution of the nerves that supply the facet joint and capsule. The resulting pain may closely simulate that of a herniated disk. Degeneration of the facet joint may contribute to hypermobility of the motion segment, resulting in pain due to intermittent nerve root compression or intermittent increase in the strain in other connective tissues at the involved joint. The hypertrophic joint may also contribute to pain by narrowing the neural foramen increasingly, until nerve root compression results. Either MR or CT effectively demonstrates pathologic changes in the fact joint, including articular cartilage destruction, subarticular erosion, sclerosis, hypertrophy, synovial cyst, and ankylosis.

Intraspinal synovial cysts represent a combination of degeneration in the facet joint and cavitation in the ligamentum flavum. With excessive fluid in the joint, the synovium

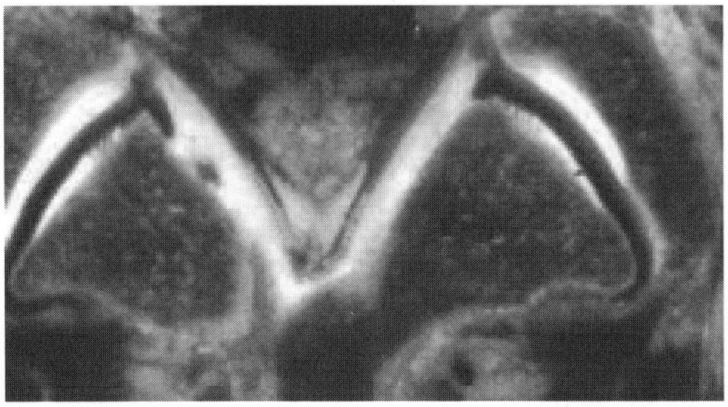

Fig. 3.9 Synovial cyst.

may herniate through a degenerated ligamentum flavum. The synovial cyst appears in images as an epidural soft tissue process adjacent to a degenerating facet joint, usually at L4-L5, and less commonly at other lumber levels, thoracic levels, or cervical levels **(Fig. 3.9).** The capsule of the cyst may be calcified. The contents of the cyst may be clear fluid, proteinaceous fluid, gas, or blood. The capsule enhances markedly after administration of intravenous contrast medium. The enhancing capsule may mimic a meningioma or schwannoma.

Vertebrae

Aging Changes The changes due to aging in the osseous spine have been extensively studied biochemically and anatomically. In terms of imaging, changes in the bone marrow produce the most conspicuous age-related changes. The conversion of cellular to fatty marrow results in a grossly inhomogeneous pattern of signal in the bone marrow that may simulate a diffuse invasive metastatic process.[54]

Degenerative Changes Spondylotic changes occur in the spine of older individuals, in response to aging and degeneration. These changes are not well characterized on MRI and therefore are not systematically considered here.

■ Magnetic Resonance Imaging Findings in Back Pain

Selection of Patients

Spinal trauma, infection, suspected tumor, cauda equina syndrome, and unexplained progressive neurologic deterioration are indications for spine imaging acutely. The onset of back pain, which usually responds to symptomatic treatment, does not warrant immediate spine imaging. In back pain persisting more than 6 weeks, MRI and CT may be used to select between surgery and other treatments. Imaging detects abnormalities in the spine effectively but fails to distinguish symptomatic from incidental changes. Because of the high incidence of asymptomatic degenerative changes in the spine, inappropriate imaging may lead to unnecessary costs for the patient and to incorrect diagnoses by physicians based on incidental degenerative changes that are confused with significant lesions.

Magnetic resonance is useful in patients with chronic radiculopathy. With its capability to produce images in multiple planes, MR effectively demonstrates the relationship of a nerve root, facet joint degenerative changes, or disk herniation. The sagittal images are especially useful in some cases such as spondylolisthesis, which may distort the anatomy of the neural foramen severely. CT, which demonstrates osseous anatomy effectively, is useful for imaging the vertebral body, facet joint, pedicle, and bony spurs. MR may be used to distinguish whether the disk herniation is sequestered, contained, or subligamentous. MRI may distinguish disk fragments that are contiguous with the disk and those that are not.

In myelopathy, MR is indicated to distinguish intrinsic processes within the cord from processes that compress the spinal cord or cauda equina. MR shows the relationship of the spinal cord and spinal nerve roots in the cauda equina and in the neural foramina to the spinal canal. The myelogram may provide additional information in selected cases because it demonstrates the relative degree of obstruction to the flow of contrast medium though a narrowed region of spine.

In patients with suspected spinal instability or internal disk disruption, MR may assist in the evaluation. For example, MR detects facet joint or disk degeneration, which may destabilize the spine. The demonstration of some degenerative changes, such as a radial tear of the annulus fibrosus, has a high predictive value for a positive diskogram at that level.[42]

Magnetic Resonance Findings in Intervertebral Disk Degeneration

On MR images, a variety of findings indicate the presence of disk degeneration. The most universal finding is loss of signal intensity on T2-weighted images **(Fig. 3.10).** In some cases, loss of signal intensity is the only indication of disk degeneration. It has been referred to as a "dehydration" of the disk, although the loss of water is only one of several chemical changes. Loss of signal intensity in the disk correlates with the development of a radial tear in the annulus fibrosus. The annular tear may not be demonstrated on the MR images, but it is demonstrated as a leakage of contrast medium from the disk if diskography is performed.[39–42] In some disks with diminished signal intensity, a high-intensity zone (HIZ) may be demonstrated in the annulus fibrosus. The HIZ results from the presence of mucoid material in the radial tear. Only approximately 70% of radial tears are detected as an HIZ on MR.[55] In some disks with reduced signal intensity, a linear region of

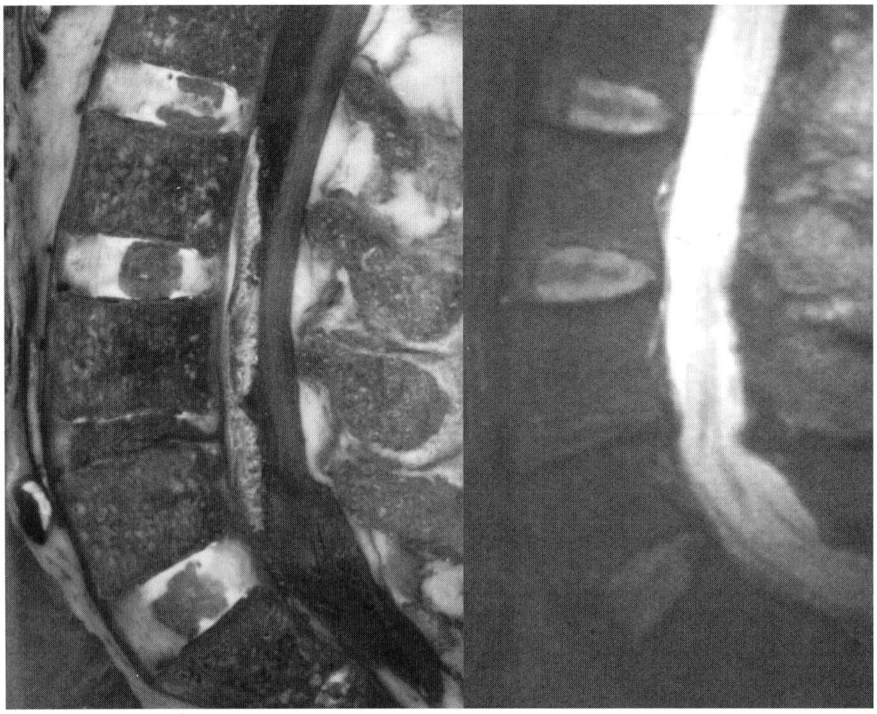

Fig. 3.10 Anatomic section **(A)** and T2-weighted MR image of a cadaver spine showing a radial tear in the L4-L5 intervertebral disk. In the anatomic image, the degenerating L4-L5 disk has a darker color than the disks above and below. The disruption of the annulus fibrosus posteriorly is evident. **(B)** In the MR image, the degenerating disk has diminished signal intensity. In this image, the radial tear is not evident.

contrast enhancement may be demonstrated, corresponding to the presence of granulation tissue in the radial tear.[56] With contrast medium, the radial tear may be demonstrated more frequently than without it, but a suspected radial tear is not customarily an indication for the administration of contrast medium. Other findings in disks with diminished signal intensity include diminished disk height, abnormal signal intensity in the adjacent end plates due to disk degeneration, and bulging of the annulus fibrosus. Adjacent to degenerating intervertebral disks, signal intensity within the bone marrow and end plate may be abnormal. Three patterns have been identified.[57] One pattern (type I) is characterized by increased signal intensity on T2-weighted images and, if contrast medium is administered, by abnormal contrast enhancement. This imaging pattern results from increased vascularity in the adjacent vertebral end plate and vertebral body. Some investigators suggest that it may be a sign of instability in the motion segment.[58] Another change (type II) is characterized by increased signal intensity on T1-weighted images. It results from a conversion of red marrow to yellow marrow near the degenerating intervertebral disk. The clinical significance is not known. A third type of change is characterized by low signal intensity on T1- or T2-weighted images and corresponds to an increase in trabecular bone adjacent to the end plate.

Complete collapse of the intervertebral disk, at the end stage of degeneration, can be demonstrated. In those cases in which nuclear material herniated through the radial tear, MR demonstrates the escaped fragment. With a combination of T2- and T1-weighted MR images in axial and sagittal projections, disk herniations can be demonstrated with close to 100% accuracy.[1] Differentiation of an asymmetrically bulging annulus and a herniated disk fragment by MR may not be perfectly accurate, although numerous criteria have been proposed. Therefore, numerous criteria have been suggested. The relationship of a disk fragment to a nerve, a much more important evaluation, can be made accurately by MR.

Magnetic Resonance Findings in Degenerative Spondylolisthesis

Degenerative spondylolisthesis is effectively demonstrated with MRI but may be underdiagnosed. The process occurs at L4-L5 typically in women in the seventh and eighth decades of life. The slippage of L4 on L5 may be minimal on MR images made with the patient placed in a comfortable supine position in the scanner. MR demonstrates severe degenerative changes in the facet joint in this condition. Spinal stenosis may be underestimated in the images obtained with the patient lying supine. Axial images demonstrate the sclerosis of the facet joints, hypertrophy, and usually fluid within the joint space. The dimensions of the subarachnoid space and spinal canal must be evaluated both in the sagittal and the axial images.

Magnetic Resonance Findings in Ankylosing Spondylitis

Magnetic resonance imaging poorly demonstrates the facet joint ankylosis. However, it effectively demonstrates the squaring of the vertebrae and the loss of bone mineral in the vertebrae. When ankylosing spondylitis is associated with the cauda equina syndrome, MR demonstrates findings of proliferative arachnoiditis, which is the cause of the neurologic deficit. The arachnoiditis appears as multiple erosions in the bony margins of the spinal canal, and in the vertebrae and neural arches. These erosions may simulate a neoplastic process. Axial images demonstrate that the nerve roots are adherent to the inflamed arachnoid and are no longer apparent within the dural sac. Abnormal contrast enhancement may be detected if contrast medium is administered.

Magnetic Resonance Findings in Diskitis and Abscess

Magnetic resonance effectively demonstrates the changes in the vertebral end plate and intervertebral disk resulting from diskitis. The hallmarks of diskitis are the destruction of the vertebral end plate, increased signal intensity in the intervertebral disk and adjacent vertebral bodies, a soft tissue mass of granulation tissue surrounding the intervertebral disk, and contrast enhancement in the disk and vertebra. Usually diskitis is easily differentiated from disk degeneration, which lacks contrast enhancement, frank destruction of the end plate, and a large soft tissue mass. Because imaging findings lag behind the pain and elevated sedimentation rate of diskitis, early cases may not have definitive findings.

Epidural Abscess

Magnetic resonance effectively shows epidural abscesses, if contrast medium is administered. The findings of osteomyelitis and diskitis on the unenhanced images are usually present on the unenhanced images. When contrast medium is administered, the thickened epidural space and the liquefied region within the enhancement are demonstrated. Diffusion weighted images show a high signal intensity due to restricted diffusion in purulent fluid collection.

Spinal Cord Abscess

Abscesses of the spinal cord are rare, but occur in the United States.[59] MR shows usually a rim-enhancing process in the spinal cord associated with edema and tumefaction of the spinal cord. The appearance may simulate that of a tumor. The onset of symptoms in a spinal cord abscess, however, is much more rapid than in a tumor. Recognition of the presence of an abscess may result in surgical procedure that preserves more spinal cord than does a procedure designed to obtain cord material for histologic examination.

Magnetic Resonance Findings in Spinal Stenosis

A combination of sagittal and axial MR images effectively shows the changes of spinal stenosis. Stenosis that results in the probable compression of spinal nerve roots in the spinal canal or neural foramen (critical stenosis) must be differentiated from stenosis that does not compress nerve tissue. On MR images, obliteration of CSF between nerve roots in the cauda equina suggests critical central spinal stenosis. Obliteration of fat and veins adjacent to nerve roots in the neural foramen suggests critical lateral stenosis. Reader agreement when grading spinal stenosis into mild, moderate, and severe categories is only fair.[60] In the assessment of spinal stenosis in the cervical and thoracic region, the presence of high signal intensity in the spinal cord suggests myelomalacia or edema secondary to stenosis.

Magnetic Resonance Findings in Tumors

Magnetic resonance effectively demonstrates tumors of the spine, involving the vertebral column, epidural space, intradural and extramedullary space, or the spinal cord. Intravenous contrast medium and T1 and T2 images are useful. Other texts should be consulted for more detailed discussion.

Magnetic Resonance Findings in Vascular Processes

Magnetic resonance provides several useful tools for the demonstration of arteriovenous malformation or arteriovenous fistulas involving the spinal cord. MR angiographic images may provide the definitive diagnosis.[61] T2-weighted MR images in most cases of arteriovenous fistula show evidence of spinal cord edema secondary to the myelopathy resulting from the venous hypertension **(Fig. 3.11)**. It often demonstrates circuitous channels of "signal void" due to the rapid flow of blood through numerous channels on the surface of the spinal cord. Undiagnosed, the arteriovenous fistula may result in progressive loss of neurologic function that could be prevented by proper intervention.

Magnetic Resonance Findings in Trauma

Ligamentous Injury

Suspected ligamentous injury of the cervical spine is a common indicator for MRI. MR shows high signal intensity in the interspinous ligament or anterior longitudinal ligament in cases of partial or complete rupture. Cases of high signal intensity in the alar ligaments secondary to whiplash injury have also been reported.[62]

Cord Injury

Magnetic resonance is the best imaging modality for the demonstration of spinal cord injury. MR images in the acute

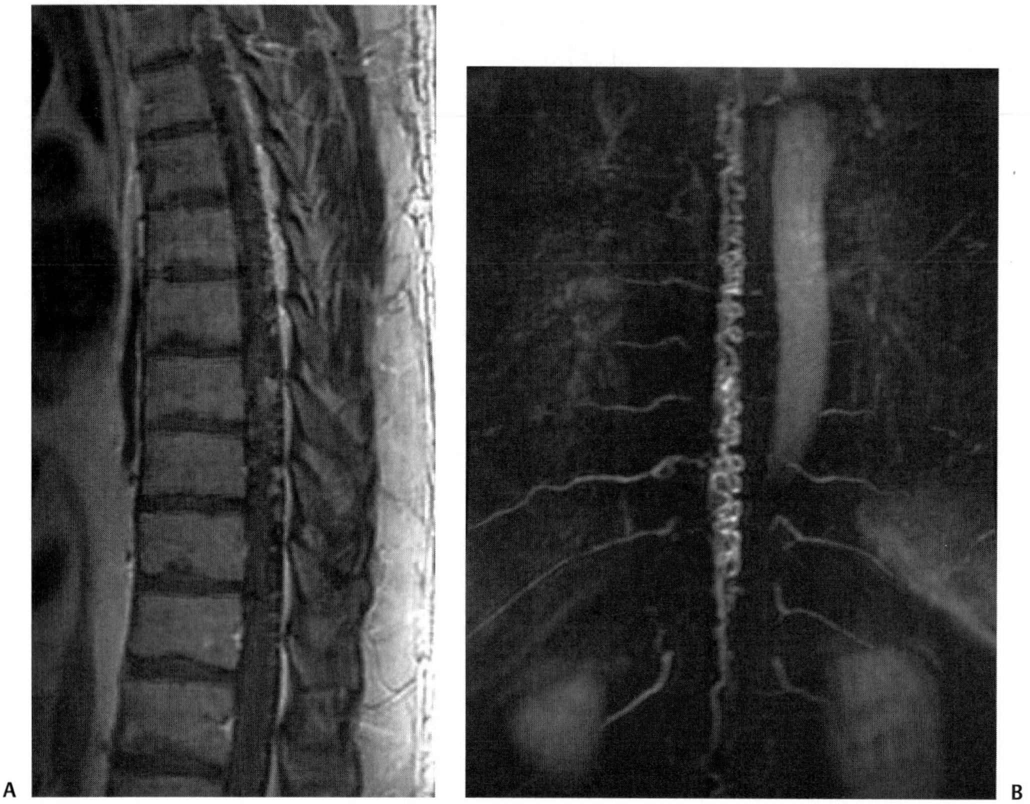

Fig. 3.11 Sagittal T2-weighted MR image **(A)** in a patient with a dural arteriovenous fistula demonstrates abnormally high signal intensity in the spinal cord and small irregular dark "signal voids" on the surface of the cord. The MR angiogram **(B)** performed with the TRICKS protocol in coronal view shows the large connection between the T9 subcostal artery on the right and a large network of serpentine arterialized veins on the surface of the cord.

case show high T2 signal intensity in the spinal cord representing edema. It may show regions of lower signal intensity in T2-weighted images secondary to bleeding in the cord. The relationship of the cord to fragments of the spinal canal can be assessed well with MR, sometimes with the addition of CT. Diffusion imaging may be used to detect infarction acutely. DTI may be used to assess the integrity of spinal fiber tracts.

Congenital Malformations of the Spine

Magnetic resonance provides an effective tool for the characterization of a spinal developmental abnormality. It can show congenital abnormalities in the spinal column and in the spinal cord. It has been applied effectively in utero to study the spine. Consult other texts for a thorough discussion of this subject.

References

1. Jarvik JG, Deyo RA. Diagnostic evaluation of low back pain with emphasis on imaging. Ann Intern Med 2002;137:586–597
2. Jensen MC, Brant-Zawadzki MN, Obuchowski N, Modic MT, Malkasian D, Ross JS. Magnetic resonance imaging of the lumbar spine in people without back pain. N Engl J Med 1994;331:69–73
3. Modic MT, Obuchowski NA, Ross JS, et al. Acute low back pain and radiculopathy: MR imaging findings and their prognostic role and effect on outcome. Radiology 2005;237:597–604
4. Ibrahim MA, Jesmanowicz A, Hyde J, Estkowski L, Haughton VM. Contrast enhancement of normal intervertebral disks: time and dose dependence. AJNR Am J Neuroradiol 1994;15:419–424
5. Nguyen CM, Ho KC, An H, Riley LH, Rongming X, Haughton VM. Ionic versus nonionic paramagnetic contrast media in differentiating between scar and herniated disk. AJNR Am J Neuroradiol 1996;17:501–505
6. Nguyen CM, Ho KC, Yu SW, Haughton VM, Strandt JA. An experimental model to study contrast enhancement in MR imaging of the intervertebral disk. AJNR Am J Neuroradiol 1989;10:811–814
7. Stabler A, Weiss M, Scheidler J, Krodel A, Seiderer M, Reiser M. Degenerative disk vascularization on MRI: correlation with clinical and histopathologic findings. Skeletal Radiol 1996;25:119–126
8. Ross JS, Modic MT, Masaryk TJ. Tears of the anulus fibrosus: assessment with Gd-DTPA-enhanced MR imaging. AJR Am J Roentgenol 1990;154:159–162
9. Schubiger O, Valavanis A. CT differentiation between recurrent disc herniation and postoperative scar formation: the value of contrast enhancement. Neuroradiology 1982;22:251–254
10. Boden SD, Davis DO, Dina TS, et al. Contrast-enhanced MR imaging performed after successful lumbar disk surgery: prospective study. Radiology 1992;182:59–64

11. Ibrahim MA, Haughton VM, Hyde JS. Effect of disk maturation on diffusion of low-molecular-weight gadolinium complexes: an experimental study in rabbits. AJNR Am J Neuroradiol 1995;16:1307–1311
12. Ibrahim MA, Haughton VM, Hyde JS. Enhancement of intervertebral disks with gadolinium complexes: comparison of an ionic and a nonionic medium in an animal model. AJNR Am J Neuroradiol 1994;15:1907–1910
13. Jinkins JR, Roeder MB. MRI of benign lumbosacral nerve root enhancement. Semin Ultrasound CT MR 1993;14:446–454
14. Willen J, Danielson B. The diagnostic effect from axial loading of the lumbar spine during computed tomography and magnetic resonance imaging in patients with degenerative disorders. Spine 2001;26:2607–2614
15. Vitzthum HE, Konig A, Seifert V. Dynamic examination of the lumbar spine by using vertical, open magnetic resonance imaging. J Neurosurg 2000;93(suppl)58–64
16. Haughton VM, Rogers B, Meyerand ME, Resnick DK. Measuring the axial rotation of lumbar vertebrae in vivo with MR imaging. AJNR Am J Neuroradiol 2002;23:1110–1116
17. Blankenbaker DG, Haughton VM, Rogers BP, Meyerand ME, Fine JP. Axial rotation of the lumbar spinal motion segments correlated with concordant pain on discography: a preliminary study. AJR Am J Roentgenol 2006;186:795–799
18. Weishaupt D, Schmid MR, Zanetti M, et al. Positional MR imaging of the lumbar spine: does it demonstrate nerve root compromise not visible at conventional MR imaging? Radiology 2000;215: 247–253
19. Pope MH, Panjabi M. Biomechnical definitions of spinal instability. Spine 1985;10:255–256
20. Panjabi MM, Thibodeau LL, Crisco JJ, White AA. What constitutes spinal instability? Clin Neurosurg 1988;34:313–339
21. Shaffer WO, Spratt KF, Weinstein J, Lehmann TR, Goel V. The consistency and accuracy of roentgenograms for measuring sagittal translation in the lumbar vertebral motion segment. An experimental model. Spine 1990;15:741–750
22. Nowicki BH, Haughton VM, Schmidt TA, et al. Occult lumbar lateral spinal stenosis in neural foramina subjected to physiologic loading. AJNR Am J Neuroradiol 1996;17:1605–1614
23. Rogers B, Wiese S, Blankenbaker D, Meyerand E, Haughton V. Accuracy of an automated method to measure rotations of vertebrae from computerized tomography data. Spine 2005;30:694–696
24. Boos N, Wallin A, Schmucker T, Aebi M, Boesch C. Quantitative MR imaging of lumbar intervertebral disc and vertebral bodies: methodology, reproducibility, and preliminary results. Magn Reson Imaging 1994;12:577–587
25. Perry J, Haughton V, Anderson PA, Wu Y, Fine J, Mistretta C. The value of T2 relaxation times to characterize lumbar intervertebral disks: preliminary results. AJNR Am J Neuroradiol 2006;27: 337–342
26. Krueger EC, Perry JO, Wu Y, Haughton V. Changes in T_2 relaxation times associated with maturation of the human intervertebral disk. AJNR Am J Neuroradiol 2007;28:1237–1241
27. Scherer A, Wittsack HJ, Engelbrecht V, et al. Proton MR spectroscopy of the lumbar spine in patients with glycogen storage disease type Ib. J Magn Reson Imaging 2001;14:757–762 DTI.
28. Baur A, Stabler A, Bruning R, et al. Diffusion-weighted MR imaging of bone marrow: differentiation of benign versus pathologic compression fractures. Radiology 1998;207:349–356
29. Hsu EW, Setton LA. Diffusion tensor microscopy of the intervertebral disc anulus fibrosus. Magn Reson Med 1999;41:992–999
30. Robson MD, Bydder GM. Clinical ultrashort echo time imaging of bone and other connective tissues. NMR Biomed 2006;19:765–780
31. Boos N, Wallin A, Gbedegbegnon T, Aebi M, Boesch C. Quantitative MR imaging of lumbar intervertebral disks and vertebral bodies: influence of diurnal water content variations. Radiology 1993;188:351–354
32. Iatridis JC, Weidenbaum M, Setton LA, Mow VC. Is the nucleus pulposus a solid or a fluid? Mechanical behaviors of the nucleus pulposus of the human intervertebral disc. Spine 1996;21: 1174–1184
33. Pfirrmann CW, Metzdorf A, Zanetti M, Hodler J, Boos N. Magnetic resonance classification of lumbar intervertebral disc degeneration. Spine 2001;26:1873–1878
34. Yu S, Sether L, Wagner M, Haughton V. Tears of the anulus fibrosus: correlation between MR and pathologic findings in cadavers. AJNR Am J Neuroradiol 1988;9:367–370
35. Resnick D, Niwayama G, Guerra J, Vint V, Usselman J. Spinal vacuum phenomena: anatomical study and review. Radiology 1981;139:341–348
36. Yu SW, Sether LA, Ho PS, Wagner M, Haughton VM. Tears of the anulus fibrosus: correlation between MR and pathologic findings in cadavers. AJNR Am J Neuroradiol 1988;9:367–370
37. Yu SW, Haughton VM, Sether LA, Wagner M. Anulus fibrosus in bulging intervertebral discs. Radiology 1988;169:761–763
38. Aprill C, Bogduk N. High-intensity zone: a diagnostic sign of painful lumbar disc on magnetic resonance imaging. Br J Radiol 1992;65:361–369
39. Buirski G. Magnetic resonance signal patterns of lumbar discs in patients with low back pain. A prospective study with discographic correlation. Spine 1992;17:1199–1204
40. Vanharanta H, Sachs BL, Spivey MA, et al. The relationship of pain provocation to lumbar disc deterioration as seen by CT/discography. Spine 1987;12:295–298
41. Osti OL, Fraser RD, Vernon-Roberts B. Annular tears and degeneration of the intervertebral disc—preliminary results of an experimental study. Spine 1990;15:762–767
42. Horton WC, Daftari TK. Which disc as visualized by magnetic resonance imaging is actually a source of pain? A correlation between magnetic resonance imaging and discography. Spine 1992;17(suppl)S164–S171
43. Goldie I. Granulation tissue in the ruptured intervertebral disc. Acta Pathol Microbiol Scand 1958;42:302–304
44. Haughton VM, Nguyen CM, Ho KC. The etiology of focal spinal arachnoiditis. An experimental study. Spine 1993;18: 1193–1198
45. Crock HV. Internal disc disruption. A challenge to disc prolapse fifty years on. Spine 1986;11:650–653
46. Smyth MJ, Wright V. Sciatica and the intervertebral disk; an experimental study. J Bone Joint Surg Am 1958;40-A:1401–1418
47. Devor M. Neuropathic pain and injured nerve: peripheral mechanisms. Br Med Bull 1991;47:619–630
48. Ho PS, Yu SW, Sether LA, Wagner M, Ho KC, Haughton VM. Ligamentum flavum: appearance on sagittal and coronal MR images. Radiology 1988;168:469–472
49. Yu SW, Sether L, Haughton VM. Facet joint menisci of the cervical spine: correlative MR imaging and cryomicrotomy study. Radiology 1987;164:79–82

50. Fletcher G, Haughton VM, Ho KC, Yu SW. Age-related changes in the cervical facet joints: studies with cryomicrotomy, MR, and CT. AJR Am J Roentgenol 1990;154:817–820
51. Ziv I, Maroudas C, Robin G, Maroudas A. Human facet cartilage: swelling and some physicochemical characteristics as a function of age. Part 2: age changes in some biophysical parameters of human facet joint cartilage. Spine 1993;18:136–146
52. Yong-Hing K, Kirkaldy-Willis WH. The pathophysiology of degenerative disease of the lumbar spine. Orthop Clin North Am 1983;14:491–504
53. Monson NL, Haughton VM, Modl JM, Sether LA, Ho KC. Normal and degenerating articular cartilage: in vitro correlation of MR imaging and histologic findings. J Magn Reson Imaging 1992;2:41–45
54. Ricci C, Cova M, Kang YS, et al. Normal age-related patterns of cellular and fatty bone marrow distribution in the axial skeleton: MR imaging study. Radiology 1990;177:83–88
55. Yu SW, Haughton VM, Sether LA, Wagner M. Comparison of MR and diskography in detecting radial tears of the anulus: a postmortem study. AJNR Am J Neuroradiol 1989;10:1077–1081
56. Ross JS, Modic MT, Masaryk TJ. Tears of the anulus fibrosus: assessment with Gd-DTPA-enhanced MR imagingAJR. AJR Am J Roentgenol 1990;154:159–162
57. Modic MT, Steinberg PM, Ross JS, Masaryk TJ, Carter JR. Degenerative disk disease: assessment of changes in vertebral body marrow with MR imaging. Radiology 1988;166(pt 1):193– 199
58. Toyone T, Takahashi K, Kitahara H, Yamagata M, Murakami M, Moriya H. Vertebral bone marrow changes in degenerative lumbar disc disease. J Bone Joint Surg Br 1994;76:757–764
59. Murphy KJ, Brunberg JA, Quint DJ, Kazanjian PH. Spinal cord infection: myelitis and abscess formation. AJNR Am J Neuroradiol 1998;19:341–348
60. Stafira JS, Sonnad JR, Yuh WT, et al. Qualitative assessment of cervical spinal stenosis: observer variability on CT and MR images. AJNR Am J Neuroradiol 2003;24:766–769
61. Bowen BC, Fraser K, Kochan JP, Pattany PM, Green BA, Quencer RM. Spinal dural arteriovenous fistulas: evaluation with MR angiography. AJNR Am J Neuroradiol 1995;16:2029–2043
62. Krakenes J, Kaale BR. Magnetic resonance imaging assessment of craniovertebral ligaments and membranes after whiplash trauma. Spine 2006;31:2820–2826

4 Imaging Modalities for Low Back Pain: Diskography

Robert F. Heary and Sanjeev Kumar

No diagnostic procedure in the field of neurosurgery has generated greater controversy than diskography. To gain an appreciation for the role of diskography in the treatment of low back pain patients, there is a need to acquire a thorough understanding of the diskography procedure itself. Proponents of diskography make two assumptions:[1] degenerative disk disease may be successfully treated,[2] and diskography is a useful diagnostic procedure. Opponents of diskography believe either that degenerative disk disease is a nonsurgical entity or that diskography is unable to accurately define this diagnosis.

This chapter provides an overview of the concept of degenerative disk disease and the diskography procedure. In addition, the history of diskography is reviewed, which includes references to numerous landmark articles and more recent studies both favoring and opposing this procedure. These varying views have led to the controversy surrounding the diskography procedure. The indications for diskography are reviewed in detail, and the specific technique of diskography is described. The results of diskography are analyzed with respect to the imaging studies generated, as well as the use of pain provocation as an interpretative factor. Comparisons are also discussed between diskography and other imaging studies used to evaluate disk abnormalities, such as plain film radiographs, computed tomography (CT) scans, and magnetic resonance imaging (MRI) studies. The reported complications of diskography are also reviewed. Finally, a rational plan is devised regarding the use of diskography in the radiographic evaluation of the patient with significant mechanical low back pain.

■ Degenerative Disk Disease

Degenerative disk disease, as a diagnostic entity, is a controversial topic. Various synonyms have been used to describe degenerative disk disease such as internal disk disruption, mechanical low back pain, black disk disease, and axial back pain. The theory, in the concept of degenerative disk disease, is that a lumbar intervertebral disk may degenerate and become a source of back pain. In this condition, the intervertebral disk loses hydration and subsequently degenerates. This degeneration is felt to be associated with low back pain. In addition, pain in the buttocks, thighs, and legs may be present; however, the classic description of degenerative disk disease says that back pain will be more severe than the extremity symptoms.

A herniated, lumbar intervertebral disk is a distinctly different entity than a degenerative disk. In the case of a herniated lumbar disk, disk material is present outside the normal confines of the annulus fibrosus. In symptomatic patients, this typically occurs in a location where a lumbar nerve root is irritated by the disk material. Not uncommonly, a herniated disk may be present simultaneously with a degenerative disk, at either the same level, or at adjacent levels, of the lumbar spine.

In pure degenerative disk disease of the lumbar spine, the patient usually presents with low back pain as the primary complaint. The degenerative disk disease patient often complains of difficulty with sitting intolerance. Frequently, patients describe their inability to sit still even for short periods of time, and they are unable to perform many activities of normal daily living. In addition, patients with degenerative disk disease often state that they are unable to ride in cars or buses for prolonged periods of time. The pain of degenerative disk disease is often worsened with changes in body position. These patients typically use external structures to attempt to gain support for their low backs. This may include leaning on tables, utilizing lumbar braces or corsets, or lying in a recumbent position to achieve relief. The neurologic examinations of the patients with classic degenerative disk disease are usually normal. Motor power, sensory examination, and deep tendon reflexes are typically normal. In addition, no nerve root tension signs are present.

When the clinical history and physical examination is consistent with degenerative disk disease of the lumbar spine, radiographic imaging studies are frequently obtained. Depending on the degree of degeneration, plain film radiographs may be completely normal or abnormalities may be demonstrated. The abnormalities may include a loss of disk space height in more degenerated cases. In addition, lateral lumbar spine radiographs, with flexion and extension views, may demonstrate evidence of dynamic instability at the level of the degenerated disk. Evidence of bony degenerative changes may also be present at the level of the facet joints, which are best visualized on oblique view x-rays of the lumbosacral spine. CT scan examinations, with or without intravenous contrast, rarely provide additional information regarding degenerative disk disease

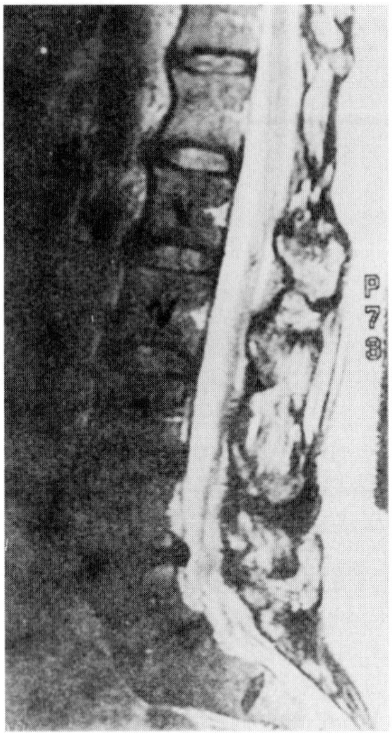

Fig.4.1 Sagittal T2-weighted magnetic resonance imaging. Black disk at L4-L5 level with modest posterior protrusion. The remaining disks appear normal.

to that which can be obtained from a high-quality lumbosacral spine plain radiograph series.

Magnetic resonance imaging is now widely used in the evaluation of patients with low back pain. Advantages of MRI include the lack of ionizing radiation, the noninvasive nature of the procedure, and the ability to accurately visualize the intervertebral disk. In degenerative disk disease of the lumbar spine, MRI may provide variable results. The classic appearance of degenerative disk disease is the loss of hydration of the intervertebral disk, which is best visualized on T2-weighted images in which the degenerative disk achieves a black appearance **(Fig. 4.1).** A normal, or nondegenerated, disk typically appears white on T2-weighted images. Significant controversy has occurred when MRI does not demonstrate any evidence of abnormal signal intensity in the intervertebral disk. In these instances, some authors recommend performance of a diskogram to attempt to define a degenerative disk.[1]

Myelography is frequently used to diagnose a herniated disk; however, myelograms do not assess the internal architecture of the disk, which is the primary abnormality in degenerative disk disease. As such, myelograms are of little use in the diagnosis of degenerative disk disease.

When clinical history, physical examination, and radiographic imaging studies are suggestive of lumbar degenerative disk disease, a course of conservative therapy is usually attempted. For patients who fail a prolonged attempt at multiple conservative treatment regimens, diskography may be considered as a further diagnostic tool to determine the diagnosis.

■ Historical Background

Holt[2] in 1968 performed a study of lumbar diskography in 30 asymptomatic volunteers from a prison population. He determined that 36% of the disk injections demonstrated an abnormal radiographic appearance and 26% of the injections were associated with pain. This led Holt to question the benefit of lumbar diskography because the false-positive rate appeared excessively high. Potential biases were present in this study. Prisoners were used as subjects, and it is unclear how thoroughly screened they were for the presence of preexisting lumbar spine conditions. In addition, Hypaque (diatrizoate) was the contrast medium used. This contrast agent came in direct contact with nerve roots, and pain may have been generated directly as a result of this highly irritant dye that leaked out of the abnormal disk. In addition, some degree of secondary gain is likely to occur among prisoners who complain of pain in a study such as this.

In 1969, Lindblom[3] published a paper on the use of diagnostic disk puncture in the evaluation of patients with suspected lumbar disk pathology. The term *diskography* was applied to this technique. Over the next 20 years, diskography became increasingly popular, particularly among orthopedic spine surgeons.

In 1970, Crock[4] defined the term *internal disk disruption.* In his article, Crock described four types of abnormality of the lumbar intervertebral disk and referred to these as disk prolapses, internal disk disruptions, isolated disk resorption, and degenerative spondylosis. His definition of internal disk disruption is currently synonymous with the definition used for degenerative disk disease.

Significant technologic advances in the field of radiology have occurred over the past few decades to improve the accuracy of needle placement in the lumbar intervertebral disk. Earlier diskograms were performed, with plain radiographs being used to confirm placement of needle tip within the disk. Advances in fluoroscopy have allowed for real-time confirmation of accurate needle placement. Biplane fluoroscopy has become a standard in the performance of modern diskograms (**Fig. 4.2**). CT scans became available in the 1970s and have been used by many authors to image the intervertebral disk following the performance of a diskogram.

In 1987, Sachs and associates[5] published the Dallas diskogram description. They classified disk disease and annular disruption as separate phenomena. They also categorized clinical information, volumes of contrast dye used, and assorted additional miscellaneous information. Important contributions made by the Dallas diskogram description include quantifying the volume of contrast dye injected into an intervertebral disk. The maximum volume

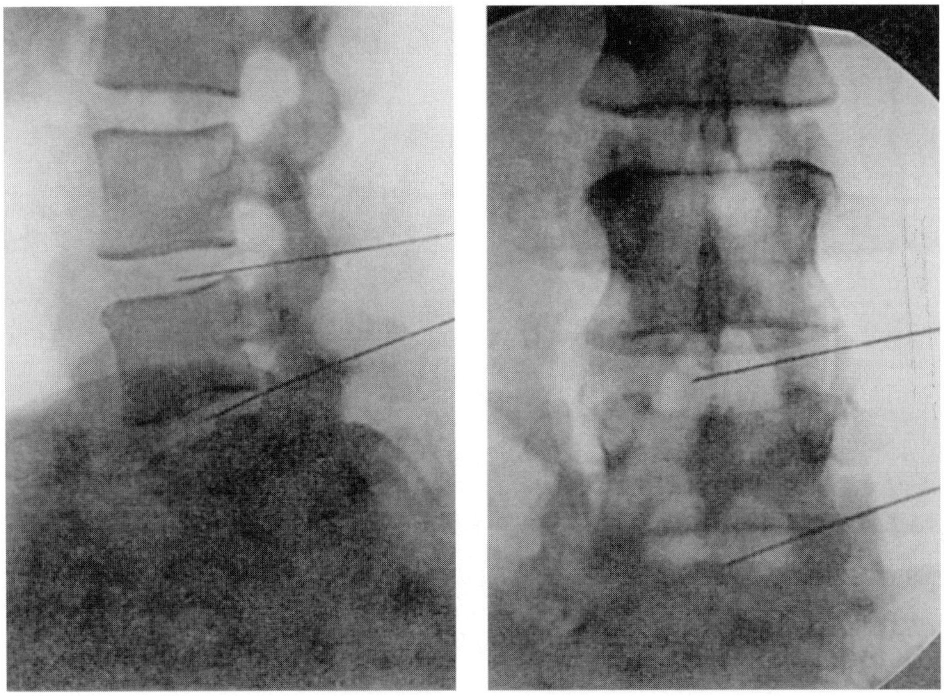

A B

Fig. 4.2 **(A)** Lateral lumbosacral radiograph demonstrates properly positioned small-bore diskography needles (22-gauge) at the L4-L5 and the L5-S1 levels (needle tip should be in the middle third of the vertebral body on this projection). **(B)** Anteroposterior (AP) lumbosacral radiograph demonstrates properly positioned diskography needles at the L4-L5 and the L5-S1 levels (needle tip should be between the pedicles on this projection).

able to be injected was recorded. The theory was that an incompetent, deteriorated disk accepts a lesser volume of contrast dye. In addition, clinical information related to the generation of pain during injection of the dye was recorded. Specifically, a comparison was made between the pain elicited by injection of the dye with the patient's original presenting complaint of pain (**Fig. 4.3**). Pain at the time of injection was rated as follows: none, dissimilar to the usual pain, similar to the usual pain, or an exact reproduction of the original pain. This definition of an exact reproduction of the patient's original pain during injection of the dye has become popularly referred to at present as concordant pain. This study was published at a time prior to the widespread use of MRI. Sachs and associates recommended diskography when revision spine surgery was considered or when the clinical information from the patient did not agree with either the myelographic or CT scan information.

In 1988, Simmons and associates[6] wrote a detailed analysis of the study performed by Holt[2] in 1968. In this critical analysis of Holt's study, Simmons and associates noted that the procedure of diskography performed in the 1980s had evolved significantly in a technologic sense. They cited the advantages of the use of fluoroscopy, different contrast dyes including contrast dyes of lower osmolarity and nonionic forms, and the use of CT scanning following the diskography. In addition, Simmons and associates were critical of the number of nondiagnostic studies obtained by Holt. They concluded that the diskography procedures performed in the 1980s were markedly different from, and superior to, the procedure as performed in the 1960s. As a result, these authors suggested that the negative impression of diskography propagated by the article by Holt in 1968 was not valid.

Nachemson,[7] in a 1989 editorial, condemned the use of diskography. He described the use of clinical judgment in the performance of diskography as "at best a disguise for ignorance, at worse, an excuse for quackery." This editorial by a well-respected member of the orthopedic spine community continued to spark significant controversy over whether diskography was a legitimate procedure for determining a painful degenerative disk in the lumbar spine that may benefit from surgical intervention. During the first 40 years diskographies were performed, the inconsistent results led to much debate regarding this procedure. Although many of the early studies were methodologically flawed and technically inadequate, a wealth of literature both supporting and refuting the procedure has been published.

Indications

Diskography is an invasive diagnostic procedure. *Provocative diskography* refers to the assessment of the pain response associated with the injection of dye during a

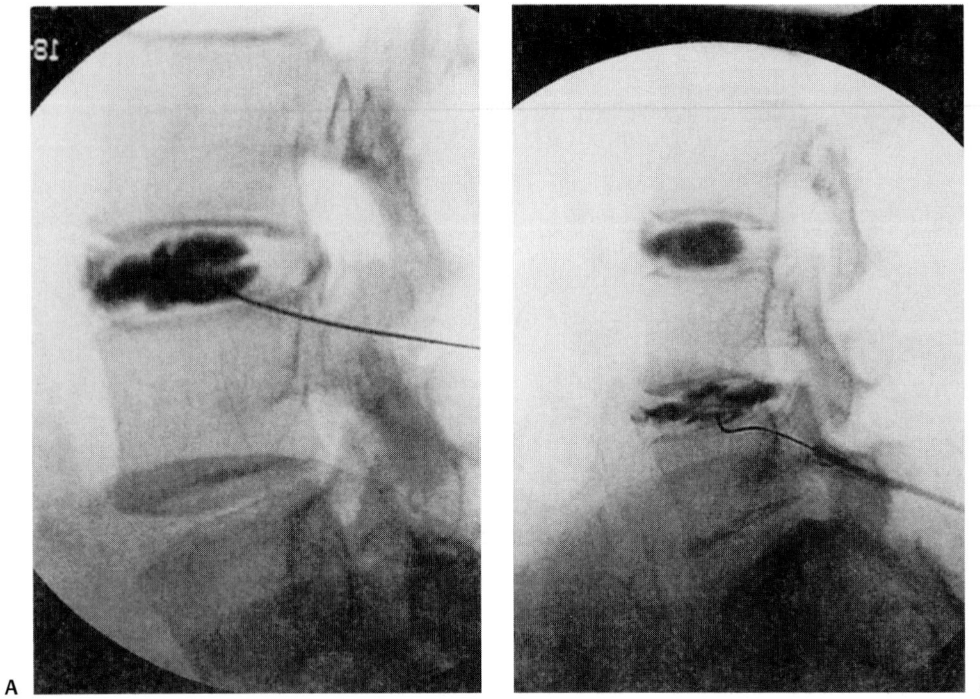

Fig.4.3 **(A)** Fluoroscopic lateral view of an L3-L4 diskogram. This "control" level shows normal pooling of contrast dye with some anterior filling and no posterior filling. **(B)** Fluoroscopic lateral view after an L4-L5 diskogram, which demonstrates a markedly degenerated disk. (Same patient as in **A.**) This L4-L5 level was accompanied by a positive "concordant" pain response.

diskography procedure. Diskography or, more appropriately, provocative diskography, is indicated to determine whether noninvasive radiographic imaging studies and appropriate history and clinical examination findings have correctly identified a painful degenerative disk. In clinical practice, provocative diskography is performed as a part of the diagnostic workup in a patient who may be a candidate for a more invasive surgical procedure.

Prior to undergoing a diskography, patients with suspected painful degenerative disk disease should have a conservative workup. The minimal time frame for conservative management has been variously reported to be between 2 and 6 months.[8–11] In the conservative treatment regimen, patients are encouraged to maintain or achieve an ideal body weight. For obese patients, this may involve referral to a medical specialist to assist in a weight loss program that may be safely performed. Physical therapy, which attempts to strengthen both back and abdominal musculature, is another standard form of conservative therapy.[12] Recently the benefits of core-strengthening exercises have been increasingly recognized. A trial of medical therapy, usually involving the use nonsteroidal antiinflammatory drugs, is also indicated.[9,10] Cyclooxygenase-2 (COX-2) inhibitors have also been used to attempt to improve medical management; however, the use of COX-2 inhibitors has recently been found to be associated with an increased risk of cardiovascular complications.[13]

As a general rule, nonnarcotic medications are preferable for the medical management of patients with suspected painful, degenerative disk disease. Well-documented problems with narcotic medications include the development of tolerance and addiction, which may limit the value of these medications in chronic low back pain patients. Additional conservative measures that have been attempted include the use of epidural steroid injections as well as trials of bracing.[9] In addition, an assortment of less invasive conservative measures including chiropractic treatment, acupuncture, and biofeedback have been attempted in conservative treatment regimens. An additional, useful, conservative treatment regimen is the performance of a formal evaluation of the psychological condition of the low back pain patient.[14] Psychological profiles help in determining which patients have somatization disorders and which patients may demonstrate secondary gain following workers' compensation cases or litigation. Among the various conservative treatment measures advocated, physical therapy remains the most commonly used and widely accepted technique.

Low back pain may be the result of degenerative disk disease. However, low back pain may also result from disease of the facet joints, the sacroiliac joint, spinal stenosis, lumbar disk herniation, and segmental instability.[15] Clinical and radiologic evaluations are used to differentiate among these other sources of low back pain and degenerative disk disease. In patients who are able to undergo MRI, this procedure has become the radiologic test of choice to evaluate the lumbar disk for signs of degeneration. A patient who has a clinical history and physical examination suggestive of degenerative disk disease and who has failed a conservative treatment regimen should be a candidate for an MRI study.

The indications for provocative diskography have been described. The most common is a painful, degenerative lumbar disk.[16–22] Numerous investigators have used diskography as a diagnostic study to determine whether the patient would benefit from a spinal fusion procedure.[9,16,18,20,23] Diskography also has been advocated for patients considering evaluation and treatment via lesser invasive methods, such as intradiskal electrothermy (IDET).[11] Some authors have used diskography to evaluate whether a disk within a previously fused segment is a pain generator.[16,19] Other authors have stated that a prior failed spinal surgery can be a serious confounding factor, and as such, diskography is not valuable in these patients.[24] An additional frequent indication for diskography is the evaluation of a disk adjacent to a successful prior spinal fusion.[16,19]

A common indication for diskography includes the patient with multiple black disks on T2 weighted MRI where an attempt is made to determine which of the black disks is a pain generator.[19,20,25] The most controversial indication for diskography is the patient with no abnormalities demonstrated on MRI where diskography is performed to attempt to determine a painful MRI-negative degenerative disk.[1,17,19]

In 1990, Boden and associates[26] investigated asymptomatic patients and found that one third of these patients, with no history of low back pain, had abnormal MRIs of the lumbar spine. This landmark study convinced the majority of spine surgeons that an abnormal MRI, in and of itself, is not sufficient for determining the presence of a painful, degenerative lumbar disk. Likewise, Buirski and Silberstein[27] have stated that MRI may only be used to assess nuclear anatomy and not to assess symptomatology of a lumbar disk. Despite these data, Horton and Daftari[25] have stated that a single-level abnormality on MRI has a high probability for provoking pain, and diskography may be avoided in these situations.

Kakitsubata and associates[28] in 2003 investigated the diagnostic capabilities of magnetic resonance diskography in the detection of tears of the annulus fibrosus, and compared the findings with those obtained from MRI. They obtained 24 intervertebral disks from cadavers and examined them using MRI and MR diskography. Magnetic resonance diskography allowed direct diagnosis of radial, transverse, and concentric tears in 100%, 57%, and 21% of specimens, respectively. With MRI, the diagnosis of radial, transverse, and concentric tears was possible in 67%, 71%, and 21% of specimens, respectively. The authors concluded that MR diskography does well in the evaluation of the clinically important radial tears of the annulus fibrosus, although not uniformly well in the identification of the other types of annular tears.

In 2003, Guyer and Ohnmeiss,[29] in a comprehensive review of literature, defined the following indications for diskography: (1) further evaluation of demonstrably abnormal disks to help assess the extent of abnormality or correlation of the abnormality with the clinical symptoms (such symptoms may include recurrent pain from a previously operated disk and lateral disk herniation); (2) patients with persistent, severe symptoms in whom other diagnostic tests have failed to reveal clear confirmation of a suspected disk as the source of pain; (3) assessment of patients who have failed to respond to surgical intervention to determine if there is painful pseudarthrosis or a symptomatic disk in a posteriorly fused segment and to help evaluate possible recurrent disk herniation; (4) assessment of disks before fusion to determine if the disks within the proposed fusion segment are symptomatic and to determine if disks adjacent to this segment are normal; and (5) assessment of candidates for minimally invasive surgical intervention to confirm a contained disk herniation or to investigate dye distribution pattern before chemonucleolysis or percutaneous procedures.

Despite conflicting reports in the literature, the optimal indications for provocative diskography include the patient with a clinical history and physical examination consistent with degenerative disk disease who also has an abnormal MRI, with a black disk demonstrated on T2-weighted imaging. These patients would also have had an appropriate, unsuccessful course of conservative therapy, as well as other causes of low back pain ruled out. Furthermore, a psychological profile that does not suggest significant secondary gain issues should be sought.

■ Technique

Diskography is an invasive diagnostic procedure that requires an appreciable degree of technical skill. There is a substantial learning curve to mastering this technique. The procedure requires an adequate understanding of the bony and soft tissue anatomy of the lumbar spine. In addition, knowledge of anesthetic and sedative techniques is useful to obtain the optimal information from the diskography procedure. The diskographer may be the spine surgeon or another health care professional skilled in the technique. The patient may be placed in either in a prone position or a lateral position.[9,15,20,22,30] Meticulous sterile technique is mandatory to prevent infectious complications.[9,15,30] To limit exaggerated pain responses from an irritated lumbar spinal nerve, most diskographers approach from the asymptomatic or less symptomatic side.[9,15,20]

Adequate use of local anesthesia on the nondiskal structures is essential.[9,22,30] It is important not to anesthetize the annulus proper; however, the skin and extraspinal soft tissues should be well anesthetized. In addition, sedation may be used.[22,30] Recently developed, very short acting sedative medication, such as propofol, allows the patient to be well sedated during the positioning of the needles. Upon discontinuation of the intravenous propofol solution, the patient completely reverses from the sedation within a few minutes. This enables the patient to be completely awake and alert to accurately monitor the pain provocation response.

The entry site on the skin typically lies between 8 and 10 cm lateral to the midline.[9,30] Either a single- or double-needle technique may be used. Of clinical importance, the needle, which perforates the annulus, should be of a small gauge. This typically involves use of a needle no larger than 22 gauge to penetrate the annulus.[9,16,20,22] McCutcheon and Thompson[31] describe the situation in which contrast extravasation occurred in a retrograde fashion through a needle tract from a 20-gauge needle, which can lead to a false-positive interpretation of the plain film images. In addition, the needle tip should attempt to reach the anatomic midline in both the sagittal and coronal planes.[9,15,20,30] The current diskography technique typically uses biplane fluoroscopy to confirm the appropriate location of the tip of the needle.[15,19,20] Numerous authors have stressed the importance of accurate needle placement in obtaining the maximal degree of diagnostic information.[15,32–34]

Once the needle is correctly positioned and the patient is fully awake and alert with no lingering effects from short-acting sedation, contrast dye is injected into the disk. During the injection of dye, a pain response is monitored from the patient.[9,15,19,20,22] In particular, the presence or absence of pain, whether it be similar or dissimilar to the usual pain, and the presence of an exact reproduction of the pain, termed concordant pain, is reported.[35] Factors that may be responsible for an inaccurate pain response by the patient include poor needle placement, an overreaction to the painful stimulus by the patient, an exaggerated pain response resulting from an extradural extravasation of dye, and pain resulting from the needle placement rather than the injection of dye.[32] An inaccurate needle placement into the annulus fibrosus may be painful and might produce atypical pain. This may result in a false-positive diskography study. Injections into the annulus fibrosus may be recognized by acceptance of a very small volume of contrast with a firm end point during injection.[15] In addition, improper needle placement may lead to nerve root sheath injection, subarachnoid injection, or irreversible damage to the disk.

In addition to recording the presence of pain, studies have documented recording the presence of resistance to injection, the volume of dye, and the pressure transduced.[9,15,19,20,22,35–37] Adams and associates[38] found that fissured and ruptured disks were more common in older spines. They determined that older disks accepted a greater volume of injected fluid and required a lower injection pressure. Derby and associates[35] performed precise manometric measurements of the pressure during diskography. They developed specific diagnostic categories for pressure measurements, including chemical, mechanical, indeterminant, and normal pressures. These parameters were defined as follows:[35]

- *Chemical:* less than 15 pounds per square inch pressure upon injection
- *Mechanical:* between 15 and 50 pounds per square inch
- *Indeterminant:* between 51 and 90 pounds per square inch
- *Normal:* greater than 90 pounds per square inch without pain

Following the injection of the dye, plain film radiographs or fluoroscopic images are taken to document the radiographic appearance of the disk.[15,20] Some investigators also perform a postdiskography CT scan **(Fig. 4.4)**.[15,22] Disk morphology can be rated as follows: normal, presence of annular tears or fissures, presence of end-plate defects, and presence or absence of leakage of contrast dye.[20]

Milette and Melanson[39] determined that technical failures were present in 2.7% of diskograms. Reasons for technical failures included impossible disk puncture, impossible contrast injection, and impossible opacification of the disk. An excessively narrow intervertebral disk space may be responsible for a technical failure. In addition, the L5-S1 disk space requires greater technical expertise and may be difficult to image, particularly with less experienced diskographers. Schellhas and Pollei[20] have emphasized the need to perform a diagnostic disk injection at a "control" disk. A control disk injection is obtained when the radiographic images are within normal limits and there is no provocation of pain with the injection. The presence of a control disk injection increases the specificity of a positive diskography result at another level.

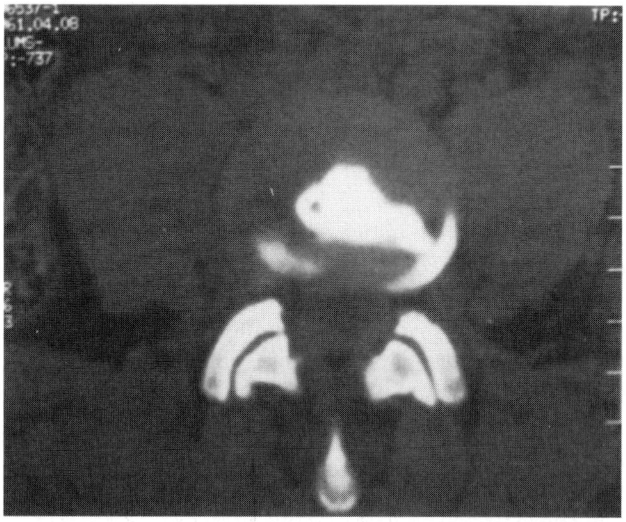

Fig. 4.4 Axial CT scan following diskogram demonstrates a left-sided annular tear with pooling of dye in multiple layers of the annulus fibrosis.

Results

Diskography results are typically classified into those related to radiographic imaging studies and those related to the provocation of pain. Both types provide useful diagnostic information for treatment planning.

Yasuma and associates[40] performed an anatomic study of radiography. They determined that the diskogram may present a false-negative result when a protrusion or prolapsed disk involved the annulus fibrosus but did not involve the nucleus pulposus. Likewise, extensive annulus fibrosus degeneration may be present in a patient who has a normal diskogram, which would result in a false-negative study. Other authors have also highlighted the importance of the annulus fibrosus with respect to pain generation.[18,41,42] In a cadaveric study of diskography, Gunzburg and associates[41] found that tears in the posterior annulus were more common than diskographic tears in the anterior annulus.

Similarly, Colhoun and associates[18] found that provocation of back pain symptoms was most common when tears were present in the posterior annulus fibrosus. Degenerative disk and internal disk disruption were less frequently associated with the provocation of pain. Moneta and associates[42] analyzed 833 diskograms in 306 patients and determined that the outer annulus fibrosus was the origin of pain reproduction during diskography. Degenerative disk changes are more common in the lower lumbar segments than in the upper lumbar segments.[43] Milette and associates[44] found that a loss of disk height or abnormal signal intensity on MRI was significantly associated with internal disk disruptions, which extended into or beyond the outer annulus on diskography, and a higher incidence of similar or exact pain reproduction was present in these cases.

Numerous investigators have found no difference between the sexes in the provocation of pain during diskography.[36,42] Some studies have demonstrated no difference in pain provocation during diskography based on the patient's age.[42] Other studies have demonstrated different patterns of pain with respect to the patient's age, with younger patients experiencing more pain.[36] There is no difference demonstrable in the average number of painful disks between smokers and nonsmokers.[9]

Provocative Diskography

In Sachs and associates[5] sentinel article in 1987 on the Dallas diskogram description, they defined the correlation between the production of pain and the injection of dye during diskographic procedures. They classified pain into the following four categories: no pain, pain dissimilar to the usual pain, pain similar to the usual pain, and pain that is an exact reproduction of the usual pain (concordant pain). This grading system has been widely accepted and is the standard used in most series of diskography.[19,21,36,45]

Some inconsistency exists in the reporting of pain provoked by diskography procedures. There is general agreement that concordant pain is a positive response; however, studies differ as to whether similar or dissimilar pain evoked by diskography is considered a positive diskographic pain response. Most studies describing the results of diskography cite a positive pain provocation response in approximately 70% of patients undergoing lumbar diskograms.[31,32,42,46] In addition to commenting on positive pain generating diskograms, most investigators also require the presence of a "control" disk injection. A control disk injection is a lumbar intervertebral disk that has dye injected that does not produce a pain response. In cases in which all disks injected invoke a pain response, meaning that no control disk injection is obtained, the diskographic procedure should be considered nondiagnostic.

Numerous factors affect whether a positive pain response occurs following diskography. When significant degenerative changes are present in a disk, the incidence of a positive pain response increases **(Fig. 4.5)**.[16,47,48] Likewise, the presence of significant annular disruptions is also associated with an increased positive pain response.[47,48] The presence of facet tropism, or asymmetry, has not been found to be associated with an increased pain response.[49] Abnormal disk protrusions, which occur centrally, paracentrally, or in an intraforaminal location, are more likely to invoke a pain response than extraforaminal disk protrusions.[36] Furthermore, pain is more likely to be found in diskograms performed at the lowest two motion segments (L4-L5 and L5-S1) than in diskograms performed at more rostral levels.[9,36] Patients with chronic somatization states or chronic pain syndromes, particularly those with active compensation claims, are more likely to report painful diskographic injections than are patients without active claims.[50] Intervertebral disks with sequestered

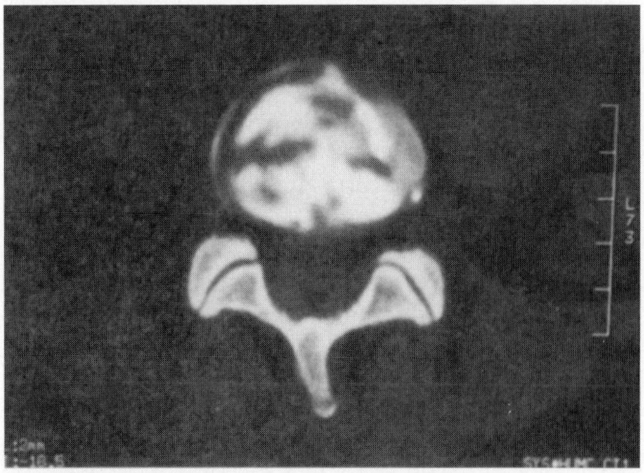

Fig. 4.5 Axial CT scan following diskogram demonstrates diffuse degenerative changes throughout the entire disk.

fragments or extraligamentous extrusions are more likely to invoke the pain response than are disk herniations that are subligamentous or merely disk protrusions.[36] Heggeness and associates[46] performed diskograms on patients following diskectomy procedures. They found that a pain response was more likely to occur in previously operated disks than in the unoperated disks. Aprill and Bogduk[16] reported a fivefold increase in the reproduction of pain in disks that were radiographically pathologic compared with disks that had a normal diskographic appearance.

Pain drawings have been used in some diskographic studies to help the patient demonstrate where pain occurs following diskographic injections. Pain drawings, which demonstrate pain in the lower extremities, are more likely to be associated with painful injections than are diskographic procedures that do not produce leg pain.[51,52] Ohnmeiss and associates[52] found that when pain radiates into the leg anteriorly, the most commonly affected level is the L3-L4 disk. When pain is in the posterior thigh or leg without pain in the anterior drawing, positive diskograms were more likely to occur in the L4-L5 or L5-S1 disk. Pain drawings, which showed pain limited to the low back and buttocks, were more often associated with the absence of disk pathology. Ohnmeiss and associates[53] have used pain drawings to help identify patients who may demonstrate an exaggerated response to diskography. Using these pain drawings, the overall accuracy of differentiating patients with false-positive pain was 78%.

In an effort to determine the prevalence of positive response to lumbar diskography in asymptomatic volunteers, controlled for pressure of injection and intensity of pain, Derby and associates[54] concluded that the pain produced in a lumbar disk in asymptomatic volunteers is mild and requires a high pressure of injection. They went on to say that if attention is paid to the pressure of injection and intensity of response, a criterion can be defined that can provide lumbar diskography with a potential false-positive rate of 0% to less than 10%.[54] Recently, Carragee and associates[55] evaluated the hypothesis that false-positive injection can effectively be eliminated by defining the positive injection criteria to include only those disks in which pain is produced with low injection pressure injections. They reached the conclusion that the rate of low-pressure painful injection in subjects without chronic low back pain illness is approximately 25% and correlates with both anatomic and psychosocial factors. In certain subgroups, this is an unacceptable risk of false positive results.

Lately, the centralization phenomenon of the pain during diskography has been published. In a prospective and blinded study by Laslett and associates,[56] they concluded that centralization is highly specific to positive diskography but specificity is reduced in the presence of severe disability or psychosocial distress. In another study in 2006, Laslett and associates[57] studied the clinical predictor of lumbar provocative diskography. They presented four clinical variables—centralization of the pain, a loss of lumbar extension, a history of persistent pain between acute episodes, and a report of vulnerability in the neutral zone—which may be used individually or in specific combinations as signs of possible discogenic pain. They concluded that other than centralization of the pain, these clinical variables have modest predictive power in relation to lumbar diskography results and two combinations of variables were highly specific to positive diskography.

Imaging Studies

Diskography typically consists of two separate phases. The imaging phase includes images obtained at the time of diskography, which may be plain film radiographs but are more frequently fluoroscopic images, as well as CT scans, which are frequently obtained following the diskography procedures. In addition, the second phase of the diskographic procedure includes the provocation of pain. As previously discussed, patients with appropriate history and physical examination findings consistent with degenerative disk disease frequently undergo an MRI. If the MRI confirms the diagnosis of degenerative disk disease, and conservative treatment has failed, then provocative diskography may be considered.

Plain film radiographs are frequently obtained in the evaluation of low back pain secondary to degenerative disk disease. In addition, dynamic imaging studies include flexion/extension lateral views of the lumbar spine looking for evidence of instability. Quinnell and Stockdale[58] performed a study comparing flexion/extension lateral lumbar spine radiographs with diskography. Interestingly, all single-level, diskographically abnormal studies were correctly diagnosed by flexion/extension radiographs. Furthermore, the presence of a single-level abnormality on flexion/extension views did not exclude the presence of another diskographically abnormal level. Some investigators have performed flexion/extension views following the contrast infusion during diskography.[59,60] Although the findings have not been consistently reported, diskograms with normal morphology demonstrate pooling of dye in a more anterior position within the disk during extension. The clinical significance of this finding is not clear.[60]

Many investigators have reported the use of CT scanning following diskography to augment the diagnostic information provided.[5,15,31,48,61–63] The abnormal images described may be consistent with either disk degeneration or disk herniations. In patients who cannot undergo an MRI, diskograms are particularly useful in diagnosing lateral disk herniations that may not be visible with myelography.[5,31,61,62] In addition, axial and sagittal reconstructed images may facilitate the precise localization of a herniated disk as being central, paracentral, lateral, or far lateral.[15] The CT scans obtained following diskography may be useful in determining the evidence of degeneration as well as in identifying annular tears. Investigators more interested in the pain provocation response may not obtain CT scans following diskography. In these instances, the images obtained by fluoroscopy will usually be sufficient.

Myelography is an invasive study that can accurately diagnose herniated lumbar intervertebral disks. Myelograms do not provide information about the internal architecture of the intervertebral disks. Whereas both myelography and diskography may be useful in diagnosing herniated lumbar intervertebral disks, in practice, myelography is usually indicated when disk herniation is the working diagnosis, and diskography is utilized when degenerative disk disease is being sought.

Significant controversy exists regarding whether MRI or provocative diskography is a more accurate test to diagnose degenerative disk disease. There are numerous published reports of patients with abnormal diskograms who had normal MRI studies. Similarly, there are numerous studies that document abnormal MRIs in patients who have normal diskograms.

Magnetic resonance imaging is a noninvasive study. As such, many surgeons prefer to use it as a screening tool prior to the more invasive diskography procedure. Boden and associates[26] documented abnormal MRI studies in one third of clinically asymptomatic patients. This study has led many investigators to consider MRI to be excessively sensitive in the diagnosis of painful degenerative disk disease. The earliest sign of a degenerated, or dehydrated, disk on MRI is black signal intensity on T2-weighted images of the intervertebral disk. Whereas MRI may be overly sensitive, numerous investigators have found that if a disk appears more degenerated on MRI, it is more likely to be associated with pain.[27,64]

In 1992, Aprill and Bogduk[16] introduced the concept of the high-intensity zone (HIZ). They defined an HIZ as a focus of high signal intensity on T2-weighted imaging within the posterior annulus of a degenerative disk. They felt that the HIZ represented inflammation in the annulus secondary to trapped nuclear material. Furthermore, they postulated that the HIZ is predictive of a painful degenerative disk responsible for low back pain.[16] Subsequently, other investigators have also found the presence of an HIZ on MRI to be a reliable marker of a painful outer annulus disruption.[59,65]

Advocates of diskography have previously claimed that diskograms are superior for determining annular pathology.[1,64,66] At the present time, it is unclear whether diskography or an HIZ on MRI is more sensitive for accurately diagnosing a painful annular disruption. Ricketson and associates[10] stated that an HIZ probably represents neovascularity or granulation tissue within the posterior annulus that is induced by inflammation. Whereas these authors stated that an HIZ was never seen in a morphologically normal disk, they cautioned that the presence of an HIZ on MRI is not necessarily associated with a positive concordant pain response. Carragee and associates[67] also evaluated the presence of HIZ on MRI in any disk, and concluded that it is weakly associated with subsequent development of low back pain episodes.

Additional advances in MRI include the use of the bony vibration test. Vanharanta and associates[68] found that pain provoked by the vibration test can improve the specificity of MRI in the diagnosis of symptomatic lumbar disk herniations. Likewise, Yrjama and associates[69] stated that the combination of an MRI with a positive bony vibration test gives more information on the origin of back pain than does MRI alone. In a recent study, Resnick and associates[70] suggested that diskography appears to have a role in evaluation of patients with low back pain, but that it is best limited to the evaluation of abnormal interspaces identified on MRI.

■ Complications of Diskography

Although diskography is an invasive procedure, its complication rate in experienced hands is quite low. The most frequently reported complication is bacterial diskitis.[19,30,39,71] Aseptic diskitis may also occur.[32] Fraser and associates[72] reported a diskitis rate of 23% when a large bore needle was used. This rate decreased to 0.7% when stiletted needles and a two-needle technique were used. Guyer and Ohnmeiss[10] in 1995 published the position statement from the North American Spine Society Diagnostic and Therapeutic Committee. They reported the overall incidence of diskitis to be 0.15%. Although rare, bacterial diskitis is a serious complication that requires prolonged antibiotic treatment.[66,71] In 2003, Klessig and associates,[73] in an in vitro study of the use of intradiskal antibiotics for diskography, supported their use for prophylaxis during diskography. They also recommended that intradiskal placement of antibiotics should eliminate the need for systemic antibiotic prophylaxis and its attendant risk of generating antimicrobial resistance. Regarding the use of prophylactic antibiotics, Willems and associates[74] studied 435 consecutive diskograms and performed a systematic review of the literature and found that there was not enough evidence to support prophylactic antibiotics for preventing diskitis.

Other than diskitis, complications related to diskography are extremely rare. Isolated reports have described the complications of retroperitoneal hemorrhage, urticaria, spinal epidural abscess, and dural violation.[15,30,75] In a recently published paper, Poynton and associates[76] have reported five cases of acute lumbar disk herniation precipitated by diskography and suggested that new-onset or persistent exacerbation of radicular symptoms following provocative diskography needs to be further investigated for diskography-induced lumbar disk herniation. Although an assortment of complications is possible following an invasive procedure in the spine, the overall complication rate in experienced hands remains extremely low with diskography. Although not truly a complication, the technical difficulty of an inability to access the L5-S1 interspace has been frequently noted in most large series. Common suggestions to avoid complications include the use of a biplane fluoroscopy to confirm needle placement, the use of a two-needle technique, the use of nonionic contrast dye, the use of antibiotic in the dye solution, and avoidance of diskography procedures in patients with known bleeding diatheses. Overall, the complication rate for provocative diskography is acceptable.

■ Conclusion

Provocative diskography remains a controversial diagnostic study. The majority of the medical literature on this subject has been reported by investigators who believe in the efficacy and use of this diagnostic tool. Detractors of provocative diskography have questioned the value of this procedure. Nachemson[7] in 1989 condemned the use of diskography. Likewise, Carragee and associates[50,77] have published reports questioning the validity of this study.

We advocate the use of "blinded" provocative diskography in selected situations. The appropriate diskography patient should have a clinical history and physical examination consistent with the diagnosis of degenerative disk disease. Specifically, useful historical information includes the presence of predominantly low back pain as well as the presence of sitting intolerance. The physical examination should not demonstrate nerve root tension signs. Appropriate candidates for diskography should have experienced a prolonged attempt at aggressive conservative therapy that failed. At a minimum, the conservative treatment regimen should include a course of physical therapy and an optimization of ideal body weight, if possible. Additional conservative measures have been previously outlined. In those patients with suggestive evidence of degenerative disk disease, an MRI of the lumbar spine, which demonstrates a black disk on T2-weighted images, is suggestive of a painful degenerative disk. Recent advances with MRI, including the presence of high-intensity zones and the use of bony vibration tests, have attempted to correlate positive MRI findings with low back pain. At the present time, the specificity and sensitivity of MRI for the diagnosis of a painful degenerative lumbar disk disease is inadequate. As such, we would not recommend a spinal fusion procedure based solely on the presence of a suggestive clinical history and physical exam and a positive MRI study.

In a patient who has failed a conservative treatment regimen with an appropriate history and physical examination, a normal psychological profile, and a positive MRI study, a "blinded" provocative diskogram is indicated. The *blinded* study refers to performance of the lumbar diskogram by a diskographer who is unaware of the results of the previously obtained MRI study. Routinely, this study evaluates the L3-L4, L4-L5, and L5-S1 disk spaces. A positive, blinded provocative diskogram will have both a positive concordant pain response and abnormal imaging at the level that matches the findings of the abnormal MRI. By having the diskographer "blinded," a potential bias in the interpretation of the diagnostic result is removed. The theory is that blinding the diskographer increases the specificity of the study. Furthermore, a control disk injection is necessary to validate a positive diskogram. If all injections evoke a positive response, with no control disk elicitable, we consider the study to be nondiagnostic. A blinded, provocative diskogram should be used only for patients who are candidates for further invasive treatment, such as a spinal fusion procedure or, possibly, the recently described procedure of intradiskal electrothermy (IDET).

If the information obtained from the history, physical examination, psychological profile, and MRI study, in a patient who has failed conservative therapy, correlates precisely with the results of a blinded provocative diskogram, then the likelihood that a degenerative lumbar intervertebral disk is a pain generator that will respond positively to further treatment is increased. As such, in appropriately selected patients, provocative diskography is a useful adjunctive diagnostic tool.

References

1. Zucherman J, Derby R, Hsu K, et al. Normal magnetic resonance imaging with abnormal discography. Spine 1988;13:1355–1359
2. Holt EP. The question of lumbar discography. J Bone Joint Surg Am 1968;50:720–726
3. Lindblom K. Diagnostic puncture of intervertebral disks in sciatica. Clin Orthop Relat Res 1969;67:6–8
4. Crock HV. A reappraisal of intervertebral disc lesions. Med J Aust 1970;1:983–989
5. Sachs BL, Vanharanta H, Spivey MA, et al. Dallas discogram description. A new classification of CT/discography in low-back disorders. Spine 1987;12:287–294
6. Simmons JW, Aprill CN, Dwyer AP, Brodsky AE. A reassessment of Holt's data on: the question of lumbar discography. Clin Orthop Relat Res 1988;237:120–124
7. Nachemson A. Lumbar discography—where are we today? Spine 1989;14:555–5572526374
8. Birney TJ, White JJ, Berens D, Kuhn G. Comparison of MRI and discography in the diagnosis of lumbar degenerative disc disease. J Spinal Disord 1992;5:417–423
9. McFadden JW. The stress lumbar discogram. Spine 1988;13:931–933
10. Ricketson R, Simmons JW, Hauser BO. The prolapsed intervertebral disc. The high-intensity zone with discography correlation. Spine 1996;21:2758–2762
11. Saal JA, Saal JS. Intradiscal electrothermal treatment for chronic discogenic low back pain: a prospective outcome study with minimum 1-year follow-up. Spine 2000;25:2622–2627
12. Wilson DH, MacCarty WC. Discography: its role in the diagnosis of lumbar disc protrusion. J Neurosurg 1969;31:520– 523

13. Cairns JA. The Coxibs and traditional nonsteroidal anti-inflammatory drugs: A current perspective on cardiovascular risks. Can J Cardiol 2007;23:125–131
14. Rankine JJ, Gill KP, Hutchinson CE, Ross ER, Williamson JB. The clinical significance of the high-intensity zone on lumbar spine magnetic resonance imaging. Spine 1999;24:1913–1919
15. Bernard TN. Lumbar discography followed by computed tomography. Refining the diagnosis of low-back pain. Spine 1990;15:690–707
16. Aprill C, Bogduk N. High-intensity zone: a diagnostic sign of painful lumbar disc on magnetic resonance imaging. Br J Radiol 1992;65:361–369
17. Brightbill TC, Pile N, Eichelberger RP, Whitman M. Normal magnetic resonance imaging and abnormal discography in lumbar disc disruption. Spine 1994;19:1075–1077
18. Colhoun E, McCall IW, Williams L, et al. Provocation discography as a guide to planning operations on the spine. J Bone Joint Surg Br 1988;70:267–271
19. Guyer RD, Ohnmeiss DD. Lumbar discography. Position statement from the North American Spine Society Diagnostic and Therapeutic Committee. Spine 1995;20:2048–2059
20. Schellhas KP, Pollei SR. The role of discography in the evaluation of patients with spinal deformity. Orthop Clin North Am 1994;25:265–273
21. Schwarzer AC, Aprill CN, Derby R, et al. The prevalence and clinical features of internal disc disruption in patients with chronic low back pain. Spine 1995;20:1878–1883
22. Simmons JW, Emery SF, McMillin JN, et al. Awake discography. A comparison study with magnetic resonance imaging. Spine 1991; 16(suppl)S216–S221
23. Weinstein J, Claverie W, Gibson S. The pain of discography. Spine 1988;13:1344–1348
24. Fairbank JC, Deans W. Discography. Spine 1990;15:839–840
25. Horton WC, Daftari TK. Which disc as visualized by magnetic resonance imaging is actually a source of pain? A correlation between magnetic resonance imaging and discography. Spine 1992;17(suppl)S164–S171
26. Boden SD, Davis DO, Dina TS, et al. Abnormal magnetic-resonance scans of the lumbar spine in asymptomatic subjects. A prospective investigation. J Bone Joint Surg Am 1990;72:403–408
27. Buirski G, Silberstein M. The symptomatic lumbar disc in patients with low-back pain. Magnetic resonance imaging appearances in both a symptomatic and control population. Spine 1993;18:1808–1811
28. Kakitsubata Y, Theodorou DJ, Theodorou SJ, et al. Magnetic resonance discography in cadavers: tears of the annulus fibrosus. Clin Orthop Relat Res 2003;407:228–240
29. Guyer RD, Ohnmeiss DD. Lumbar discography. Spine J 2003;3(suppl)11S–27S
30. McCulloch JA, Waddell G. Lateral lumbar discography. Br J Radiol 1978;51:498–502
31. McCutcheon ME, Thompson WC. CT scanning of lumbar discography. A useful diagnostic adjunct. Spine 1986;11:257–259
32. Brodsky AE, Binder WF. Lumbar discography. Its value in diagnosis and treatment of lumbar disc lesions. Spine 1979;4:110– 120
33. Ito S, Muro T, Urasaki T, Ozaki S. Reevaluation of discograms not classified into usual classifications. J Spinal Disord 1999;12:151–156
34. Urasaki T, Muro T, Ito S, Hattori Y, Ozaki S. Consistency of lumbar discograms of the same disc obtained twice at a 2-week interval: influence of needle tip position. J Orthop Sci 1998;3:243–251
35. Derby R, Howard MW, Grant JM, et al. The ability of pressure-controlled discography to predict surgical and nonsurgical outcomes. Spine 1999;24:364–371
36. Maezawa S, Muro T. Pain provocation at lumbar discography as analyzed by computed tomography/discography. Spine 1992;17:1309–1315
37. Southern EP, Fye MA, Panjabi MM, Patel TC, Cholewicki J. Disc degeneration: a human cadaveric study correlating magnetic resonance imaging and quantitative discomanometry. Spine 2000;25:2171–2175
38. Adams MA, Dolan P, Hutton WC. The stages of disc degeneration as revealed by discograms. J Bone Joint Surg Br 1986;68: 36–41
39. Milette PC, Melanson D. A reappraisal of lumbar discography. J Can Assoc Radiol 1982;33:176–182
40. Yasuma T, Ohno R, Yamauchi Y. False-negative lumbar discograms. Correlation of discographic and histological findings in postmortem and surgical specimens. J Bone Joint Surg Am 1988;70: 1279–1290
41. Gunzburg R, Parkinson R, Moore R, et al. A cadaveric study comparing discography, magnetic resonance imaging, histology, and mechanical behavior of the human lumbar disc. Spine 1992;17:417–426
42. Moneta GB, Videman T, Kaivanto K, et al. Reported pain during lumbar discography as a function of anular ruptures and disc degeneration. A re analysis of 833 discograms. Spine 1994;19:1968–1974
43. Soini J, Antti-Poika I, Tallroth K, et al. Disc degeneration and angular movement of the lumbar spine: comparative study using plain and flexion-extension radiography and discography. J Spinal Disord 1991;4:183–187
44. Milette PC, Fontaine S, Lepanto L, et al. Differentiating lumbar disc protrusions, disc bulges, and discs with normal contour but abnormal signal intensity. Magnetic resonance imaging with discographic correlations. Spine 1999;24:44–53
45. Vanharanta H, Sachs BL, Ohnmeiss DD, et al. Pain provocation and disc deterioration by age. A CT/discography study in a low-back pain population. Spine 1989;14:420–423
46. Heggeness MH, Watters WC, Gray PM. Discography of lumbar discs after surgical treatment for disc herniation. Spine 1997;22:1606–1609
47. Schechter NA, France MP, Lee CK. Painful internal disc derangements of the lumbosacral spine: discographic diagnosis and treatment by posterior lumbar interbody fusion. Orthopedics 1991;14:447–451
48. Vanharanta H, Sachs BL, Spivey MA, et al. The relationship of pain provocation to lumbar disc deterioration as seen by CT/discography. Spine 1987;12:295–298
49. Vanharanta H, Floyd T, Ohnmeiss DD, et al. The relationship of facet tropism to degenerative disc disease. Spine 1993;18:1000–1005
50. Carragee EJ, Tanner CM, Khurana S, et al. The rates of false-positive lumbar discography in select patients without low back symptoms. Spine 2000;25:1373–1380
51. Ohnmeiss DD, Vanharanta H, Ekholm J. Degree of disc disruption and lower extremity pain. Spine 1997;22:1600–1605
52. Ohnmeiss DD, Vanharanta H, Ekholm J. Relationship of pain drawings to invasive tests assessing intervertebral disc pathology. Eur Spine J 1999;8:126–131
53. Ohnmeiss DD, Vanharanta H, Guyer RD. The association between pain drawings and computed tomographic/discographic pain responses. Spine 1995;20:729–733

54. Derby R, Lee SH, Kim BJ, et al. Pressure-controlled lumbar discography in volunteers without low back symptoms. Pain Med 2005;6:213–221
55. Carragee EJ, Alamin TF, Carragee JM. Low-pressure positive Discography in subjects asymptomatic of significant low back pain illness. Spine 2006;31:505–509
56. Laslett M, Oberg B, Aprill CN, McDonald B. Centralization as a predictor of provocation discography results in chronic low back pain, and the influence of disability and distress on diagnostic power. Spine J 2005;5:370–380
57. Laslett M, Aprill CN, McDonald B, Oberg B. Clinical predictors of lumbar provocation discography: a study of clinical predictors of lumbar provocation discography. Eur Spine J 2006;15:1473– 1484
58. Quinnell RC, Stockdale HR. Flexion and extension radiography of the lumbar spine: a comparison with lumbar discography. Clin Radiol 1983;34:405–411
59. Saifuddin A, Braithwaite I, White J, Taylor BA, Renton P. The value of lumbar spine magnetic resonance imaging in the demonstration of anular tears. Spine 1998;23:453–457
60. Schnebel BE, Simmons JW, Chowning J, Davidson R. A digitizing technique for the study of movement of intradiscal dye in response to flexion and extension of the lumbar spine. Spine 1988;13:309–312
61. Kornberg M. Computed tomography of the lumbar spine following discography. Clinical application in selective cases. Spine 1987;12:823–825
62. Linson MA, Crowe CH. Comparison of magnetic resonance imaging and lumbar discography in the diagnosis of disc degeneration. Clin Orthop Relat Res 1990;250:160–163
63. Tervonen O, Lahde S, Rydberg J. Lumbar disc degeneration. Correlation between CT and CT/discography. Acta Radiol 1990;31:551–554
64. Ito M, Incorvaia KM, Yu SF, et al. Predictive signs of discogenic lumbar pain on magnetic resonance imaging with discography correlation. Spine 1998;23:1252–1258
65. Schellhas KP, Pollei SR, Gundry CR, Heithoff KB. Lumbar disc high-intensity zone. Correlation of magnetic resonance imaging and discography. Spine 1996;21:79–86
66. Osti OL, Fraser RD. MRI and discography of annular tears and intervertebral disc degeneration. A prospective clinical comparison. J Bone Joint Surg Br 1992;74:431–435
67. Carragee EJ, Barcohana B, Alamin T, van den Haak E. Prospective controlled study of the development of lower back pain in previously asymptomatic subjects undergoing experimental discography. Spine 2004;29:1112–1117
68. Vanharanta H, Ohnmeiss DD, Aprill CN. Vibration pain provocation can improve the specificity of MRI in the diagnosis of symptomatic lumbar disc rupture. Clin J Pain 1998;14:239–247
69. Yrjama M, Tervonen O, Kurunlahti M, Vanharanta H. Bony vibration stimulation test combined with magnetic resonance imaging. Can discography be replaced? Spine 1997;22:808–813
70. Resnick DK, Choudhri TF, Dailey AT, et al. Guidelines for the performance of fusion procedures for degenerative disease of the lumbar spine. Part 17: bone growth stimulators and lumbar fusion. J Neurosurg Spine 2005;2:737–740
71. Guyer RD, Collier R, Stith WJ, et al. Discitis after discography. Spine 1988;13:1352–1354
72. Fraser RD, Osti OL, Vernon-Roberts B. Discitis after discography. J Bone Joint Surg Br 1987;69:26–35
73. Klessig HT, Showsh SA, Sekorski A. The use of intradiscal antibiotics for discography: an in vitro study of gentamicin, cefazolin, and clindamycin. Spine 2003;28:1735–1738
74. Willems PC, Jacobs W, Duinkerke ES, De Kleuver M. Lumbar discography: should we use prophylactic antibiotics? A study of 435 consecutive discograms and a systematic review of the literature. J Spinal Disord Tech 2004;17:243–247
75. Junila J, Niinimaki T, Tervonen O. Epidural abscess after lumbar discography. A case report. Spine 1997;22:2191–2193
76. Poynton AR, Hinman A, Lutz G, Farmer JC. Discography-induced acute lumbar disc herniation: a report of five cases. J Spinal Disord Tech 2005;18:188–192
77. Carragee EJ, Tanner CM, Yang B, Brito JL, Truong T. False-positive findings on lumbar discography. Reliability of subjective concordance assessment during provocative disc injection. Spine 1999;24:2542–2547

5 Biomechanics and Technique Selection for Lumbar Fusion

Eve Tsai, Kene T. Ugokwe, and Edward C. Benzel

Lumbar fusion can be used to restore stability, which may decrease pain and improve early function. A key component to a successful spinal fusion is an understanding of how various fusion techniques can be used to craft a biomechanically stable architecture. Biomechanics is the application of the principles of physics to biologic systems. Although personal experience and skillful assembly of the mechanical construct certainly influence technique selection, the experience of others and laboratory data aid in the choice of the optimal technique. Several biomechanical factors have been identified: (1) applied forces at the disk interspace, (2) subsidence, (3) restoration of disk height, (4) angular deformation and sagittal balance, (5) graft bed preparation, (6) strut position, (7) strut integrity, (8) strut geometry, (9) ligamentous disruption, and (10) load sharing versus load bearing.[1] This chapter discusses the biomechanical principles that are applicable to lumbar spine fusion.

■ Biomechanical Factors to Consider in Lumbar Fusion

Applied Forces at the Disk Interspace

Spine motion can occur along (translation) or around (rotation) the three axes of the Cartesian coordinate system **(Fig. 5.1)**.[2] The underlying orientation of the spinal elements affects the magnitude of each applied force vector. For example, because the end plates at the L5-S1 disk interspace are not aligned perpendicular to an axial load, increased shear stresses are applied to the disk interspace. This is associated with an increased likelihood of translation at the L5-S1 interspace. This should be considered during construct planning. For example, interbody struts, including cages, are typically not effective in preventing translation. Although cages have been designed as interference screws to decrease translational motion, they are usually not effective for this purpose **(Fig. 5.2)**. Thus the additional measures, such as the use of dorsal fixation strategies, should be considered to supplement the use of interbody struts or cages.

Subsidence

A decrease in disk space height is a major contributor to subsidence. This can occur following anterior interbody fusion. Excessive subsidence is associated with vertebral body endplate and bone-graft factors. In the case of excessive end-plate removal or end-plate fracture, the interbody strut can piston into the vertebral body. The end plate or the graft can also fracture if the modulus of elasticity of the interbody strut and vertebral body is not matched. If the area of contact between the graft and the vertebral body is inadequate, excessive pressure can be exerted on the end plate. Likewise, subsidence can also occur if the geometrical interface between the strut and the graft bed is poor or if the graft dislodges. The use of instrumentation that is too rigid can also lead to subsidence secondary to stress shielding; thus leading to graft absorption.

Restoration of Disk Height

Restoration of disk height can expand the neural foramina and decompress the neural structures. Because the spine has a predisposition to subsidence until fusion is achieved, increased distraction of the disk interspace may be desirable to achieve adequate decompression once fusion transpires. Therefore, one of the primary intraoperative objectives when using a threaded interbody fusion cage (TIFC) or other interbody strut is to restore the intervertebral disk height to a normal or supranormal height.[3,4]

With repetitive cyclical axial loading, subsidence is inevitable but not necessarily undesirable. Cyclical loading increases pressure within an interbody cage.[5,6] Two different outcomes may occur as a result. One is that the bone within the cage "sees" the pressure forces that enhance fusion according to Wolff's law. In this case, compression forces optimize healing. The other potential outcome is that "excessive" motion prevails and the incidence of fusion is diminished. Therefore, a construct that simultaneously permits enough subsidence to facilitate fusion, but not too much so that excessive motion exists, is desirable.

Angular Deformation and Sagittal Balance

When designing a spinal fusion construct, it is important to consider restoring and maintaining sagittal balance to prevent further deformity and to eliminate a potential source of persistent axial pain.[1] With the placement of a cylindrical TIFC into a disk interspace, the normal trapezoidal relationship of the end plates can be rendered parallel **(Fig. 5.2)**. With multiple level interbody cylindrical

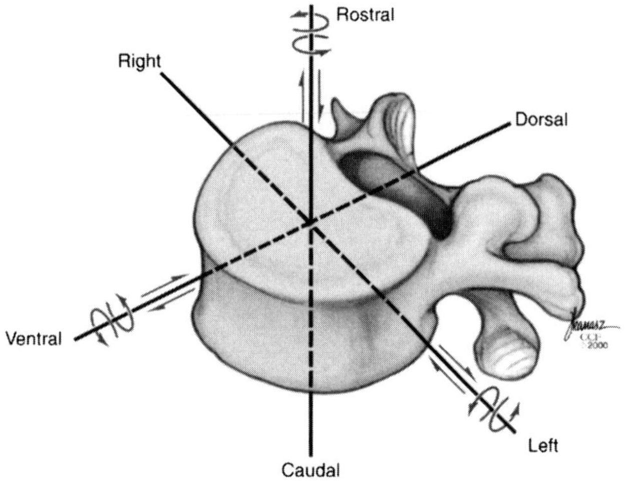

Fig. 5.1 The Cartesian Coordinate system centered on the vertebral body. Motion occurs in a bidirectional manner along *(straight arrows)* and about *(curved arrows)* each axis. (Permission granted, Cleveland Clinic Medical Illustrations Department, 2006.)

implants, a more dramatic loss of lordosis and sagittal balance can result. If lumbar lordosis is lost, a moment arm is created that further encourages kyphotic deformation by moving the instantaneous axis of rotation (IAR) ventrally. Thus, for a given axial load, the kyphotic deformity increases the length of the moment arm of the applied force. This results in a greater bending moment, thereby aggravating the preexisting deformity.[7]

Graft Bed Preparation

Careful preparation of the graft bed and strut is essential for successful lumbar fusion. With excessive end-plate debridement, end-plate fractures may occur. This may lead to increased subsidence and possible progressive kyphotic deformation, as discussed. Inadequate debridement of the end plates, on the other hand, may result in pseudarthrosis.

As interbody struts by themselves provide little translational resistance, deep mortises in the vertebral bodies have been utilized to increase translational resistance **(Fig. 5.3)**. Although these deep mortices may decrease translation, the technique also damages the end plates and decrease axial load-bearing capacity. An appreciation of the anticipated applied load vectors, whether axial or shear in nature, provides additional vital information that facilitates appropriate preparation of the graft bed and mortise.

Strut Position

The IAR is the axis about which each vertebral segment rotates at any given instant. It is truly dynamic in nature. For example, with spinal flexion, the IAR tends to move

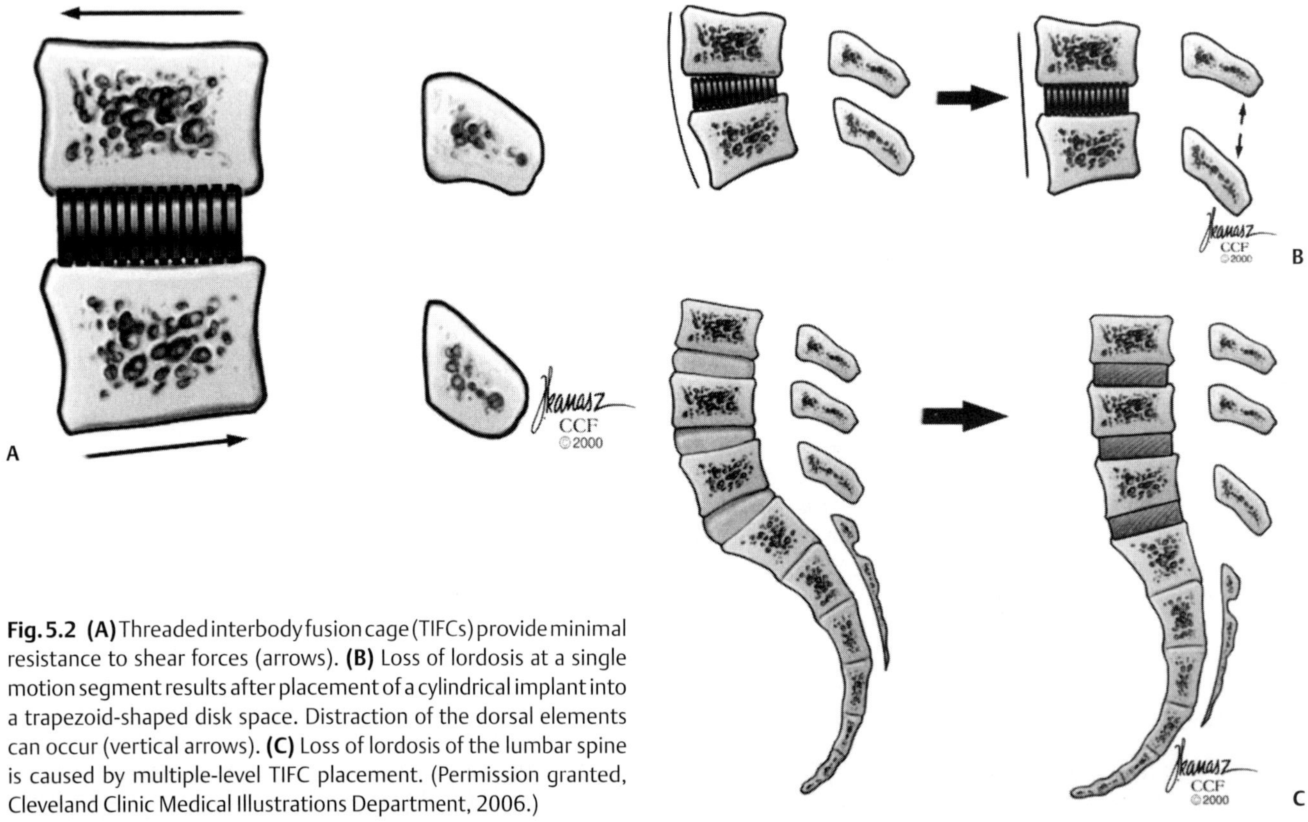

Fig. 5.2 **(A)** Threaded interbody fusion cage (TIFCs) provide minimal resistance to shear forces (arrows). **(B)** Loss of lordosis at a single motion segment results after placement of a cylindrical implant into a trapezoid-shaped disk space. Distraction of the dorsal elements can occur (vertical arrows). **(C)** Loss of lordosis of the lumbar spine is caused by multiple-level TIFC placement. (Permission granted, Cleveland Clinic Medical Illustrations Department, 2006.)

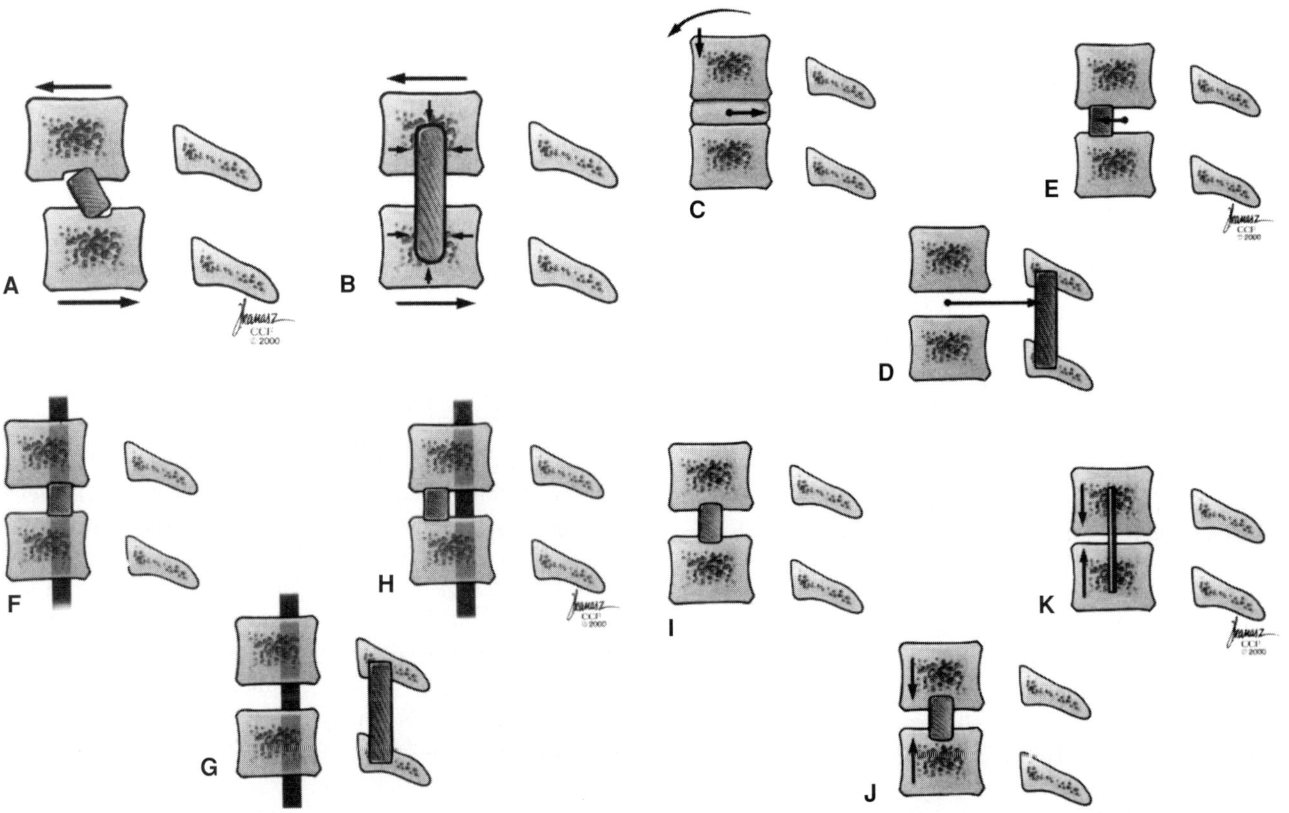

Fig. 5.3 **(A)** Shallow mortices do not effectively resist significant translational forces *(horizontal arrows)*. **(B)** Deep mortices resist translational forces *(small horizontal arrows)* but have reduced axial load-bearing capacity *(vertical arrows)*. **(C)** The instantaneous axis of rotation (IAR) *(dot)* shifts dorsally when an axial load is applied ventral to the IAR, creating a bending moment *(curved arrow)*. **(D,E)** A solid fusion causes the IAR to move toward the fusion mass. **(F)** Bone graft placement close to the IAR *(thick black line)* improves axial load-bearing capacity. **(G)** A graft placed ventral to the IAR improves resistance to flexion, whereas a graft placed dorsal to the IAR improves resistance to extension. **(H)** Angular motion resistance is improved the farther the fusion mass is from the IAR, as in the dorsal onlay fusion. **(I,J)** A strut with a high modulus of elasticity will piston through a soft end plate and vertebral body. **(K)** Pistoning is encouraged if a strut has a small area of contact with the end plate. (Permission granted, Cleveland Clinic Medical Illustrations Department, 2006.)

dorsally, and with extension, the IAR tends to move moves ventrally **(Fig. 5.3)**.

An axial load applied ventral to the IAR generates a flexion bending moment about the IAR. Likewise, an axial load applied dorsally to the IAR generates an extension bending moment about the IAR. Spinal instrumentation or spinal fusion tends to move the IAR toward the spinal implant. To provide superior axial load-bearing capacity, a strut should be placed in line with the preexisting IAR (e.g., midvertebral bodies). However, the strut in this position provides little resistance to angular deformation from applied bending moments. A strut placed at a distance from the IAR improves resistance to applied bending moments **(Fig. 5.3)**. Although a dorsal onlay fusion has poor axial load-bearing capacity, it resists bending moments and angular deformation well by acting as a tension band fixator. Improved resistance to applied bending moments can be enhanced by increasing the distance from the fusion mass to the IAR. This increases the moment arm length and is clinically efficacious, providing that the middle column is intact and adequate axial load-bearing capacity is present.

Strut Integrity

Careful consideration of strut integrity is essential in minimizing interbody fusion construct collapse, fracture, or reabsorption.[1] The integrity or the mechanical nature of a strut can be measured by the modulus of elasticity. The modulus of elasticity is defined as the ratio between the extent of deformation a solid body undergoes in response to an applied load (the stress/strain ratio). A material that is stiff has a greater modulus of elasticity than does a material that is less stiff. In choosing a strut for a fusion construct, the modulus of elasticity of the strut and the graft bed should be matched appropriately. If the stiffness of the strut is greater than that of the graft bed, the strut may piston through the end plate into the vertebral body or dislodge **(Fig. 5.3)**. Pistoning may be minimized by increasing the surface area of contact between the strut and the graft bed (see below). If the modulus of elasticity of the strut is less than that of the graft bed, the strut may collapse, fracture, and reabsorb.

Strut Geometry

Increasing the surface area of contact between the bone graft and the graft bed increases the capacity of an interbody fusion strut to resist axial loads, minimize micromotion,[1] and increase fusion rates. The surface area can be increased by matching the contour of the graft bed to that of the strut contact surface **(Fig. 5.4).** In the lumbar spine, it should mimic the wedge-shaped lumbar intervertebral space.

Struts or cages can be grouped by the way they interface with the graft bed: flat- or round-faced. Flat-faced struts present a relatively large surface area of contact with the graft bed **(Fig. 5.5A,B).** They can be square, rectangular, circular, or oval. Their flat surface, however, is presented to the graft bed. Due to the flat surface contact with the end plate, the struts can resist compressive, angular, and translation deformation.

Round-faced struts, conversely, present a round surface to the graft bed. The TIFC is a prototypical round-faced strut. A single round-faced cage poorly resists angular deformation **(Fig. 5.5C,D).** Placement of two rounded cages improves resistance to angular deformation. Care must be taken to ensure that the cage is placed properly, lest suboptimal contact with the graft bed results **(Fig. 5.5E,F).**

As a cylindrical strut is placed into an elliptical wedge-shaped lumbar interspace, the area of contact between the cage and the graft bed is not uniform **(Fig. 5.6A).** Coronal cross-sectional views are demonstrated in planes A, B, and C. In plane A, there is minimal contact between the implant and the end plate. The decreased bone-to-bone contact decreases fusion rates. There may be some load-bearing resistance in flexion. However, excessive micromotion across the interspace may further contribute to fusion failure. In plane B, there is optimal contact, although the width of the contact of the implant with the end plate is still narrow. In plane C, the implant sits deep in the end plate and invades the vertebral cancellous bone. This location increases the tendency to piston and also decreases the capacity to bear axial loads, compared with plane B.

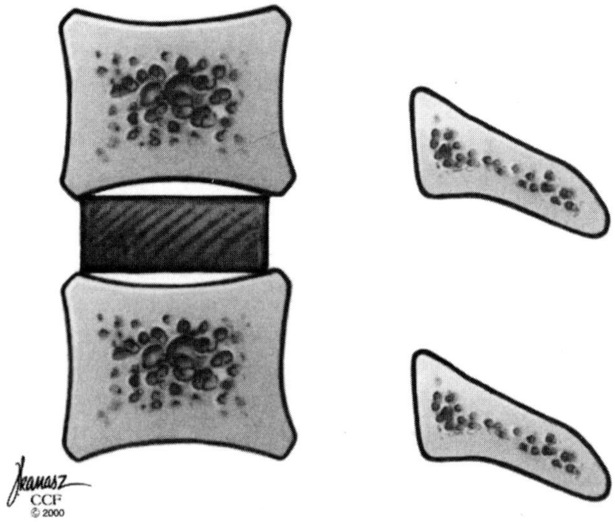

Fig. 5.4 Uniform contact between an intervertebral strut and elliptically shaped vertebral end plates. (Permission granted, Cleveland Clinic Medical Illustrations Department, 2006.)

Ligamentous Disruption

To dorsally place (via a posterior lumbar interbody fusion [PLIF] technique) a large enough interbody strut to achieve interspace distraction, the disruption of the dorsal ligaments and bony elements, including the facet joints, is required **(Fig. 5.6).** With disruption of the facet joints, the significant loss of stiffness with respect to flexion and rotation may cause progressive postoperative deformity. Increased interspace height is desired because this places the ligamentous tissues in tension and increases the overall stiffness of the construct.

Load Sharing Versus Load Bearing

Load sharing is achieved when multiple components of a construct bear a portion of the overall load, thus sharing the load between components, for example, when a construct's applied load is borne by an interbody strut and by another implant or by the native spine itself.[1] Thus, if an interbody strut is used with dorsal instrumentation, the applied axial load is shared between the strut and the dorsal instrumentation. Conversely, when an interbody strut is used without dorsal instrumentation, the interbody strut must bear the majority of the axial load.

The extent that the axial load is transferred through the interbody strut varies with intraoperative preloading of the dorsal instrumentation. When the dorsal construct is preloaded under compression, the graft is loaded and the dorsal instrumentation unloaded when the patient is upright. Loading the graft encourages bone fusion and reduces the load applied to the dorsal implant. If the dorsal construct is not preloaded, the interbody strut and the dorsal instrumentation share the applied axial load. If the dorsal construct is preloaded in distraction, the dorsal construct bears both the preloaded forces and the applied axial loads. Thus the interbody strut is effectively shielded from axial loading and bone-fusion forces. A balance must be struck between too much motion and not enough motion. The result of excessive motion may be pseudarthrosis, construct failure, and persistence of low back pain. Too little motion may result in the shielding of the bone graft from bone healing enhancing forces. Obviously, the type of motion is also important. The axial loading of a bone graft via

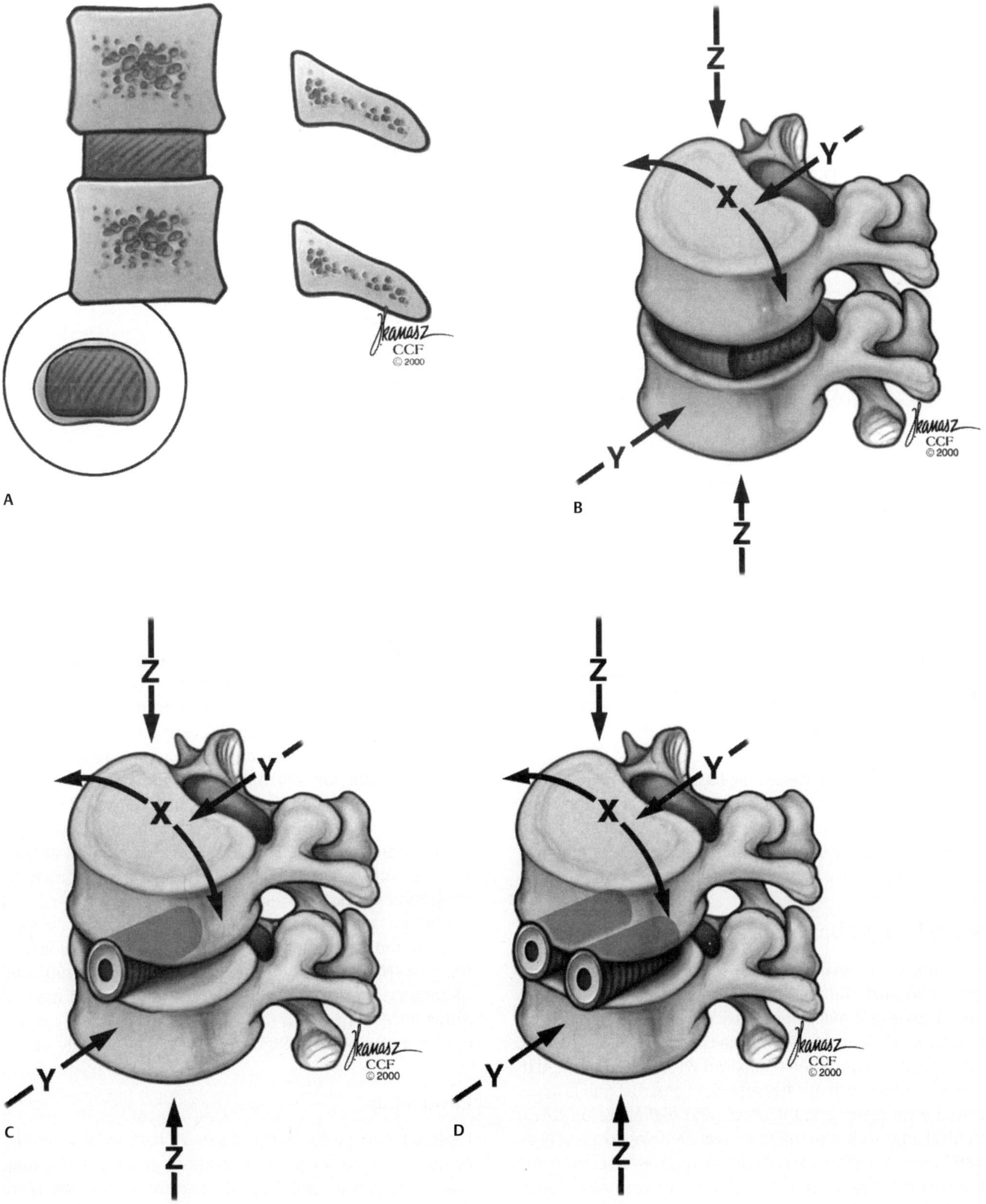

Fig. 5.5 **(A)** Flat-faced struts present a large surface area of contact to the graft bed (inset: axial view). **(B)** Flat-faced struts resist angular "x," shear "y," and axial "z" forces. **(C)** A single round-faced cage functions poorly in resisting angular "x," shear "y," and axial "z" forces. **(D)** Paired cages have improved load-bearing capacity in all planes. (*Continued on next page*)

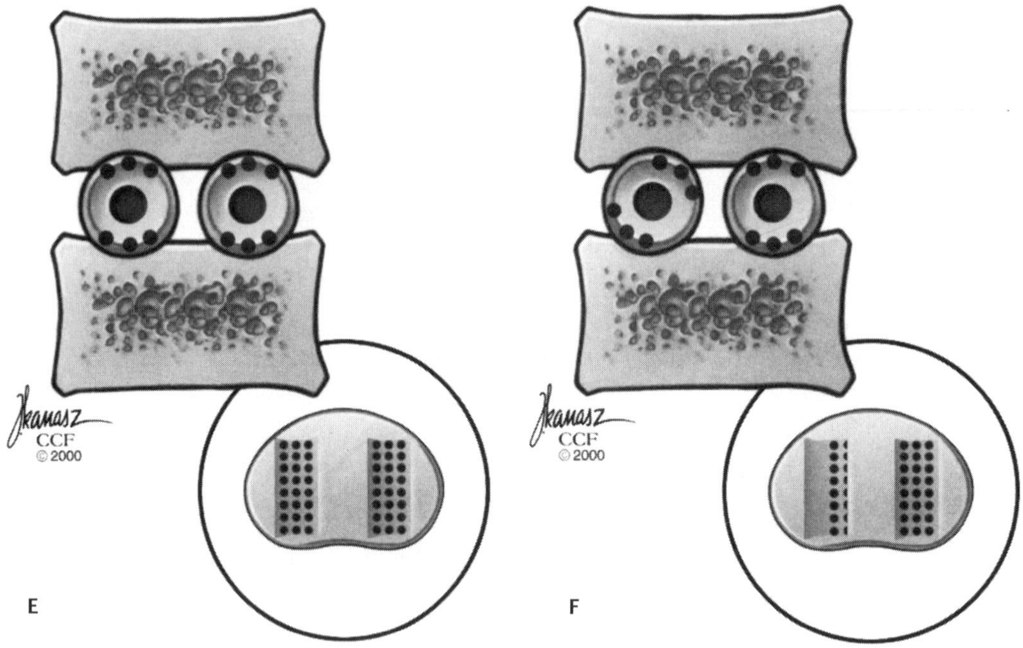

Fig. 5.5 *(Continued)* **(E)** Area of contact between bone graft and vertebral end plate through holes *(dots)* in the TIFCs. **(F)** Reduced area of contact if placed improperly (insets: axial views). (Permission granted, Cleveland Clinic Medical Illustrations Department, 2006.)

subsidence may be beneficial, whereas flexion-extension motion inhibits bone fusion.

■ Surgical Procedures for Lumbar Fusion

Now that we have described the basic biomechanical principles as they apply to spinal fusion, we can turn to the surgical procedures for mechanical back pain, which should be considered for patients only after aggressive and appropriate nonoperative management has failed.

Anterior Lumbar Interbody Fusion

The anterior lumbar interbody fusion (ALIF) approach is used to improve lumbar lordosis and to treat degenerative disk disease and mechanical back pain. It is also employed to enlarge the neuroforamina via the elevation of the disk interspace height. When compared with the PLIF, the ALIF provides a biomechanically superior construct and is associated with fewer complications and higher fusion rates. Ventral approaches to the spine were employed as early as 1892 when Vincent[8] described a costotransversectomy for the treatment of tuberculosis of the ventral lumbar spine. In 1934, Ito et al[9] described a transperitoneal approach to the lumbar spine with fusion. The indications for ALIF include degenerative disk disease with back pain, failure of prior dorsal surgery, and failure of a prolonged trial of conservative management.[10,11] As with any surgical procedure, absolute and relative contraindications exist. The only absolute contraindication to ALIF is severe osteoporosis, to the extent that it prevents the vertebral bodies from supporting a bone graft.[12] Relative contraindications include neural compression from disk pathology, obvious peritoneal or pelvic infection, gross obesity, prior retroperitoneal surgery, previous laparotomy, severe peripheral vascular disease,[12–14] an infrarenal aortic aneurysm, an active disk space infection, and a neoplasm.[15] Prior to performing an ALIF, it is important for the surgeon and the patient to agree on realistic goals. It is also important to note that surgical outcome cannot be completely evaluated until at least 6 to 12 months after surgery. A detailed preoperative radiographic workup is required, including plain x-rays of the lumbosacral spine with flexion and extension views.[16] A computed tomography (CT) scan and magnetic resonance imaging (MRI) should also be done. In patients who have undergone a prior instrumented fusion, the MRI may be difficult to interpret due to artifact. In this situation, a myelogram with a postmyelogram CT should be considered.

Positioning

Most ALIFs are performed at the two most caudal segments of the spine. As with any operation, general positioning practices such as padding all pressure points and bony prominences should be employed. With ALIF, visualization is obtained both directly and fluoroscopically and, as such, the operating table must facilitate both anterior/posterior and lateral fluoroscopy. The optimal intraoperative posture is lordosis. This is best achieved by reversing the flexion of the operating table and placing a bump or roll in the low

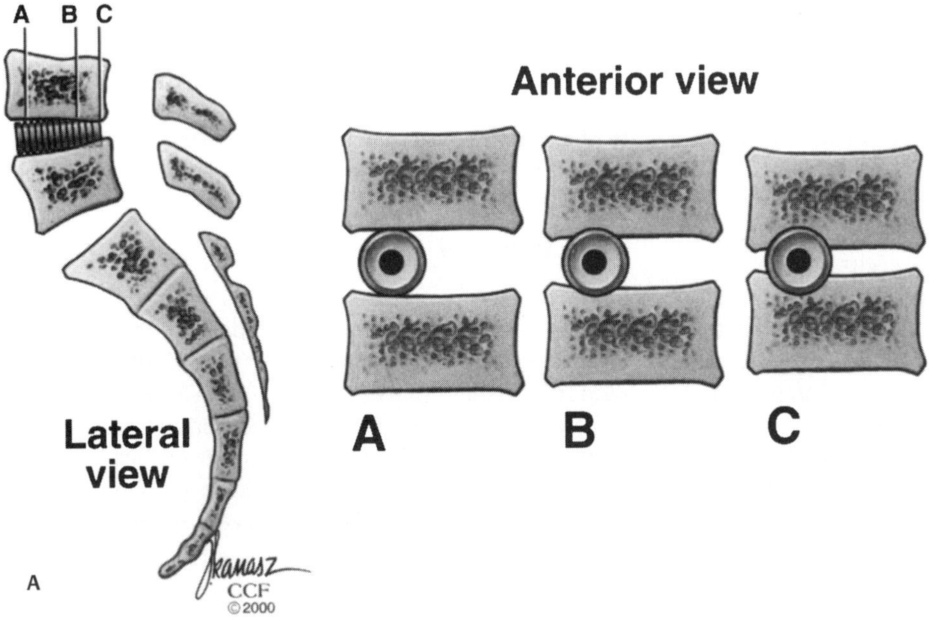

A

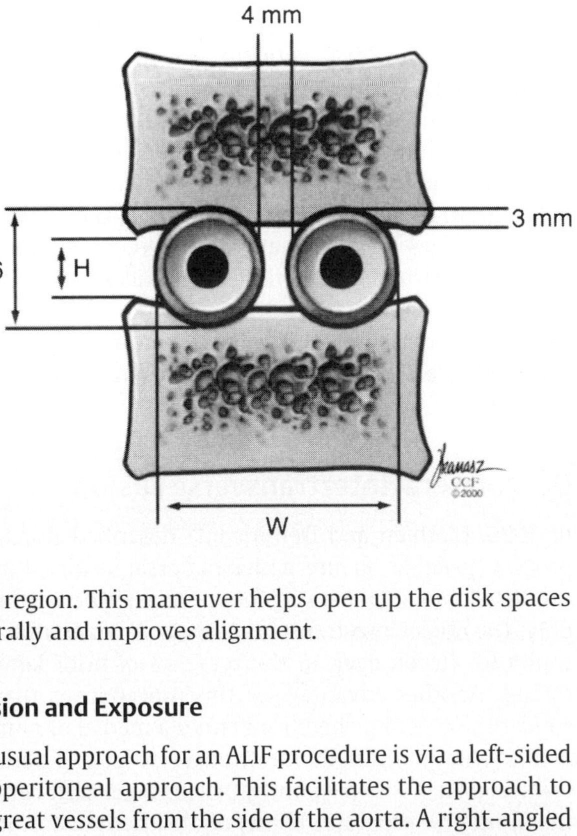

B

Figure 5.6 **(A)** Depiction of three regions of contact of a cylindrical implant in relation to the vertebral body cancellous bone and end plate (planes A, B, and C). Plane A: minimal implant–end-plate contact. Plane B: optimal contact. Plane C: excessive penetration into cancellous bone. **(B)** In order for TIFCs to achieve the desired disk interspace distraction, excessive resection of the dorsal elements is required. The width (W) necessary to achieve this interspace distraction is $2(H + 6\text{ mm} + 4\text{ mm} = 2H + 16\text{ mm}$, where H is the desired interspace distraction height. A penetration of 3 mm of the implant in the end plate and a distance of 4 mm between the implants is assumed. (Permission granted, Cleveland Clinic Medical Illustrations Department, 2006.)

back region. This maneuver helps open up the disk spaces ventrally and improves alignment.

Incision and Exposure

The usual approach for an ALIF procedure is via a left-sided retroperitoneal approach. This facilitates the approach to the great vessels from the side of the aorta. A right-angled incision is often used. The horizontal limb extends from the midline to the lateral border of the rectus abdominis muscle, and the vertical limb extends up to the linea semilunaris. The exposure should be performed by a surgeon who harbors a clear foundation of knowledge regarding the retroperitoneal region and one who can manage complications that may arise. It is important to identify and protect the ureter. If the peritoneum is violated, it should be repaired immediately to prevent the formation of a hernia.[17] If, however, the bowel is perforated, the ALIF procedure should be aborted and the bowel should be irrigated and closed in a layered fashion. Intraoperative radiographs must be obtained and compared with preoperative imaging to confirm the appropriate levels.[18,19]

Diskectomy and Fusion

Lateral fluoroscopy is used to reconfirm the appropriate level, and anterior/posterior fluoroscopy is used to mark the midline. Prior to the diskectomy, all tissues overlying the disk should be swept laterally and monopolar cautery should be avoided because it increases the incidence of retrograde ejaculation. In general, disk material is removed to 25 to 30 mm in depth and 30 to 35 mm in width. These figures are only a guide. In particular, the depth should be confirmed with fluoroscopy. After the diskectomy is performed, disk space distractors with calibrated tips are used to distract the disk space. Spacers are then placed. A variety of materials are currently used as spacers. These include iliac crest autograft, donor femoral ring, tibia, and humerus. More recently, threaded allograft dowels have been employed. Likewise, titanium and carbon fiber cages have gained increased popularity.[20,21] The spacer functions to restore lumbar lordosis and improve sagittal plane alignment. In order for a fusion to be successful, compression and appropriate immobilization are necessary. Compression is best achieved by using a slightly oversized spacer in the disk space. It is nearly impossible to maintain a dorsally placed interbody graft in compression. A dorsal onlay graft provides minimal compressive forces. Immobilization is achieved by using a firm fitting spacer in the disk space and using postoperative external orthosis. Once the spacers have been placed, fluoroscopic confirmation of placement should be obtained.[18,19]

Posterior Lumbar Interbody Fusion

The posterior lumbar interbody fusion (PLIF) is a popular procedure, but it is moderately difficult to perform. In addition, it is associated with significant complications. Ralph Cloward[22–25] was the first to perform this operation in 1940. The indications for PLIF include spondylolisthesis, degenerative scoliosis, degenerative disk disease, and recurrent disk herniations. Compared with a ventral ALIF approach, PLIF facilitates an improved exposure and decompression of the neural structures.[26] A PLIF procedure allows fusion to occur at approximately the center of the axis of rotation. Therefore, it subjects the graft to compressive rather than tensile forces. This is superior to dorsolateral (intertransverse) fusion. A PLIF also protects the nerve roots, maintains disk height, immobilizes the unstable disk area, and restores weight-bearing capacity to the ventral spinal structures.[27] The early operations performed by Cloward involved subtotal diskectomy with decompression of the dorsal elements and interbody fusion of the vertebral bodies. Today, several variations of the original operation exist, including unilateral or bilateral facetectomies for ample disk access lateral to the exiting nerve root (TLIF).

Positioning and Exposure

The patient is placed prone on an operating table that allows the abdomen to hang freely. This helps to prevent venous engorgement and thereby decreases bleeding. The Jackson table is very useful because it also facilitates hip extension, thus maximizing lumbar lordosis, in addition to facilitating the minimization of intraabdominal pressure. After the skin incision is marked, prepped, and draped, the incision is made and the dissection is carried to the lumbodorsal fascia. The fascia is opened in the midline, exposing the spinous processes and lamina at the levels rostral and caudal to the pathologic levels. Partial laminectomies are performed and the lower third of the caudal facet and the medial two thirds of the rostral facet are also removed to improve the exposure. Commercially available disk interspace distractors may be used to better expose the intervertebral space.

Diskectomy and Fusion

Commercially available disk shavers with cutting sides may be placed into the intervertebral space to achieve disk interspace decompression. It is advisable to begin with the smallest shaver, which is often 7 mm, and to alternate the sides of shaver insertion and shaver size by 2-mm increments. Once 90% of the dorsal disk material is removed, the end plates should be prepared for fusion. Interbody grafts are then placed. In the past, this "stand-alone" PLIF was sufficient. Today, most surgeons augment their PLIF procedures with pedicle screw fixation, which helps prevent interbody graft displacement. Cloward originally used rectangular tricortical grafts for his interbody fusion, but the cortical surfaces integrated very slowly and it was very cumbersome to shape these grafts. Branch and Branch[28,29] reported the use of vertical support columns in the interspace, in addition to packing the interspace with cancellous bone chips. More recently, a plethora of interbody cages have become available. Brantigan et al[30,31] developed a carbon fiber cage that has ridges or teeth that resist dislodgment. In 1988, Ray[32,33] used threaded titanium cages packed with cancellous bone for a PLIF. After placement of the interbody graft, the distractor is removed to allow for compression, and the transpedicular fixation is also performed to provide further compression.

Dorsolateral Intertransverse Fusion

In 1936, Mathieu and Demirleau[34] described transverse process fusion as an alternative to dorsal fusions. Prior to this development, most surgeons performed dorsal fusions only. The dorsal intertransverse fusion provides an opportunity for fusion even in the presence of prior laminectomies. Another advantage of this procedure is that the spine can be approached from either a medial or paramedian orientation. Initially, intertransverse fusions were performed in an in-situ fashion, by placing bone graft between the transverse processes bilaterally (without instrumentation). More recently, the use of internal fixation has helped improve the fusion rate and has also improved the surgeon's ability to correct deformity.[35,36]

Positioning, Exposure, and Fusion

The positioning for a dorsolateral intertransverse fusion is similar to that for an ALIF. Again, it is recommended that a Jackson or equivalent table be used. As previously stated, it is important to position the patient prone with the abdomen hanging freely. Also, as with all operations, all pressure points must be adequately padded. The midline approach allows bilateral exposure of the dorsal elements of the spine, whereas a paramedian approach requires two separate incisions. Once the fascial dissection is complete, the soft tissue exposure is carried laterally to expose the transverse processes. During the exposure, it is important to preserve the facet capsule at levels that will not be fused. Also, a subperiosteal dissection leads to less bleeding in the operative field. At this point, if a decompression is warranted, the surgeon may proceed with it. If only an onlay in-situ fusion is performed, the bone obtained from the decompression is placed between the transverse processes and into the dorsal facet joints (after denuding the synovium) bilaterally. If an instrumented fusion is to be performed, the instrumentation is placed prior to the placement of the bone graft.

Posterior Lumbar Interbody Fusion Versus Dorsolateral Intertransverse Fusion

More muscle dissection and retraction is required for a dorsolateral intertransverse fusion than for a PLIF. However, it is important to note that a PLIF provides a circumferential spinal fusion and helps restore ventral interbody height.

Posterior Lumbar Interbody Fusion Versus Anterior Lumbar Interbody Fusion

In terms of ease of operation, an ALIF facilitates the performance of a diskectomy and the placement of the interbody graft without traction on the nerve roots. In a study by Voor et al,[37] comparing ALIF and PLIF with dorsal instrumentation, ALIF was noted to be slightly superior, especially regarding torsion.

References

1. Benzel EC, Lastra JJ, Kalfas I, et al. The biomechanics of interbody fusion and the shortcomings of lumbar fusion with cages and interbody bone dowels. Clin Neurosurg 2000;47:557–588
2. White AA, Panjabi MM. Biomechanical considerations in the surgical measurement of the spine. In: Clinical Biomechanics of the Spine, 2nd edition. Philadelphia: JB Lippincott, 1990:511–631
3. Chen D, Fay LA, Lok J, et al. Increasing neuroforaminal volume by anterior interbody distraction in degenerative lumbar spine. Spine 1995;20:74–79
4. Vamvanij V, Ferrara LA, Hai Y, et al. Quantitative changes in spinal canal dimensions using interbody distraction for spondylolisthesis. Spine 2001;26:E13–E18
5. Bourn SM, Ghanayem AJ, et al. Hydrostatic forces within intervertebral fusion cages. North American Spine Society 12th Annual Meeting, New Orleans, 1997:18–19
6. Parten P, Ghanayem AJ, et al. Hydrostatic loads within a cervical interbody fusion cage: An in vitro model. Cervical Spine Research Society, Atlanta, GA, 1998, paper 13
7. Kitchel SH. Improvement in sagittal plane alignment following anterior lumbar interbody fusion with threaded titanium cages. North American Spine Society Proceedings 12th Annual Meeting, New Orleans, 1997:108–109
8. Vincent E. Contribution a la chirurgie. Rev Chir Orthop Reparatrice Appar Mot 1892;12:273
9. Ito H, Tsuchiya J, Asami G. A new radical operation for Pott's disease. J Bone Joint Surg Br 1934;16:499–515
10. Chow SP, Leong JCY, Ma A, Yau AC. Anterior spinal fusion for deranged lumbar intervertebral disc: a review of 97 cases. Spine 1980;5:452–458
11. Leong JCY. Anterior interbody fusion. In: Lin P, Gill K, eds. Lumbar Interbody Fusion. Rockville, MD: Aspen, 1989:133–148
12. Collis JS, Rojas C, Janack M. Anterior total disc replacement: a modified anterior lumbar interbody fusion. In: Lin P, Gill K, eds. Lumbar Interbody Fusion. Rockville, MD: Aspen, 1989:149–152
13. Dodge LD, Bohlman HH, Rhodes RS. Concurrent lumbar spinal stenosis and peripheral vascular disease: a report of nine patients. Clin Orthop Relat Res 1988;230:141–148
14. Gill K. Technique and complications of anterior lumbar interbody fusion. In: Lin P, Gill K, eds. Lumbar Interbody Fusion. Rockville, MD: Aspen, 1989:95–106
15. Watkins RG. Anterior approaches to the lumbar spine. In: Torrens MJ, Dickson RA, eds. Operative Spinal Surgery. New York: Churchill Livingstone, 1991:161–171
16. Harmon PH. Anterior lumbar disc excision and fusion: operative technique including observations upon variations in the left common iliac veins and thir connections. Clin Orthop Relat Res 1960;18:185–198
17. Southwick WO, Robinson RA. Surgical approaches to the vertebral bodies in the cervical and lumbar regions. J Bone Joint Surg Am 1957;39A:631–644
18. Crock HV. Lumbar vertebral interbody fusion. In: Lin P, Gill K, eds. Lumbar Interbody Fusion. Rockville, MD: Aspen, 1989:115– 125
19. Hodgson AR, Wong SK. A description of a technique and evaluation of results in anterior spinal fusion for deranged intervertebral disc and spondylolisthesis. Clin Orthop Relat Res 1968;56:133–162
20. Brantigan JW, Steffee AD. A carbon fiber implant to aid interbody lumbar fusion: two year clinical results in the first twenty-six patients. Spine 1993;18:2106–2117
21. Enker P, Steffee AD. Interbody fusion and instrumentation. Clin Orthop Relat Res 1994;300:90–101
22. Cloward RB. The treatment of ruptured lumbar intervertebral disc by vertebral body fusion II. Method of use of banked bone. Ann Surg 1952;136:987–992
23. Cloward RB. Lumbar intervertebral disc surgery. Description of a new instrument, the vertebral spreader. Surgery 1952;32:852–857
24. Cloward RB. The treatment of ruptured lumbar intervertebral disc by vertebral fusion. Indications, operative technique, aftercare. J Neurosurg 1953;10:154–166
25. Cloward RB. History of PLIF. Forty years of personal experience. In: Thomas CC, Lin PM, eds. Posterior Lumbar Interbody Fusion. Springfield, IL: Charles C. Thomas, 1982
26. Rish BL. A critique of posterior lumbar interbody fusion: twelve years experience with two hundred and fifty patients. Surg Neurol 1989;31:281–289

27. Brantigan JW, McAfee PC, Cunningham BW, et al. Interbody lumbar fusion using a carbon fiber cage implant versus allograft bone. An investigational study in the Spanish goat. Spine 1994;19:1436–1444
28. Branch CL, Branch CL. Posterior lumbar interbody fusion with the keystone graft: technique and results. Surg Neurol 1987;27:449–454
29. Branch CL, Branch CL Jr. Posterior lumbar interbody fusion: the keystone technique. In: Lin P, Gill K, eds. Lumbar Interbody Fusion. Rockville, MD: Aspen, 1989
30. Brantigan JW, Steffee AD, Geiger JM. A carbon fiber implant to aid interbody lumbar fusion. Mechanical testing. Spine 1991;16(suppl)S277–S282
31. Brantigan JW, Cunningham BW, Warden PC, et al. Compression strength of donor bone for posterior lumbar interbody fusion. Spine 1993;18:1213–1221
32. Ray CD. Transfacet decompression with dowel fixation: a new technique for lumbar lateral spinal stenosis. Acta Neurochir Suppl (Wien) 1988;43:48–54
33. Ray CD. Lumbar interbody threaded prostheses. In: Brock M, Mayer HM, Weigel K, eds. The Artificial Disc. Berlin: Springer-Verlag, 1991:53–67
34. Mathieu P, Demirleau P. Traitement chirurgical du spondylolisthesis douloureaux. Rev Orthop 1936;23:352
35. Grubb SA, Lipscomb HJ. Results of lumbosacral fusion for degenerative disc disease with and without instrumentation. Two and five year follow up. Spine 1992;17:349–355
36. Schwab FJ, Nazarian DG, Mahmud F, Michelsen CB. Effects of spinal instrumentation on fusion of the lumbosacral spine. Spine 1995;20:2023–2028
37. Voor MJ, Mehta S, Wang M, et al. Biomechanical evaluation of posterior and anterior lumbar interbody fusion techniques. J Spinal Disord 1998;11:328–334

6 Measuring, Preserving, and Restoring Sagittal Balance in Reconstructive Spinal Surgery

Brian A. O'Shaughnessy and Stephen L. Ondra

The importance of sagittal balance and its implications in reconstructive spinal surgery have gained significant attention over the past decade. Despite marked progress, our understanding of sagittal spinal contour and its relationship to posture, locomotion, and energy expenditure continues to evolve. A great deal of practical and conceptual information and data have been accrued through focused research. In a recent retrospective analysis of 752 patients with adult spinal deformity, Glassman and colleagues[1] showed that the severity of symptoms increases linearly with progressive worsening of sagittal plane imbalance. They determined that while proximal thoracic kyphosis is often tolerable, sagittal deformity in the lumbar spine is associated with very poor clinical performance. This has important implications for clinicians when making decisions regarding the most effective clinical care of symptomatic spine patients. Such information provides guidance into the appropriate use and efficacy of treatment alternatives as well as the goals of surgical intervention.

In this chapter we review the concepts of global, regional, and local sagittal balance. We describe the role of the pelvis with a particular focus on changes in pelvic orientation that accompany compensatory behaviors in sagittal imbalance. We discuss the proper technique for measurement and assessment of sagittal alignment. We review how patient positioning and basic strategies for preserving sagittal balance are critical when performing lumbar and lumbosacral fusion procedures for the maintenance of sagittal alignment. Finally, in the event that surgical restoration of sagittal spinal balance is required, osteotomy techniques are reviewed as well as principles that underpin their selection. This is critical because spinal osteotomy is the primary method of spinal mobilization that allows sagittal as well as coronal plane manipulation and correction.

■ Measuring Sagittal Alignment

Global Sagittal Balance

The most common technique to measure sagittal alignment is to drop a plumb line from the middle of the C7 vertebral body down to the sacrum on a 14- × 36-inch lateral scoliosis radiograph. This is also known as the sagittal vertical axis (SVA) and is a measurement of global sagittal alignment.[2–4] The SVA typically falls anterior to the thoracic spine and through the apical lumbar vertebral body and superior sacrum. By convention, a plumb line falling anterior to the posterior-superior corner of the sacrum is considered positive **(Fig. 6.1)**. If the plumb line falls dorsal to this point, the patient is said to have negative sagittal alignment. Some studies have utilized the center of the dens as the superior reference point instead of the C7 vertebral body;[5] however, the inability to consistently visualize this structure with clarity on routine long cassette radiographs has limited its routine use. More importantly, the dens plumb line has not been validated as a measure of sagittal balance. Recent work at our institution has suggested that the dens falls anterior to the SVA.[6] It appears that cervical alignment is more powerfully influenced by the need to align the cranial center of mass over the femoral axis and body center of mass. This seems to be the most important driver for cervical sagittal alignment.

Many authors have studied the sagittal plane in healthy subjects in an attempt to elucidate a set of normative values. These normal values appear to be age dependent, with children having slightly more negative balance than adults. Vedantam et al[3] showed that the SVA was −5.7 ± 3.5 cm in the pediatric population. In an analysis by Gelb et al,[4] adults were found to be slightly less negative in their sagittal balance with a mean SVA measuring −3.2 ± 3.2 cm. Interestingly, in their study of asymptomatic adult volunteers, Jackson and McManus[2] found a wide range of normative SVA values (range, −6.0 to +6.5 cm). This paper stands in contradistinction to the work of Farcy and Schwab,[7] who examined sagittal alignment in the context of lumbar flatback deformity and determined that deviation of the SVA over 4 cm from the anterior sacral promontory was associated with pain and poor response to nonoperative therapy. Recent work by Schwab and colleagues[8] has focused on center-of-gravity analysis using a force plate and has shown that the SVA approximates a more important global balance parameter, namely the center of gravity line. In fact, a decade ago, Dubousset[9] proposed the concept of the "cone of stability" to illustrate the narrow range within which the center of gravity must fall in the standing patient

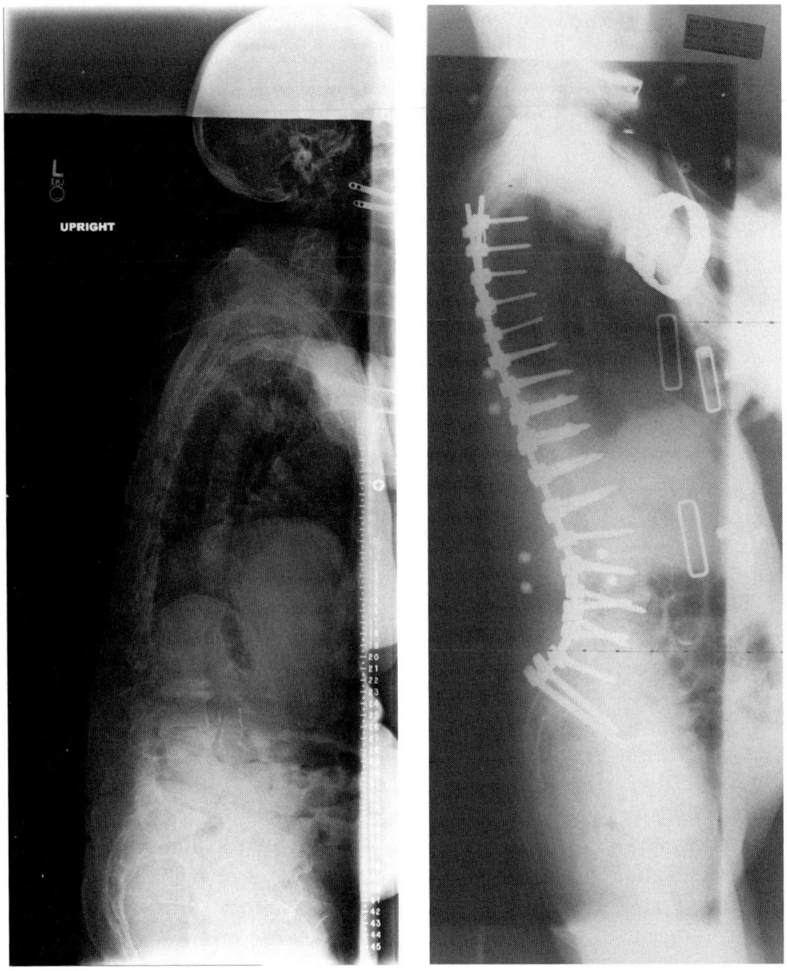

A, B

Fig. 6.1 **(A)** Preoperative lateral scoliosis x-ray of an osteoporotic patient with a degenerative flat back deformity resulting in a positive sagittal balance. **(B)** Postoperative x-ray demonstrates restoration of normal sagittal alignment.

to minimize energy consumption and maintain overall balance.

Of additional importance in global assessment of spinal balance is recognizing the dynamic interplay between regions of the spinal column as well as the pelvis. A patient with thoracic hyperkyphosis attempts to maintain global sagittal balance initially by hyperlordosing the lumbar spine. As mentioned, the concept of normal cervical lordosis is erroneous. Cervical alignment seems determined more by head alignment over the femoral axis and body center of mass. In fact, according to the work of Koski et al[6] and Kuntz et al,[10] the cervical spine can range from slightly kyphotic to lordotic in the normal state (**Fig. 6.2**).

There is a reciprocal relationship between the various regions of the spine to maintain global balance. For example, patients with adolescent idiopathic scoliosis often have a hypokyphotic thoracic contour, which is balanced by a straight to kyphotic cervical spine. In their analysis of 38 subjects with idiopathic scoliosis, Hilibrand et al[11] found a subaxial cervical kyphosis of $+6 \pm 11$ degrees, which was significantly correlated with preoperative hypokyphosis of the thoracic spine. The orientation of the various spine regions, particularly the cervical, may be more complicated than simply counterbalancing other regions of the spine. Although without experimental or clinical validation as yet, it is theorized that alignment of the spinal column may be most critical in generating appropriate position of the cranium in space such that vestibulo-ocular equilibrium is achieved.

With specific regard to the role of the pelvis in global sagittal balance, important work has been put forth by Labelle et al,[12–14] Duval-Beaupere et al,[15] and Jackson and McManus.[2,16,17] In a methodologically sound analysis, Jackson and McManus found a significant correlation, in both healthy and diseased subjects, between sacral inclination and segmental lumbar lordosis. With the patient's knees fully extended, the correlations indicated that as segmental lordosis decreases, the pelvis rotates posteriorly around the hip axis, thereby resulting in a more vertical sacral inclination. This concept has been extended to take into account the pelvic incidence. This angle is the measure of the arc created by a line from the femoral axis to the center of the S1 end plate and the line perpendicular to that end plate. This angle gradually increases until a person reaches skeletal maturity and then becomes a stable, relatively fixed, value. Labelle and others[12–15] have shown

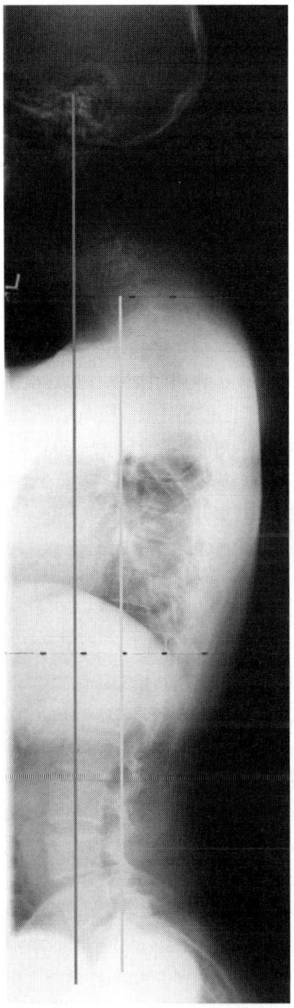

Fig. 6.2 Normal asymptomatic 30-year-old patient's 36-inch scoliosis x-ray demonstrates normal spinal alignment with a C7 plumb line over the S1 end plate. Note that C1 is not located in the spinal balance line. The head center of mass is in alignment with the femoral axis.

that the pelvic incidence is the primary driver and determining value of lumbar lordosis. Patients with a high pelvic incidence must have a comparatively high lumbar lordosis to balance their spine and body center of mass over the femoral axis. Conversely, low pelvic incidence necessitates a decreased lumbar lordosis. This level of sophistication has important clinical implications when a surgeon analyzes preoperative imaging. It helps guide the analysis of pathology and the surgical goals by allowing the surgeon to understand the relative need for lordosis restoration based on the pelvic incidence, which gives clues as to the degree of premorbid lordosis. This then guides balance restoration goals.

These concepts are also important in understanding the primary mechanism by which the pelvis can be effectively utilized to compensate for otherwise abnormal sagittal spinal alignment. When performing reconstructive spinal surgery, it is important to consider that a fusion to the sacropelvis precludes the ability to perform this compensatory pelvic rotation, underscoring the importance of optimizing sagittal alignment when performing a lumbosacral fusion. In our practice, sacral inclination on preoperative radiographs is carefully accounted for and taken into consideration when computing the degrees of correction required to restore sagittal spinal balance.

Regional and Local Sagittal Balance

In addition to global sagittal balance, regional and local alignment is important for normal pain-free activity because a normal SVA is not always consistent with acceptable sagittal balance. For instance, a patient can achieve normal global sagittal balance in the face of a profound focal thoracic kyphosis by lumbar hyperlordosis and retroversion of the pelvis. Such compensatory behaviors are typically painful over time and can lead to muscle fatigue, accelerated hip degeneration, and structural changes in the osseous spinal anatomy. Normative values for each region of the spinal column have been studied as well as the role certain spinal segments play in establishing regional contour.

Hardacker et al[5] noted that 40 degrees of lordosis occurs between the occiput and C7, 30 degrees of which is generated from the occiput to C2. By default, the subaxial cervical spine therefore contributes approximately 10 degrees of lordosis to overall cervical lordosis and does so by the wedge shape of the vertebral bodies in concert with disk morphology. Numerous studies have analyzed sagittal thoracic and thoracolumbar alignment.[2,3,18] The range of thoracic kyphosis in normal patients of all ages has been reported from 9 to 63 degrees; however, mean thoracic kyphosis appears to be fairly consistently in the range of 30 to 40 degrees. From a technical standpoint with regard to measurement, the ideal method is a Cobb angle from the superior end plate of T1 to the inferior end plate of T12; however, because the proximal thoracic segments are often poorly visualized on lateral radiographs, many studies use T4 or T5 as the upper measured vertebra. As determined by Bernhardt and Bridwell,[18] the segmental contribution of the upper thoracic vertebrae to overall thoracic kyphosis is approximately 1 to 3 degrees per level, allowing one to infer overall thoracic kyphosis without measuring the upper segments per se.

As one moves caudally down the spinal column to encounter the thoracolumbar junction, T10 to L2, a sagittal alignment and anatomic transition occurs as the structural support of the rib cage ceases. The more rigid thoracic spine transforms into the more flexible lumbar spine marked by larger vertebrae, lordotic disks, and sagittal facet orientation. Gelb et al[4] showed that the disk at L1-L2 is the first lordotic segment and that the thoracolumbar junction is therefore usually neutral or slightly kyphotic in normal healthy patients. When measured from the top of the L1 vertebral body to the superior sacral end plate, a smooth lordotic sagittal contour is noted in healthy subjects. According to Gelb et al, segmental measurements in the lumbar spine are as follows: L1-2, -4 ± 5 degrees; L2-3, -10 ± 5 degrees; L3-4, -14 ± 17 degrees; L4-5, $24^\circ \pm 7$ degrees; and L5-S1, $-24^\circ \pm 7$ degrees. Similar values were discovered by Bernhardt and Bridwell[18] in a study where they determined the mean lumbar lordosis as measured from T12-S1 to be 61 degrees.

Wambolt and Spencer[19] examined the roles of the lumbar vertebral bodies and disks and their relative contribution to overall lumbar lordosis. In a population with a mean lumbar lordosis of 59 degrees, these authors determined that 47 degrees of lordosis was contributed by the disks and only 12 degrees by the vertebral shape. Studies have demonstrated that the sagittal apex of lordosis in the lumbar spine is usually at L3, L4, or the intervening disk space. Of profound clinical importance, the segments L4-5 and L5-S1 together contribute over 60% of the overall lumbar lordosis. Given that this is the most common region of symptomatic degenerative spinal pathology and therefore surgical intervention, understanding this concept is critical to the preservation of sagittal balance.

■ Preserving Sagittal Alignment

Preservation of sagittal alignment during spinal surgery can be accomplished by proper patient positioning as well as sound surgical technique. From the standpoint of patient positioning, one should never perform a lumbar or lumbosacral fusion procedure with the patient placed on a kyphosing frame or in a knee-chest position. Prone positioning on a Jackson table (Orthopedic Systems, Inc., Union City, CA) with approximately 30 degrees of hip flexion and 70 to 90 degrees of knee flexion is ideal and routinely employed in our fusion cases. Using the Jackson table, the chest pad can be built up with towels to even further accentuate the natural lumbar lordosis.

With regard to the surgical technique used to preserve sagittal alignment, one must be particularly careful to avoid destabilizing the segment rostral to a fusion in any manner, particularly the lamina and facet joints. Failure to adhere to this principle, particularly in cases where a long fusion exists below a violated posterior tension band, can result in dramatic loss of sagittal alignment due to postoperative proximal junctional kyphosis. Strategies are ideally used to reconstitute collapsed disk spaces from degenerative disease. This can be performed from an anterior approach using lordotic threaded cages or custom-cut allograft wedges. Alternatively, segmental lordosis can be preserved and enhanced using interbody devices placed anterior in the disk space through a transforaminal posterior approach. Using this technique, we frequently perform a Smith-Petersen osteotomy at the level of surgery and compress across the interbody to close the osteotomy. We have found this strategy very valuable at preserving segmental lordosis in patients without an ankylosed anterior spinal column.

■ Restoring Sagittal Alignment

Principles of Sagittal Correction

Osteotomies are the primary tool in the surgical armamentarium by which the surgeon can introduce mobility into the spinal column and effectively restore sagittal balance. The three most commonly implemented osteotomies in deformity surgery are the Smith-Petersen osteotomy (SPO), pedicle subtraction osteotomy (PSO), and vertebral column resection (VCR). The choice of osteotomy is dependent on the goals of the procedure, the correction requirements, the native bone quality of the patient, and anatomic variations that may be present. Each of the osteotomy techniques has specific advantages as well as inherent limitations. They can be used individually or together in combination to achieve the desired correction.

In theory, the SPO offers up to 10 degrees of correction per level; however, 5 to 7 degrees per level is more commonly achieved. It can be performed at any level in the thoracolumbar spine and is best accomplished at a level where there is a disk that is not ankylosed. This is usually clearly visualized on a preoperative computed tomography (CT) scan. We also frequently order lateral scoliosis radiographs with the patient positioned supine over a bolster to get an idea prior to surgery about the sagittal curve flexibility. The taller the disk, the more effective the osteotomy because this technique requires posterior osteotomy closure and simultaneous anterior opening. If the disk is collapsed, placement of an interbody graft anterior in the disk space can restore disk space height and allow posterior closure. This is a strategy to maximize the angular restoration provided by a Smith-Petersen osteotomy. In doing this, it is important that the interbody graft not only restore disk height but also end at or anterior to the midvertebral body to allow it to act as a fulcrum for sagittal plane restoration by posterior closure. Large interbody spacers can block posterior closure and result in limited sagittal plane correction **(Fig. 6.3)**.

The PSO, a far more powerful technique that hinges on the anterior column and involves middle and posterior column shortening, can reliably achieve between 30 and 40 degrees of correction at a single segment. This technique removes a pedicle and its associated facets, creating a large combined foramen. A wedge is then removed from the vertebral body. Closure of this vertebral body osteotomy wedge results in a sagittal plane correction angle that matches the degrees of the osteotomy wedge closure. This technique is useful from T10 or T11 to L5. At the thoracolumbar junction, we often also remove the disk at the superior edge of the PSO and close the inferior end plate of the body above onto the osteotomy for added correction.

A, B

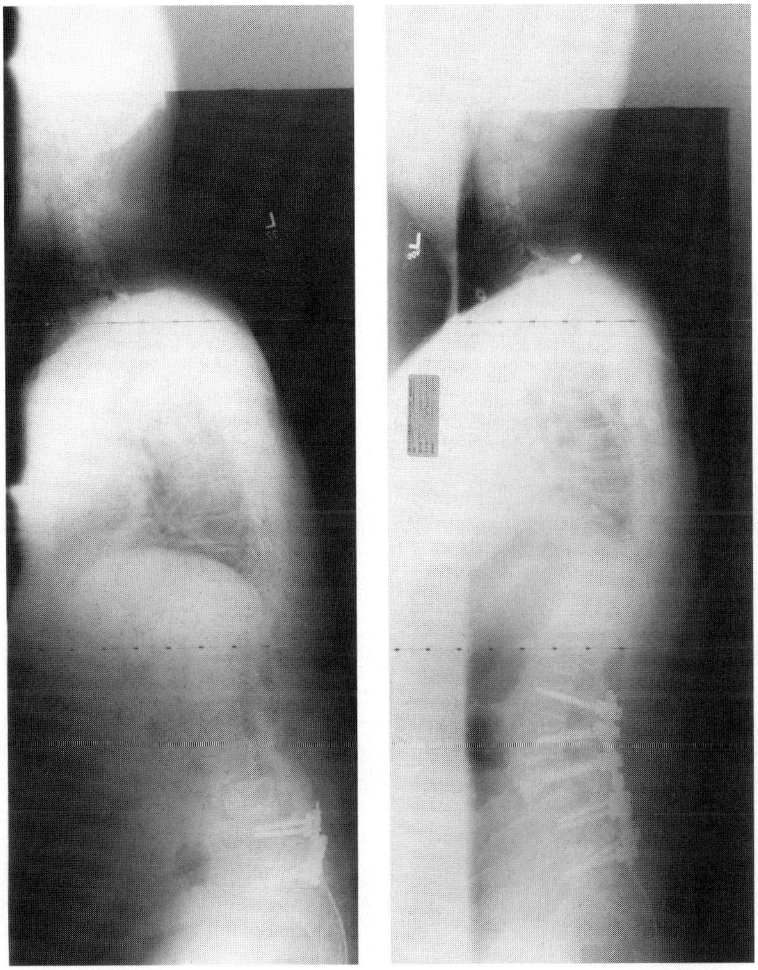

Fig. 6.3 (A) Patient with prior lumbar fusion from L4 to S1 now with degeneration above the fusion and positive sagittal imbalance, causing difficulty standing and walking due to sagittal imbalance as well as pain. **(B)** To achieve acceptable correction, anterior interbody devices were placed anteriorly in the disk space to allow disk height restoration and maximum correction with the Smith-Petersen osteotomy (SPO). This avoided the need for a pedicle subtraction osteotomy (PSO) and extension of the construct to the structural thoracic spine.

This is in part necessary due to the more narrow space available for vertebral body resection in this area **(Fig. 6.4).**

The VCR, an extension of the pedicle subtraction technique, typically yields a bit more correction than a standard PSO due to the distance and height of the anterior pivot, which places the correction arc point anterior to the vertebral body. This technique is best suited for the thoracic spine where PSO is less effective due to the more triangular shape of the thoracic bodies, which limit a bony pivot point, and the shorter nature of the thoracic bodies, which limits the extent of resection amount. We utilize this technique from T2 to L1. Below L1, we find PSO to be more practical.

The indications for each of these osteotomy techniques include a fixed segmental kyphosis or a globally positive sagittal imbalance. The SPO is best suited for a mobile anterior column, which is not always the case. A PSO, by contrast, does not have the same limitation because the bony resection is carried through into the anterior column. Although a PSO is commonly performed for fixed sagittal correction, it can also be used for coronal correction or combined sagittal–coronal correction. The PSO can also be utilized in a nonfixed deformity if one prefers a single osteotomy over multiple SPOs to achieve the desired correction. A VCR, the most powerful osteotomy technique, is particularly valuable in the setting of sharp, angular deformities.

The choice of osteotomy is based on the bone quality, patient needs, local anatomy, the pathology being treated, and the amount of correction needed. We have developed a method that allows rapid, easy, and precise mathematical calculation of the degrees of correction needed in any plane. Our method, which takes advantage of simple trigonometry, has had a high level of correlation among the calculated degrees, the bony resection based on these parameters, and the clinical result.[20,21] The distance from the planned osteotomy to C7 is measured. The distance from C7 to the S1 plumb line on a standing 36-inch film is then measured. This establishes a right triangle and a simple trigonometric calculation is performed: $(\text{Opposite}/\text{Adjacent})^{-1} = \text{Angle}$. In this case it is $(\text{C7-S1 Plumb Line Distance}/\text{Osteotomy to C7 Distance})^{-1} = \text{Angle Needed for Correction}$.

Once the degrees of needed correction are known, the surgeon can factor in the postural corrections based on sacropelvic parameters and ascertain the surgical correction needed. The surgeon can then make the decision regarding what single osteotomy or combination of

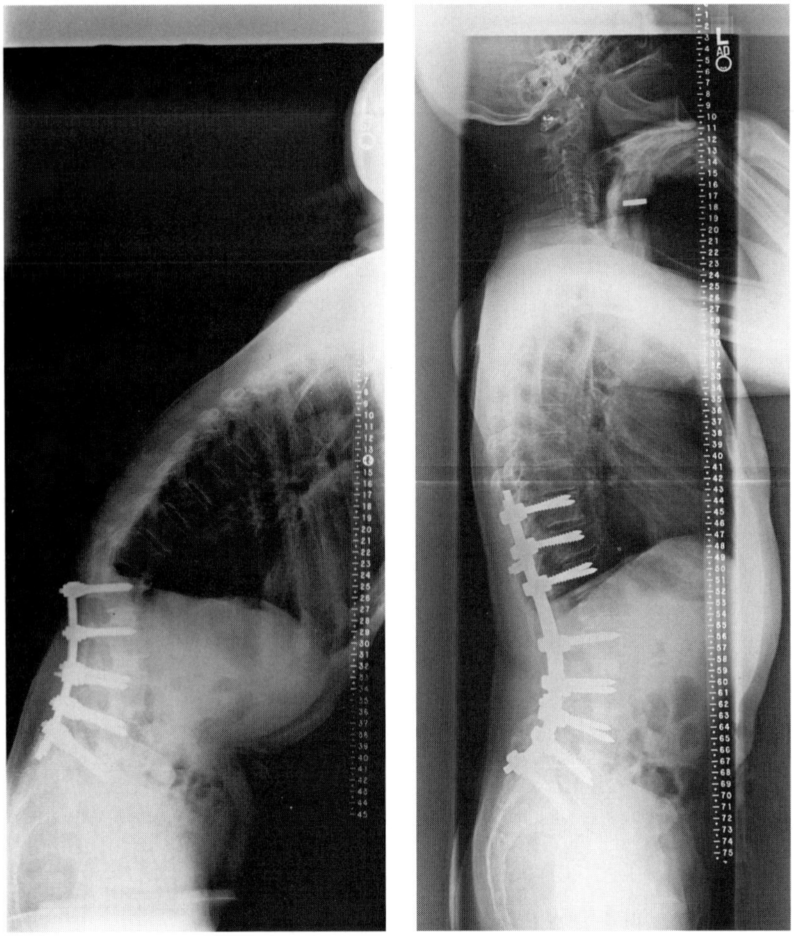

A, B

Fig. 6.4 (A) Preoperative lateral scoliosis film of an iatrogenic flat back and a proximal junction kyphosis. **(B)** Postoperative lateral scoliosis film demonstrates the restoration of sagittal balance with a pedicle subtraction osteotomy that removed the cephalad disk and placed a spacer to retain a closure pivot without collapse of the disk space and osteotomy. This allows the desired angular closure.

osteotomies is needed to accomplish the planned correction based on the expected correction with each type of osteotomy and the unique patient characteristics that may enhance or limit an osteotomy correction. For instance, if the surgeon knows that 45 degrees of correction are needed, it is unlikely to be achieved by three or four SPOs. More likely, a single PSO with one or two SPOs would be adequate. This type of calculation and information enables the surgeon to develop a comprehensive surgical plan that will realistically achieve the goals of correction.

Techniques

Smith-Petersen Osteotomy

The most important aspect of this osteotomy is removal of the superior facet. The osteotomy is begun by using an osteotome to resect the inferior facet of the cephalad vertebra the desired number of millimeters. A drill or rongeur is then utilized to create a chevron-like resection of the inferior and superior facet complex and the inferior edge of the superior lamina of the osteotomy level **(Fig. 6.5)**. The ligamentum flavum is then resected to expose the dura. Gelfoam is used to deal with epidural bleeding. Once all osteotomies are completed, the pedicle screws or other implants are placed into screw holes that have been previously prepped prior to the osteotomies. Closure of the osteotomy is achieved by compression, postural effects, table manipulation, cantilever correction, or some combination of these.

At times, to maximize the correction at a level and to improve fusion, an interbody device is placed in the anterior one third of the disk space. This increases the height of the disk and provides an anterior pivot. The axis of rotation moves forward to the pivot, increasing the correction angle of closure. It also has the advantage of providing graft in the anterior column for fusion. This can be done using a unilateral or bilateral TLIF technique as the facets are already resected by the osteotomy. It is important not to place an implant that does not taper or that covers a large part of the end plate because this has the potential to block the closure of the posterior disk space and, as a result, the osteotomy.

Pedicle Subtraction Osteotomy

After placing pedicle screws above and below the osteotomy level, the PSO begins with placement of a pedicle preparatory hole. With no implant in place, a prepped and tapped pedicle is very useful to maintain orientation while the bone removal is taking place. The bone removal of the posterior elements then begins. The removal should be centered at the pedicle that is to be removed. The amount of bone to be removed should be calculated to match the amount of closure needed. It should involve the superior and inferior facet of the osteotomy level and the inferior facet of the cephalad level and the superior facet of the level below. In the case of a prior posterior fusion mass, removal of the fusion mass is performed. This is done with osteotomes, rongeurs, and curettes to save all bone for later fusion. The osteotomy can be fine-tuned with a high-speed drill. It is helpful to undercut the posterior bone edge centrally in a "keystone" fashion. This decreases any dural impingement risk upon closure. Others surgeons cut a small hole in the bone overlying the dura at the level of closure.

The pedicle is then fully removed with a rongeur and a drill. Care should be taken to fully remove the pedicle base. Small spicules of bone can result in a radiculopathy once the osteotomy is closed. In revision cases, it is also important to remove all scar tissue from the dura to avoid soft tissue crowding once closure has been done. Once the pedicle has been removed, dissection of the lateral vertebral body wall is performed bilaterally. Penfield dissectors and elevators are used, with the dissection being carried out

A
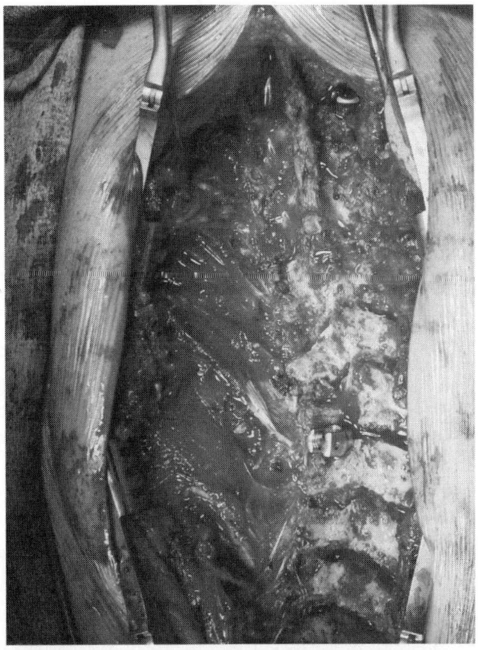

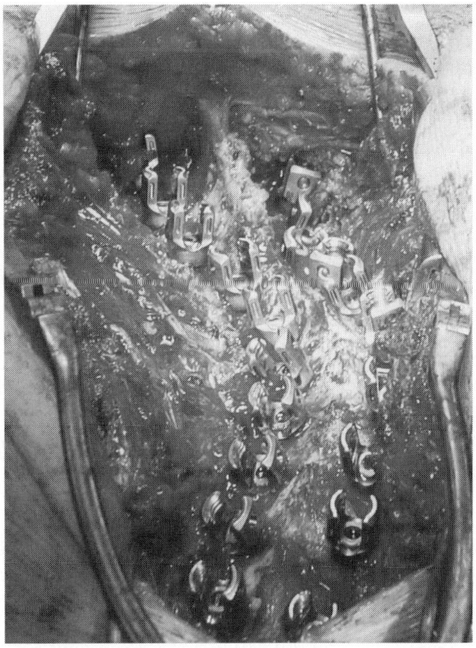
B

C
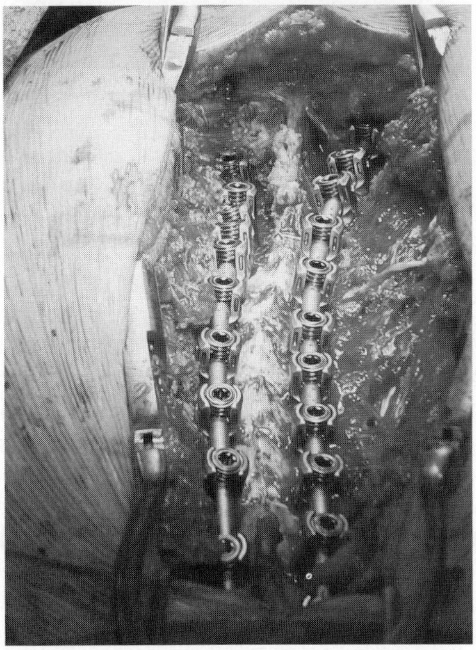

Fig. 6.5 Intraoperative photos of Smith-Petersen type osteotomies in a case of degenerative scoliosis. **(A)** Osteotomies cut. **(B)** Instrumentation in place. **(C)** Postcorrection (*Continued*).

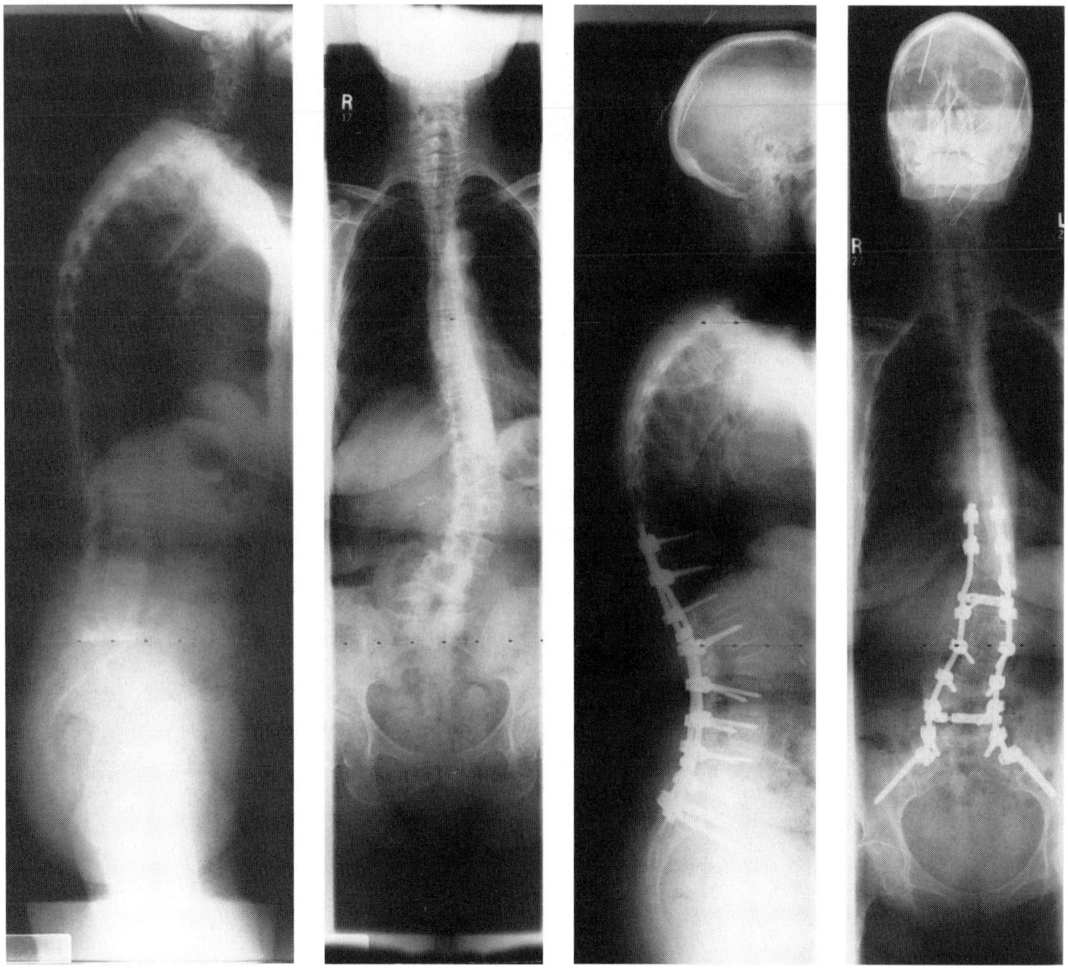

D–G

Fig. 6.5 (*Continued*) Pre- **(D,E)** and postoperative **(F,G)** X-rays of an adult degenerative scoliosis with junctional kyphosis and positive sagittal balance corrected with segmental instrumentation and lumbar PSO.

from the level of the disk that immediately lies above the removed pedicle moving caudally until the desired exposure is achieved. The body should be dissected all the way to the anterior vertebral body to get adequate exposure and resection. The segmental artery is swept caudally subperiosteally. This can typically be done without difficulty over two thirds of the vertebral body. If the vessel begins to bleed, bipolar cautery can be used. If this does not work, the area can be packed with hemostatic agents. Bleeding typically resolves with osteotomy closure. We have not had to extend our exposure or alter the procedure due to segmental bleeding. If bleeding is profuse and unable to be controlled by the above steps, it would be reasonable to consider performing a flank incision for control of the segmental at the aorta should all else fail.

The bone of the vertebral body is removed with rongeurs and a drill in a precise wedge shape, based on the calculated degrees of closure. The apex of the wedge is at the anterior vertebral body wall. This wall should be preserved as a pivot point. The base of the osteotomy is at the floor of the spinal canal. This is more easily done today with specialized vertebral body retractors to assist in exposure. The cancellous bone is then removed with curettes and rongeurs in a wedge-shaped fashion matching the cuts on the lateral walls. Again, all bone is saved for later grafting. Drills can be used for final shaping. The final bone resection is the posterior vertebral body wall, or the floor of the spinal canal. The lateral edge can be removed with rongeurs. The final removal is an impaction technique into the vertebral body cavity created by the resection. This can be done with curettes or with specialized impactors that facilitate the procedure **(Fig. 6.6)**.

It is important to place a temporary holding rod to maintain vertebral body orientation and prevent early collapse and closure of the osteotomy when the posterior wall is removed. This is occasionally necessary earlier in the procedure should the osteotomy begin to sag closed. With all bone resected and the canal and root exit zones inspected for any tissue that could impinge on neurologic structures, the osteotomy is closed. Typically, very little compressive pressure is needed on the screws above and below the osteotomy. The osteotomy is closed by gentle pressure on

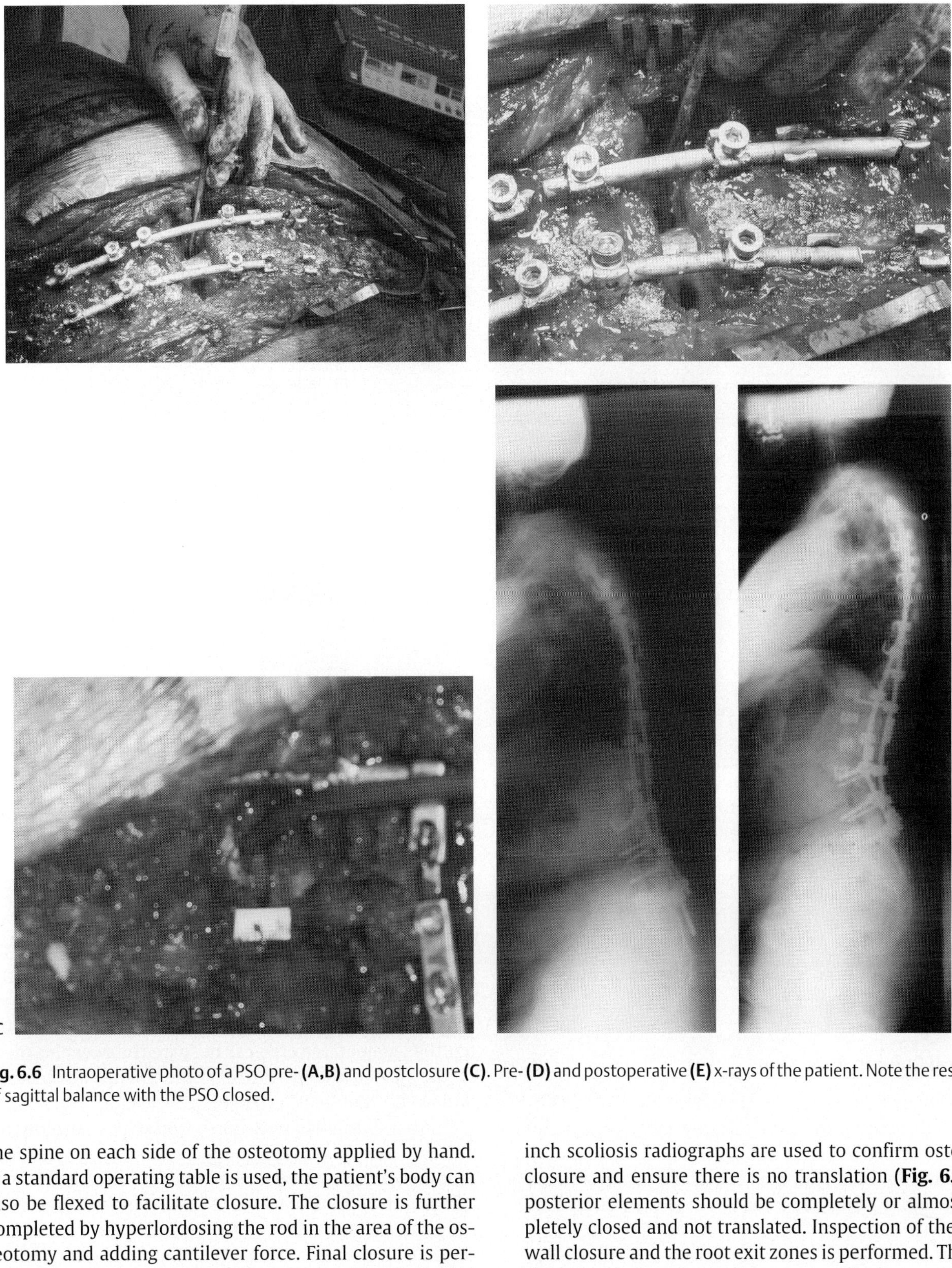

A B C D, E

Fig. 6.6 Intraoperative photo of a PSO pre- **(A,B)** and postclosure **(C)**. Pre- **(D)** and postoperative **(E)** x-rays of the patient. Note the restoration of sagittal balance with the PSO closed.

the spine on each side of the osteotomy applied by hand. If a standard operating table is used, the patient's body can also be flexed to facilitate closure. The closure is further completed by hyperlordosing the rod in the area of the osteotomy and adding cantilever force. Final closure is performed by gentle rod compression. If more force is needed and posterior elements are available, a compression hook combination can be put in the bone above and below the osteotomy. A third rod can be used for added compression. Once the final rod is in place, the third rod and hooks are generally removed. Anteroposterior and lateral 14- × 36-inch scoliosis radiographs are used to confirm osteotomy closure and ensure there is no translation **(Fig. 6.7).** The posterior elements should be completely or almost completely closed and not translated. Inspection of the lateral wall closure and the root exit zones is performed. The roots above and below the pedicle are now both contained in a combined single foramen. Attention should also be given to ensuring that there has been no translation or subluxation at the level of the osteotomy closure. If subluxation occurs, it is typical that the spine caudal to the osteotomy subluxes anteriorly relative to the spine cephalad to the

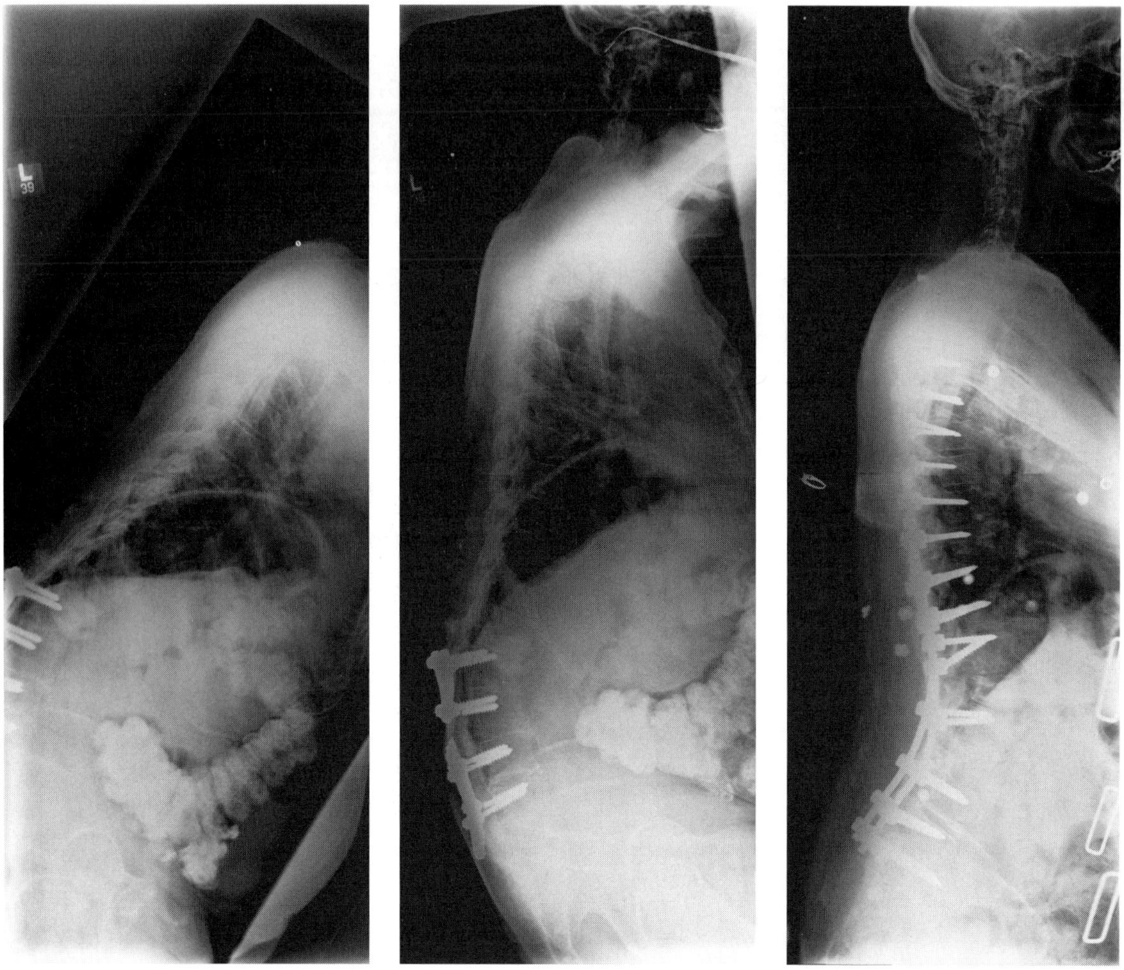
A-C

Fig. 6.7 **(A)** X-ray of a patient with an iatrogenic fixed lumbar kyphosis and a profound positive sagittal balance of 23 cm. **(B)** Note the posterior rotation of the pelvis and retroversion of the sacrum in an attempt to compensate for the imbalance. **(C)** Postoperatively, both sagittal balance and normalized sacral-pelvic orientation are restored with two pedicle subtraction osteotomies achieving almost 70 degrees of correction in the sagittal plane.

closure. When this occurs, the closure should be manipulated to restore alignment.

Vertebral Column Resection

This technique is an extension of the PSO. The distinct difference is that the entire vertebral body and both adjacent disks are resected. As with a PSO, all implants are placed via a midline incision with the exception of the osteotomy levels. Access is gained, and dissection of the ribs that articulate with the disks above and below the osteotomy level is then performed; 2 to 3 cm of the rib should be removed from both sides of the vertebra to be resected to enhance closure of the osteotomy. This is typically done for the ribs intersecting the disk spaces cephalad and caudal to the body that is to be resected. This helps provide access for resection and exposure of the lateral disk, which facilitates arthrodesis of the end plates as well as closure. A lateral extracavitary dissection is then performed to the anterior vertebral body. It may be necessary to coagulate one or both segmentals at the level of resection. More often, the segmental arteries can be spared by sweeping them off the bone in a subperiosteal fashion. With the rib heads removed, attention is turned to the vertebral resection.

The bony vertebral resection begins with a posterior removal of the lamina or fusion mass and the pedicles. This is done with a rongeur, saving bone for fusion and a drill. Often, both of the thoracic roots at the cephalad end of the resection site are sacrificed by tying them off proximal to the ganglia with 2-0 silk ties and then transecting them. This facilitates access to the vertebral body. In many cases, the nerves can be spared. Vertebral body wall retractors from the PSO set can then be inserted to facilitate vertebral body resection. The vertebral body is then fully resected to include the disks above and below the body. Temporary holding rods are important early in this procedure due to

A, B

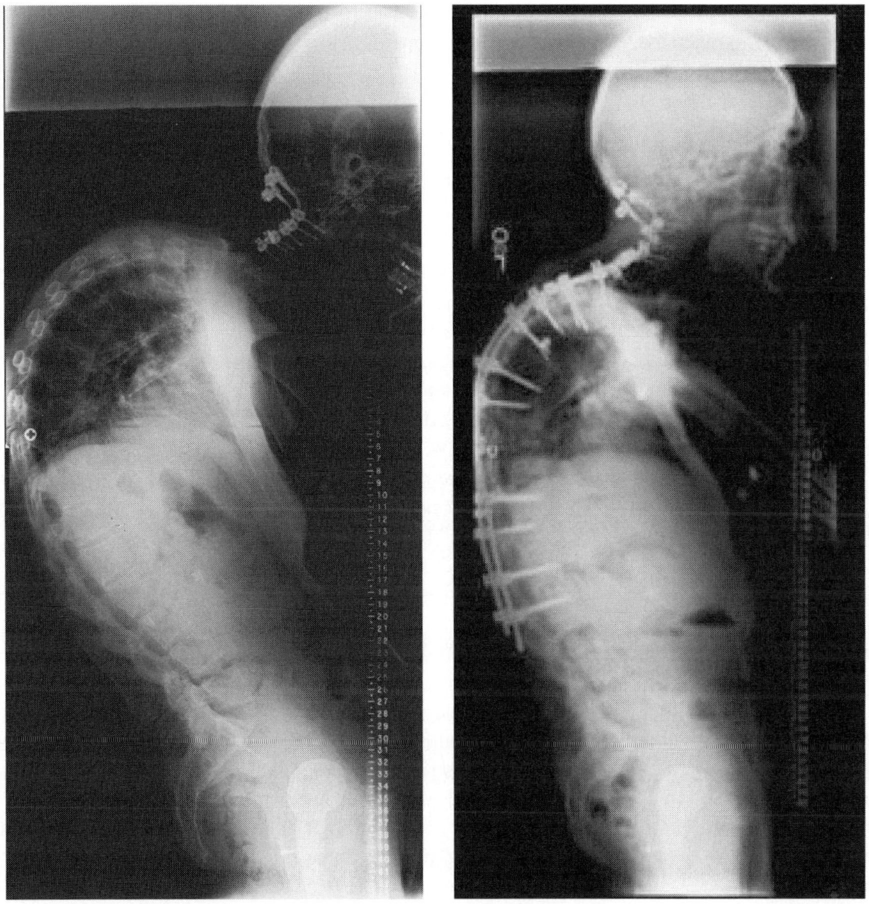

Fig. 6.8 **(A)** X-ray of a patient with ankylosing spondylitis who previously underwent an occipital cervical fusion. He presented with severe upper thoracic kyphosis and the inability to lift his head. Ambulation was limited by his positive sagittal balance. **(B)** Scoliosis x-ray of the patient after undergoing a T4 VCR and a T8 PSO to achieve the desired correction.

the complete instability created by a total vertebra removal. This reduces the risk of subluxation or translation.

The vertebral body resection is begun by using a specialized osteotome to resect the lateral one third of the vertebral body above and below the disks that are caudal and cephalad to the body that is being resected. Curettes are used to resect the cancellous bone, and rongeurs and drills are used to remove the cortical bony shell completely. The end plates of the disks above and below the resected vertebra are removed. A No. 15 blade scalpel is used to resect the lateral annulus at the remaining end plate and the posterior lateral aspect of the disk. Curettes and pituitary rongeurs are used to remove the disks completely. The end plates of the vertebral bodies above and below the resection are arthrodesed with curettes, rasps, and drills. The posterior vertebral body wall is then carefully removed with PSO impactors. Care must be taken to completely remove all bone and disk material.

Closure is more complex due to the complete instability of the spine. We prefer to perform a construct-to-construct closure through a domino connector. In this technique, temporary rods are placed through two or three screws above the osteotomy and a second rod is placed similarly below the osteotomy. Both rods pass through a domino connector at the site of the closure. Once this is secured, the temporary holding rod on the opposite side is removed and replaced with a similar construct. Closure is then begun with compressors closing the two constructs through the domino. If the closure is an end-plate to end-plate closure, it is done until bony approximation occurs. More commonly, an anterior cage is placed as a pivot point after partial closure. This cage should be an anterior pivot only and it should cover a minimal amount of the end plate to allow continued sagittal correction and closure of the posterior aspects of the vertebral bodies. After the closing vertebral bodies engage the cage, a gradual posterior closure is performed while pivoting on the cage. When the desired correction is obtained, permanent rods are placed and final arthrodesis is performed. The spine is always secured with at least one rod (**Fig. 6.8**).

Conclusion

The last decade has witnessed dramatic improvement in both the understanding and treatment of sagittal plane deformity. We have reviewed several studies that have clarified normative values for sagittal plane geometry as well as the role of the pelvis as we understand it today. In the treatment of lumbar degenerative disease with a fusion procedure, proper patient positioning and adherence to a thoughtful surgical plan are critical in the preservation of sagittal balance. In the event that restoration of sagittal alignment is required, it is best accomplished by the use of osteotomies, the techniques for which have been described.

References

1. Glassman SD, Bridwell KH, Dimar JR. The impact of positive sagittal balance in adult spinal deformity. Spine 2005;30:2024–2029
2. Jackson RP, McManus AC. Radiographic analysis of sagittal plane alignment and balance in standing volunteers and patients with low back pain matched for age, sex, and size. A prospective controlled clinical study. Spine 1994;19:1611–1618
3. Vedantam R, Lenke LG, Keeney JA, et al. Comparison of standing sagittal spinal alignment in asymptomatic adolescents and adults. Spine 1998;23:211–215
4. Gelb DE, Lenke LG, Bridwell KH, et al. An analysis of sagittal spinal alignment in 100 asymptomatic middle and older aged volunteers. Spine 1995;20:1351–1358
5. Hardacker JW, Shuford RF, Capicotto PN, et al. Radiographic standing cervical segmental alignment in adult volunteers without neck symptoms. Spine 1997;22:1472–1480
6. Koski TR, Salehi SA, Ondra SL. Analysis of cranio-cervical sagittal balance and their relationship to the remainder of the spinal column. Presentation No. 88, 12th Annual International Meeting on Advanced Spinal Techniques, 2005
7. Farcy JP, Schwab FJ. Management of flatback and related kyphotic decompensation syndromes. Spine 1997;22:2452–2457
8. Schwab F, Lafage V, Boyce R, et al. Gravity line analysis in adult volunteers: age-related correlation with spinal parameters, pelvic parameters, and foot position. Spine 2006;31:E959–E967
9. Dubousset J. Pelvic obliquity correction in lumbosacral and spinopelvic fixation. In: Marguiles JY, Floman Y, Farcy JP, eds. Lumbosacral and Spinopelvic Fixation. Philidelphia: Lippincott-Raven, 1996:40
10. Kuntz C, Levin LS, Ondra SL, et al. Neutral upright sagittal spinal alignment from the occiput to the pelvis in asymptomatic adults: a review and resynthesis of the literature. J Neurosurg Spine 2007;6:104–112
11. Hilibrand AS, Tannenbaum DA, Graziano DP, et al. The sagittal alignment of the cervical spine in adolescent idiopathic scoliosis. J Pediatr Orthop 1995;15:627–632
12. Labelle H, Roussouly P, Berthonnaud E, et al. The importance of spino-pelvic balance in L5–S1 developmental spondylolisthesis: a review of pertinent radiologic measurements. Spine 2005;30:S27–S34
13. Berthonnaud E, Dimnet J, Roussouly P, et al. Analysis of the sagittal balance of the spine and pelvis using shape and orientation parameters. J Spinal Disord Tech 2005;18:40–47
14. Labelle H, Roussouly P, Berthonnaud E, et al. Spondylolisthesis, pelvic incidence, and spinopelvic balance: a correlation study. Spine 2004;29:2049–2054
15. Duval-Beaupere G, Marty C, Barthel F, et al. Sagittal profile of the spine prominent part of the pelvis. Stud Health Technol Inform 2002;88:47–64
16. Jackson RP, Peterson MD, McManus AC. Compensatory spinopelvic balance over the hip axis and better reliability in measuring lordosis to the pelvic radius on standing lateral radiographs of adult volunteers and patients. Spine 1998;23:1750–1767
17. Jackson RP, Kanemura T, Kawakami N, et al. Lumbopelvic lordosis and pelvic balance on repeated standing lateral radiographs of adult volunteers and untreated patients with constant low back pain. Spine 2000;25:575–586
18. Bernhardt M, Bridwell KH. Segmental analysis of the sagittal plane alignment of the normal thoracic and lumbar spines and thoracolumbar junction. Spine 1989;14:717–721
19. Wambolt A, Spencer DL. A segmental analysis of the distribution of lumbar lordosis in the normal spine. Orthop Trans 1987;11:92–93
20. Yang BP, Ondra SL. A Method for calculating the exact angle required during pedicle subtraction osteotomy for fixed sagittal deformity: comparison with the trigonometric method. Neurosurgery 2006;59(suppl 2):ONS458–ONS463
21. Yang BP, Ondra SL, Chen LA, et al. Clinical and radiographic outcomes of thoracic and lumbar pedicle subtraction osteotomy for fixed sagittal imbalance. J Neurosurg Spine 2006;5:9–17

7 Patient Selection: Who and How Do We Fuse?

Jason M. Highsmith and Gerald Rodts Jr.

Lumbar fusion for trauma, infection, and tumors is a relatively accepted practice. However, indications for fusion of the degenerative lumbar spine are more controversial.

Low back pain (LBP) is well known to be one of the most significant causes of disability in the United States. Unfortunately, no specific diagnosis can be made in 80 to 90% of patients with LBP.[1,2] Furthermore, with several studies questioning the benefit of fusion,[3] the surgical treatment of LBP has come under significant scrutiny. In fact, cognitive intervention and exercises proved equally efficacious as lumbar fusion in a series from Norway.[4,5] Although later studies questioned the findings,[6] Fritzell et al[7] concluded that lumbar fusion in a well-informed and selected group of patients with severe LBP can diminish pain and decrease disability more efficiently than commonly used nonsurgical treatment in their 2001 Volvo Award paper.

Proper patient selection remains the greatest barrier to favorable outcome data for the surgical treatment of LBP. Improper patient selection can yield unfavorable results despite a technically splendid procedure. Traditionally, outcome data from spine fusions have focused on neurologic recovery and fusion rates. Now, lifestyle outcomes, as measured by the Oswestry Low Back Pain Questionnaire and the Short Form–36 (SF-36), are critical indicators of patient satisfaction, and ultimately the success and efficacy of surgery.

Unfortunately, as clinicians we have failed to construct prospective, randomized studies in our assessment of LBP. This lack of solid data confuses patients, confounds our medical colleagues, and threatens proper reimbursement by third carriers and government agencies. With increasing pressure from pay for performance medicine, proper patient selection remains paramount in the surgical treatment of LBP.

The indications for fusion in lumbar degenerative disk disease (DDD) are quite varied. Many surgeons simply use fusion as the last step in a treatment algorithm. Other surgeons choose to operate aggressively in a situation where nonfusion surgeries such as laminectomy or diskectomy may be indicated. One study attempted to establish an outlined classification scheme for surgical indications and found significant variability in surgeon responses. The study concluded that surgical indications were only moderately agreed upon among the responders.[8]

History

Understanding the pain generators of the spine is essential to directing the patient interview. Important components of the history include the chronicity and distribution of pain as well as modifying factors. Spinal sources of pain in the low back are typically described as discogenic, radicular, or facet-based.

Typically the pain from an annular tear is worse with activity and relieved by rest. These patients cannot tolerate prolonged sitting. Their pain is a deep midline ache that extends into the gluteal region and occasionally into the posterior thighs, but seldom past the knee. Discogenic pain is often worse when the patients flex their trunk, as when ascending a staircase. Sitting is also a painful position. Discogenic pain can often result from direct sensitization of the annular nerve fibers.

Discogenic pain can precede more typical radicular pain, especially in light of a disk herniation. These patients develop LBP as a result of dorsal root ganglion (DRG) and spinal root irritation, which often resolve before the classic radiculopathy that follows. Many of these patients report improvement in their LBP before the onset of leg pain. Radicular pain may be exacerbated by Valsalva maneuvers. Some theorize that the internal pressure on the annular pain fibers decreases with the herniation.[9] The extreme case of radicular LBP is that associated with cauda equina syndrome. The onset is rapid and the presentation is alarming. These patients typically have a mixture of bowel/bladder symptoms, saddle anesthesia, leg pain, and weakness.

Facet-based back pain is also related to activity, but typically is worse in extension as when descending a staircase. It is also exacerbated by twisting. Important factors to consider in the history are which activities of daily living elicit the pain.

Before attributing back pain to any of these degenerative conditions, other diagnoses should be excluded. This is especially true for younger patients in whom the degenerative process may play less of a role. Pain from infection is typically not relieved with rest and is not activity dependent. Infectious pain can arise from diskitis, vertebral osteomyelitis, and epidural abscesses. Although infection more often occurs in the patients who are diabetic or immunosuppressed, osteomyelitis or diskitis can arise in patients with no known risk factors. Recent urinary tract infection, hemodialysis, dental work, or a history of intravenous (IV) drug abuse should also raise suspicion. Recent spine surgery is a warning sign for postoperative diskitis, which typically presents with worse or subacute postoperative back pain.

Recent weight loss should raise a red flag for a metastatic process and warrants further workup. Often these patients present with pathologic fractures and the acute onset of pain from the highly innervated periosteum. Typically patients with LBP from degenerative changes report weight gain, from pain and lack of activity. Other characteristics of patients with primary or metastatic spine tumors include pain unrelieved by bed rest, failure to improve with conservative therapy, and age greater than 50 years.[10]

Traumatic fractures are another known source of acute back pain. Younger patients should be questioned about a history of trauma, a recent motor vehicle accident, or a fall. In the elderly, even a ground-level fall may cause significant fractures, especially in the osteoporotic patient. Heavy lifting and coughing have also been implicated. Chronic steroid use is a known risk factor for traumatic vertebral body fractures.

A patient's past medical history should be addressed as well. Medical conditions to note include osteoarthritis, rheumatoid arthritis, peripheral vascular disease, and peripheral neuropathy. Patients with ankylosing spondylitis typically exhibit improvement with exercise, whereas symptoms in the morning and at rest are the worst.[11] The use of statins to treat hypercholesterolemia can also induce myalgias of the lumbar spine. Other medical sources of LBP include ankylosing spondylitis (with erosion of the sacroiliac [SI] joint and positive human leukocyte antigen [HLA] B27) and Paget disease.

Past surgical history should focus not only on spinal surgeries but also on orthopedic surgeries related to the hip and knees. Prior surgeries and their associated recuperation yield important information about patients' tolerance of surgery in general. It also may reveal their pain threshold.

Although elderly patients have significantly poorer osteoblast proliferation, that does not always correlate with decreased rates of fusion.[12] Some scoliosis series showed significantly worse fusion with increasing age.[13] Other studies have demonstrated that elderly patients can tolerate the procedure quite well.[14]

Patients' social history can reveal warning signs such as alcohol and substance abuse. Their use of long-term narcotics and prior narcotic history are equally important factors. Preoperative tobacco consumption had no discernible effect on osteoblast proliferation, and no correlation between smoking and fusion was found in one series of patients.[12] However, smoking alone has been shown to have a significant adverse impact on both employment and pain outcomes despite high fusion rates, particularly in patients under the age of 55 years.[15] Conversely, Silcox et al[16] and others have clearly demonstrated a negative effect of smoking on the success of arthrodesis. Multiple failed attempts at smoking cessation and weight loss are problematic. Family support can help the physician assess the likelihood of treatment plan compliance. The surgeon should evaluate the patient's work status and expectations regarding the surgery. In many cases, the goal may be a return to functionality rather than achieving a completely asymptomatic state. In such cases, shared expectations between the physician and the patient are vital.[17]

Patients often report their pain using a pain diagram. One study looked at whether the pain drawing was an accurate predictor of the outcome for patients with LBP.[18] The concept of organic/nonorganic pain in conjunction with chronic low-back pain is not supported by the results of the study.

The quantification of pain through scales such as the Visual Analogue Pain Scale is difficult to assess. Objective criteria for the measure of pain are elusive. However, assessment of disability is more reliable. A patient's work status and the activities that they can tolerate are valuable indicators. In our opinion, it is better to evaluate patients based on the pleasurable and leisure activity they can tolerate rather than on their occupational roles.

■ Prior Surgery

Failed back surgery syndrome (FBSS) is a condition in which patients fail to improve after previous back surgery and are left with intractable pain. Its incidence has been estimated at 5 to 10% of spinal surgeries.[19] The major causes of FBSS are fibrosis and adhesions, spinal instability, recurrent herniated disk, and inadequate decompression.[19] Repeated operation should be performed only if an obvious abnormality is found.[20] Although some authors report a successful revision outcome in 92% of patients with FBSS,[19] others conclude "salvage" surgery is not recommended.[21]

A panel symposium at North American Spine Society (NASS) in 2002 concluded that a diagnosis can be reached in over 90% of patients with FBSS. This claim was based on a careful history, examination, imaging studies, psychological evaluation, and diagnostic injections (**Table 7.1**).[22]

Pseudarthrosis can be a costly and disabling complication of lumbar spinal fusion.[23] Although its incidence is reported to be only 14% in failed back surgery, the outcome from repair of pseudarthrosis is the most difficult to predict.[24]

If the decision is made to reoperate, it is important to have clearly defined pathology and clear expectations from the patient. The prognosis for a revision surgery can be predicted best by the patient's outcome after the primary surgery.[25] The single most important factor in achieving a successful clinical outcome in revision spine surgery is patient selection.[24]

Table 7.1 Specific Diagnoses Resulting in Failed Back Surgery Syndrome[59]

Foraminal stenosis	25–29%
Painful disk	20–22%
Pseudarthrosis	14%
Neuropathic pain	10%
Recurrent disk herniation	7–12%
Facet joint pain	3%
Sacroiliac joint pain	2%

Physical Exam

The physical exam is also important to delineate the cause of LBP. Patients' general stamina can be assessed throughout the exam from the initial encounter. For example, whether they rise from the seated position or not provides important information.

A patient's vital signs can direct the diagnosis as well. An elevated body temperature may be a warning sign of central fever, diskitis, or osteomyelitis. Acute pain may present with tachycardia, although chronic patients may have subdued this response.

Obesity is a significant risk factor. Logistic regression revealed that the probability of a significant complication was related to the body mass index (BMI) ($p <.04$); the chance of a significant complication was 14% with a BMI of 25, 20% with a BMI of 30, and 36% with a BMI of 40 in a series of obese patients.[26] Positioning-related palsies were only found in extremely obese patients (BMI $\geq$40).

Although many surgeons choose not to operate on obese patients, one study found no significant difference between obese and control patients in terms of functional outcome, blood loss, operative time, hospital stay, and rate of complications.[27] These authors went on to say that with proper indications, surgery should not be withheld from obese patients. Regardless, certainly the benefit of weight loss in terms of reducing back pain, facilitating the surgical procedure, and expediting recovery cannot be overlooked.

Manual palpation of the spine and paravertebral musculature is an important early step in the exam. Although spine tenderness has an 86% sensitivity in bacterial infections, the specificity is only 60%.[10] Splaying or palpable step-off of the spinous processes should be noted. Palpation of the facets, sacroiliac joint, ischial tuberosity, and trochanteric bursa as well as the sciatic nerve itself should be performed. Palpation of the buttocks and thigh may reveal underlying soft tissue tumor or enlarged pyriformis.

Also, the surgeon should evaluate the range of motion of the spine, preferably with the patient in a standing position. Pain with extension typically occurs in patients with facet arthropathy or spondylolisthesis. A careful orthopedic examination of the hips and knees can localize pathology. Examination of the extremities can reveal signs of peripheral vascular disease such as hair loss, diminished capillary refill, and pulses. A motor and sensory exam can reveal radicular signs, such as focal weakness or sensory loss, which point to selective nerve root involvement.

Finally, the physical exam should include assessment of gait. A waddling gait may reveal weakness in hip abduction as seen in L5 involvement. Heel walking can reveal dorsiflexion weakness in the tibialis anterior (L4). Likewise toe walking can reveal weakness in the gastrocnemius (S1).

Imaging

More than ever, surgeons are armed with an arsenal of diagnostic imaging options. In addition to evaluating disk height and spondylosis, plain film imaging is important in evaluating coronal and sagittal balance, which is vitally important in achieving optimal results with deformity surgery.[28] Flexion-extension plain films can be used to rule out instability and likewise to determine whether arthrodesis has already occurred. Although the parameters of instability remain a subject of debate, many authors consider the criteria 4 to 5 mm of translation and 15 degrees of relative angulation.[29]

Although not routinely obtained for the evaluation of LBP, computed tomography (CT) of the lumbar spine provide additional details. It can evaluate the paraspinous tissue for tumor or abscess. Likewise it can provide additional bony detail such as fractures or pars defects. CT is also invaluable in determining the presence of a successful posterolateral or interbody arthrodesis.[30]

Although the presence of a dark disk has been a focus of much debate, some suggest that the specifics of the diagnosis be refined. Chataigner et al[31] suggest that the common "black disk" phenomenon be carefully differentiated from Modic type I changes. The latter are endplate changes (decreased signal on T-1–weighted images and increased signal on T-2–weighted images) seen with disk narrowing and anterior condensation of the vertebral plates on magnetic resonance imaging (MRI). They suggest that these patients respond better to anterior fusion because that is the location of the pathology. Modic type II cases indicate use of the posterior approach as well, because the risk of pseudofusion is increased by fatty degenerative involution.

Magnetic resonance imaging can also reveal other sources of back pain, although caution should be used in interpretation as many asymptomatic patients show pathology. In a series of 98 asymptomatic patients, only a third had normal disks at all levels.[32] The nucleus pulposus has been implicated as a toxic inflammatory agent of the lumbar epidural space.[33] However, annular tears have been described in 40% of asymptomatic patients in their 50s and

75% of asymptomatic patients in their 60s.[34] MRI can also reveal the presence of a Schmorl node, or intravertebral herniation of a disk. Up to 19% of asymptomatic patients have this finding, however.[32]

Although it has grown out of favor in light of less invasive testing, myelography is still a valuable tool. It is particularly beneficial to diagnose positional stenosis in high-degree blocks.

Diskography is another invasive technique that has been met with mixed feelings. It is an exquisitely sensitive but not specific diagnostic test for the diagnosis of discogenic LBP. The restriction of the definition of a positive diskographic study to one that elicits concordant pain from a morphologically abnormal disk improves the definition's accuracy. Only 36% of patients with LBP have a provocative diskogram.[35] Equally problematic is that significantly painful injections were as common in patients with annular disruption as those with abnormal psychometric testing. In this study 83% of patients with somatization disorder had painful injections.[36] Fusion surgery based on diskography alone, however, is not reliably associated with clinical success.[37] The positive predictive value of diskography has been calculated at 50 to 60%.[38]

Diskography is best limited to the evaluation of abnormal interspaces identified on MRI, the investigation of adjacent-level disk disease, and as a means to rule out cases of nonorganic pain from surgical consideration.[37]

Assessment

Once a history has been obtained and a patient has been examined, it is important to assess the patient's overall health status. Psychological distress deteriorates the subjective outcome of lumbosacral spine fusion.[39] Furthermore, psychological screening should be included in the global assessment of patients for whom surgery is considered.[39]

Psychological distress had a profound effect on patient's disability score and on their satisfaction ratings.[21] Medical and psychological risk levels were significantly related to outcome, with the poorest results obtained by patients having both high psychological and medical risk. A battery of psychological screening tests were performed and found to predict overall outcome by 82%.[40]

Waddell et al[41] suggested that three of five screening parameters suggest psychological distress **(Table 7.2)**. Although some authors[42] have criticized the validity of the later two, a more recent study reconfirmed these findings.[8]

After assessing patients' overall health status, their social history in terms of secondary gain should be scrutinized. Compensation status was a significant prognostic factor in the surgical treatment of LBP.[21] Compensation claims have been shown to negatively impact return-to-work rates and pain, even in light of solid bony fusion, particularly in young to middle-aged patients.[15] Successful outcome appears to be limited in the subset of patients receiving workers' compensation and those chronically disabled.[44] Many surgeons consider this phenomenon a financial disincentive to heal.

Table 7.2 The Signs of Psychological Distress[67]

- Pain on simulated axial loading (pressing on top of head)
- Inconsistent performance (difficulty tolerating straight leg raising [SLR] while supine, but no difficulty sitting)
- Overreaction during the physical exam
- Inappropriate tenderness that is superficial or widespread
- Motor or sensory abnormalities not corresponding to anatomic confines

Regression analyses have shown that tobacco use, depression, and litigation were the most consistent presurgical predictors of poor patient outcome.[45] The factors that significantly increased the likelihood of an optimal result—defined as patient satisfaction, return to work, and reduced medication—were male gender, being employed prior to surgery, and being a nonsmoker.[46]

In a case series of 45 patients undergoing redo decompression and uninstrumented fusion for failed back surgery, the authors found several negative predictive factors. Those factors that were found to correlate with a poor result were workers' compensation cases, less than 6 months' pain free interval from the previous operation, male sex, history of psychiatric illness, and predominant diagnosis of perineural fibrosis.[47]

Treatment Plan

Subacute LBP typically lasts >6 weeks and <3 months. Pain lasting >3 months is considered chronic and is typically the basis for referral from primary care. As patient-directed imaging and referrals increase, it is important for the surgeon to diligently pursue nonoperative management first. As such, many surgeons advocate at least 4 to 6 weeks of conservative treatment under their own care.

Noninterventional measures are typically exhausted first in the treatment algorithm. Although initial studies[48] suggested limited bed rest (<4 days), more recent studies, even those by the same author,[49] suggest minimal if any best rest. As part of conservative care, patient exercise should be encouraged. For the first 2 weeks, walking, swimming, or another minimal stress exercise is typically encouraged. When the pain worsens, studies have shown it is better to slowly increase the duration rather than stopping entirely.[50] Other activity modifications should be addressed as well. For example, patients should reduce prolonged sitting, heavy lifting, and repetitive bending, lifting, and twisting. A host of other noninvasive treatments are available that are beyond the scope of this chapter, such as physical therapy, transcutaneous electrical nerve

Table 7.3 The Ideal Surgical Candidate for Lumbar Fusion Treatment of Degenerative Disk Disease (DDD)

• Age 30 to 50, with significant LBP with or without leg symptoms
• Does not use nicotine
• Symptoms interfere significantly with lifestyle
• Failed a minimum of 6 months of aggressive conservative treatment
• Imaging studies reveal one or two adjacent levels of DDD (usually L4-L5 and L5-S1) with remaining disk spaces healthy and no significant osteoporosis
• Minimal psychosocial pathology

stimulation (TENS) units, nonsteroidal antiinflammatory drugs (NSAIDs), oral steroids, and cognitive therapy. Temporary bracing improved patient selection and was concluded to be a valid prognostic instrument in a case series from Sweden.[51] Substantial pain relief from a pantaloon cast test in chronic LBP patients without prior spine surgery suggested a favorable outcome of lumbar fusion compared with conservative management in another series.[52] When these methods fail, a more aggressive approach is warranted.

Invasive treatments include facet blocks and epidural steroid injections. Injections can be both therapeutic and diagnostic. They also provide a means to evaluate patient tolerance of surgical pain and patient compliance. In a retrospective review of 126 patients with facet blocks, the authors concluded that lumbar facet joint injections cannot be used to determine appropriate patient treatment because they are not predictive of either surgical of nonsurgical success.[53] Although facet injections can predict the response to radiofrequency ablation, they are not recommended as a diagnostic tool to predict response to fusion.[54]

Intradiskal electrothermy (IDET) has been met with mixed results. Provider self-referral and narcotic use before IDET are significant risk factors for poor outcomes.[55] Randomized controlled trials are needed to determine whether there is a subset of patients with discogenic back pain who derive substantial and sustained benefit from this procedure.

Synthesis of all factors in the patient's history and exam is essential before committing a patient to surgery. The key factors are listed in **Table 7.3**.

■ Decision for Surgery

Once the decision for surgery has been made, several surgical options must be considered before fusion. In many cases, a lumbar decompression may be all that is needed. In a series of 119 patients with lumbar stenosis over a 7-year period, no patient went on to need fusion.[56] Other nonfusion alternatives include interspinous process decompression, nucleoplasty, and disk or facet. Finally, alternative surgical techniques should be investigated. Some patients, especially those with metastatic disease, may benefit from intrathecal pump implantation. Epidural spinal cord stimulator may help those with nerve root injury or pain from arachnoiditis.

Once fusion has been selected, there are several other decisions to be made. The surgeon must consider the availability of local bone and the need to harvest autologous hip graft. In patients with multiple surgeries or those with thin paraspinous tissue, protrusion of hardware may be a concern. Likewise, pseudomeningocele and arachnoiditis should be approached with caution.

In patients with existing hardware, it is helpful to know the manufacturer. If adjacent level disease is involved, it is helpful to know whether the existing hardware can be extended or whether explantation needs to be performed. In patients who have new hardware placed, it is important to evaluate the size of the pedicles for upsizing of the screws.

The patient's overall health status as assessed above should be evaluated. Recent infections such as a urinary tract infection (UTI), diabetic foot ulcers, or venous stasis ulcers may warrant delay of surgery. Patients on antiplatelet agents or anticoagulants need a medication-free interval. Cytotoxic medications such as methotrexate and chemotherapy may very well impede bone healing. Patients with a history of deep venous thrombosis (DVT) may be treated preoperatively with subcutaneous heparin. Women who are pregnant may wish to postpone surgery given the risks of anesthesia and the use of intraoperative fluoroscopy.

A patient's body habitus can limit the extent of surgical treatment available. The anatomy of an obese or very muscular patient may preclude the use of sacral fixation from a midline approach. In this case percutaneous screws may be an option.

The number of affected levels to cover with fusion remains an area of great debate. We are seeing high rates of adjacent segment disease in a phenomenon that can be attributed to the natural progression of the disease or the supraphysiologic forces induced by long rigid construct. One study that used a strict protocol of provocative diskography and completion of a preoperative conditioning program found no difference in the clinical outcome of patients undergoing short-segment (one or two levels) and long-segment (three to five levels) fusions.[57] The Joint Spine Section of the Congress of Neurological Surgeons and the American Association of Neurological Surgeons limits their recommendation to patients with one or two levels of DDD.[58]

The use of cages in lumbar surgery has become a treatment option aimed at restoring disk height, although these efforts may not be warranted.[59] While disk space height was increased and better maintained in posterior lumbar interbody fusion (PLIF) patients, no differences in clinical and functional outcomes were noted. The authors conclude that disk space height did not seem to impact clinical outcome in lumbar fusion.

Many surgeons advocate the use of cages to improve fusion rates and clinical outcomes. Posterior fusion with cages (BAK®) was shown to have significantly lower operative time; blood loss, hospitalization time, and total costs were significantly different. There was a quicker return to work and closure of workers' compensation claims for the posterior lumbar interbody fusion–BAK group compared with those undergoing 360-degree fusion.[60] Anotherx study showed that circumferential fusion improves outcomes.[61] Poor patient selection and technical difficulties with implantation were blamed for most reported cage failures.[62] Other authors report worse outcomes with interbody fusion despite better correction and fusion rates.[63]

In a large review of the literature for the treatment of low-grade spondylolisthesis, the authors could not identify the best surgical technique (posterior lumbar function [PLF], PLIF, anterior lumbar interbody fusion [ALIF], instrumentation) to perform the fusion.[64] In a prospective study comparing ALIF and PLIF, the authors found no significant difference in radiographic or clinical outcomes.[65] The Joint Spine Section Guidelines do not recommend the use of multiple approaches (anterior and posterior) to accomplish lumbar fusion in patients with LBP without deformity.[66]

A 5-year review of the surgical treatment of spinal instability concluded that pedicle screw fixation was a safe and effective procedure with minimal complications. The proper selection of patients for surgery is probably the most important factor associated with good outcomes.[67] The use of unilateral[68] or bilateral[69] pedicle screws has been reported to be effective in conjunction with minimally invasive TLIF.

■ Conclusion

As the treatment and implant options expand at a rate greater than the body of supporting literature, it is important to establish strict criteria for fusion. The proper selection of patients should remain the paramount factor guiding our practices.

The Cochrane Reviews from 2000 concluded that there was no scientific evidence to support surgical decompression or fusion for degenerative lumbar spondylosis compared with natural history, placebo, or conservative treatment.[70] While the 2005 Cochrane Review was somewhat more optimistic, concluding that limited evidence is now available to support some aspects of surgical practice,[71] clearly a more solid body of evidence is needed.

References

1. Bigos SJ, Davis GE. Scientific application of sports medicine principles for acute low back problems. The Agency for Health Care Policy and Research Low Back Guideline Panel (AHCPR, Guideline #14). J Orthop Sports Phys Ther 1996;24:192–207
2. Turner JA, Ersek M, Herron L, et al. Patient outcomes after lumbar spinal fusions. JAMA 1992;268:907–911
3. Frymoyer JW. Back pain and sciatica. N Engl J Med 1988;318:291–300
4. Brox JI, Reikeras O, Nygaard O, et al. Lumbar instrumented fusion compared with cognitive intervention and exercises in patients with chronic back pain after previous surgery for disc herniation: a prospective randomized controlled study. Pain 2006;122:145–155
5. Brox JI, Sorensen R, Friis A, et al. Randomized clinical trial of lumbar instrumented fusion and cognitive intervention and exercises in patients with chronic low back pain and disc degeneration. Spine 2003;28:1913–1921
6. Kwon B, Katz JN, Kim DH, et al. A review of the 2001 Volvo Award winner in clinical studies: lumbar fusion versus nonsurgical treatment for chronic low back pain: a multicenter randomized controlled trial from the Swedish lumbar spine study group. Spine 2006;31:245–249
7. Fritzell P, Hagg O, Wessberg P, et al. 2001 Volvo Award Winner in Clinical Studies: Lumbar fusion versus nonsurgical treatment for chronic low back pain: a multicenter randomized controlled trial from the Swedish Lumbar Spine Study Group. Spine 2001;26:2521–2532
8. Glassman SD, Carreon LY, Dimar JR, et al. Lumbar degenerative classification study. Am J Orthop 2006;35:175–179
9. Yonemura KS, Yuan HA. The black disc. In: Benzel EC, ed. Spine Surgery—Techniques, Complication Avoidance, and Management, vol 1, 2nd ed. Philadelphia: Elsevier, 2005:626–631
10. Deyo RA, Rainville J, Kent DL. What can the history and physical examination tell us about low back pain? JAMA 1992;268:760–765
11. Calin A, Porta J, Fries JF, et al. Clinical history as a screening test for ankylosing spondylitis. JAMA 1977;237:2613–2614
12. Christensen FB, Lind M, Eiskjaer SP, et al. Can autologous bone culture predict spinal fusion capacity? Eur Spine J 1999;8:54–60
13. Goldstein JM, Nash CL, Wilham MR. Selection of lumbar fusion levels in adult idiopathic scoliosis patients. Spine 1991;16:1150–1154
14. Vitaz TW, Raque GH, Shields CB, et al. Surgical treatment of lumbar spinal stenosis in patients older than 75 years of age. J Neurosurg 1999;91:181–185
15. Schnee CL, Freese A, Ansell LV. Outcome analysis for adults with spondylolisthesis treated with posterolateral fusion and transpedicular screw fixation. J Neurosurg 1997;86:56–63
16. Silcox DH, Daftari T, Boden SD, et al. The effect of nicotine on spinal fusion. Spine 1995;20:1549–1553
17. Bambakidis NC, Feiz-Erfan I, Klopfenstein JD, et al. Indications for surgical fusion of the cervical and lumbar motion segment. Spine 2005;30:S2–S6
18. Hagg O, Fritzell P, Hedlund R, et al. Pain-drawing does not predict the outcome of fusion surgery for chronic low-back pain: a report from the Swedish Lumbar Spine Study. Eur Spine J 2003;12:2–11

19. Skaf G, Bouclaous C, Alaraj A, et al. Clinical outcome of surgical treatment of failed back surgery syndrome. Surg Neurol 2005;64:483–488
20. North RB, Campbell JN, James CS, et al. Failed back surgery syndrome: 5-year follow-up in 102 patients undergoing repeated operation. Neurosurgery 1991;28:685–690
21. Greenough CG, Peterson MD, Hadlow S, et al. Instrumented posterolateral lumbar fusion. Results and comparison with anterior interbody fusion. Spine 1998;23:479–486
22. Schofferman J, Reynolds J, Herzog R, et al. Failed back surgery: etiology and diagnostic evaluation. Spine J 2003;3:400–403
23. Larsen JM, Capen DA. Pseudarthrosis of the Lumbar Spine. J Am Acad Orthop Surg 1997;5:153–162
24. Etminan M, Girardi FP, Khan SN, et al. Revision strategies for lumbar pseudarthrosis. Orthop Clin North Am 2002;33:381–392
25. Eichholz KM, Ryken TC. Complications of revision spinal surgery. Neurosurg Focus 2003;15:E1
26. Patel N, Bagan B, Vadera S, et al. Obesity and spine surgery: relation to perioperative complications. J Neurosurg Spine 2007;6:291–297
27. Andreshak TG, An HS, Hall J, et al. Lumbar spine surgery in the obese patient. J Spinal Disord 1997;10:376–379
28. Kuklo TR. Principles for selecting fusion levels in adult spinal deformity with particular attention to lumbar curves and double major curves. Spine 2006;31:S132–S138
29. Spratt KF, Weinstein JN, Lehmann TR, et al. Efficacy of flexion and extension treatments incorporating braces for low-back pain patients with retrodisplacement, spondylolisthesis, or normal sagittal translation. Spine 1993;18:1839–1849
30. Burkus JK, Foley K, Haid RW, et al. Surgical Interbody Research Group–radiographic assessment of interbody fusion devices: fusion criteria for anterior lumbar interbody surgery. Neurosurg Focus 2001;10:E11
31. Chataigner H, Onimus M, Polette A. [Surgery for degenerative lumbar disc disease. Should the black disc be grafted?] Rev Chir Orthop Reparatrice Appar Mot 1998;84:583–589
32. Jensen MC, Brant-Zawadzki MN, Obuchowski N, et al. Magnetic resonance imaging of the lumbar spine in people without back pain. N Engl J Med 1994;331:69–73
33. McCarron RF, Wimpee MW, Hudkins PG, et al. The inflammatory effect of nucleus pulposus. A possible element in the pathogenesis of low-back pain. Spine 1987;12:760–764
34. Hirsch C, Schajowicz F. Studies on structural changes in the lumbar annulus fibrosus. Acta Orthop Scand 1953;22:184–231
35. Carragee EJ, Alamin TF, Miller J, et al. Provocative discography in volunteer subjects with mild persistent low back pain. Spine J 2002;2:25–34
36. Carragee EJ, Tanner CM, Khurana S, et al. The rates of false-positive lumbar discography in select patients without low back symptoms. Spine 2000;25:1373–1380
37. Resnick DK, Choudhri TF, Dailey AT, et al. Guidelines for the performance of fusion procedures for degenerative disease of the lumbar spine. Part 6: magnetic resonance imaging and discography for patient selection for lumbar fusion. J Neurosurg Spine 2005;2:662–669
38. Carragee EJ, Lincoln T, Parmar VS, et al. A gold standard evaluation of the "discogenic pain" diagnosis as determined by provocative discography. Spine 2006;31:2115–2123
39. Van Susante J, Van de Schaaf D, Pavlov P. Psychological distress deteriorates the subjective outcome of lumbosacral fusion. A prospective study. Acta Orthop Belg 1998;64:371–377
40. Block AR, Ohnmeiss DD, Guyer RD, et al. The use of presurgical psychological screening to predict the outcome of spine surgery. Spine J 2001;1:274–282
41. Waddell G, McCulloch JA, Kummel E, et al. Nonorganic physical signs in low-back pain. Spine 1980;5:117–125
42. McCombe PF, Fairbank JC, Cockersole BC, et al. 1989 Volvo Award in clinical sciences. Reproducibility of physical signs in low-back pain. Spine 1989;14:908–918
43. Blom A, Taylor A, Whitehouse S, et al. A new sign of inappropriate lower back pain. Ann R Coll Surg Engl 2002;84:342–343
44. Parker LM, Murrell SE, Boden SD, et al. The outcome of posterolateral fusion in highly selected patients with discogenic low back pain. Spine 1996;21:1909–1916
45. LaCaille RA, DeBerard MS, Masters KS, et al. Presurgical biopsychosocial factors predict multidimensional patient: outcomes of interbody cage lumbar fusion. Spine J 2005;5:71–78
46. Gehrchen PM, Dahl B, Katonis P, et al. No difference in clinical outcome after posterolateral lumbar fusion between patients with isthmic spondylolisthesis and those with degenerative disc disease using pedicle screw instrumentation: a comparative study of 112 patients with 4 years of follow-up. Eur Spine J 2002;11:423–427
47. Biondi J, Greenberg BJ. Redecompression and fusion in failed back syndrome patients. J Spinal Disord 1990;3:362–369
48. Deyo RA, Diehl AK, Rosenthal M. How many days of bed rest for acute low back pain? A randomized clinical trial. N Engl J Med 1986;315:1064–1070
49. Atlas SJ, Deyo RA. Evaluating and managing acute low back pain in the primary care setting. J Gen Intern Med 2001;16:120–131
50. Lindstrom I, Ohlund C, Eek C, et al. The effect of graded activity on patients with subacute low back pain: a randomized prospective clinical study with an operant-conditioning behavioral approach. Phys Ther 1992;72:279–290
51. Axelsson P, Johnsson R, Stromqvist B, et al. Temporary external pedicular fixation versus definitive bony fusion: a prospective comparative study on pain relief and function. Eur Spine J 2003;12:41–47
52. Willems PC, Elmans L, Anderson PG, et al. The value of a pantaloon cast test in surgical decision making for chronic low back pain patients: a systematic review of the literature supplemented with a prospective cohort study. Eur Spine J 2006;15:1487–1494
53. Esses SI, Moro JK. The value of facet joint blocks in patient selection for lumbar fusion. Spine 1993;18:185–190
54. Resnick DK, Choudhri TF, Dailey AT, et al. Guidelines for the performance of fusion procedures for degenerative disease of the lumbar spine. Part 13: injection therapies, low-back pain, and lumbar fusion. J Neurosurg Spine 2005;2:707–715
55. Webster BS, Verma S, Pransky GS. Outcomes of workers' compensation claimants with low back pain undergoing intradiscal electrothermal therapy. Spine 2004;29:435–441
56. Tuite GF, Stern JD, Doran SE, et al. Outcome after laminectomy for lumbar spinal stenosis. Part I: Clinical correlations. J Neurosurg 1994;81:699–706
57. Lettice JJ, Kula TA, Derby R, et al. Does the number of levels affect lumbar fusion outcome? Spine 2005;30:675–681
58. Resnick DK, Choudhri TF, Dailey AT, et al. Guidelines for the performance of fusion procedures for degenerative disease of the lumbar spine. Part 7: intractable low-back pain without stenosis or spondylolisthesis. J Neurosurg Spine 2005;2:670–672
59. Lidar Z, Beaumont A, Lifshutz J, et al. Clinical and radiological relationship between posterior lumbar interbody fusion and posterolateral lumbar fusion. Surg Neurol 2005;64:303–308

60. Hacker RJ. Comparison of interbody fusion approaches for disabling low back pain. Spine 1997;22:660–665
61. Rousseau MA, Lazennec JY, Bass EC, et al. Predictors of outcomes after posterior decompression and fusion in degenerative spondylolisthesis. Eur Spine J 2005;14:55–60
62. Zdeblick TA, Phillips FM. Interbody cage devices. Spine 2003;28: S2–S7
63. Madan S, Boeree NR. Outcome of posterior lumbar interbody fusion versus posterolateral fusion for spondylolytic spondylolisthesis. Spine 2002;27:1536–1542
64. Jacobs WC, Vreeling A, De Kleuver M. Fusion for low-grade adult isthmic spondylolisthesis: a systematic review of the literature. Eur Spine J 2006;15:391–402
65. Madan SS, Boeree NR. Comparison of instrumented anterior interbody fusion with instrumented circumferential lumbar fusion. Eur Spine J 2003;12:567–575
66. Resnick DK, Choudhri TF, Dailey AT, et al. Guidelines for the performance of fusion procedures for degenerative disease of the lumbar spine. Part II: interbody techniques for lumbar fusion. J Neurosurg Spine 2005;2:692–699
67. Masferrer R, Gomez CH, Karahalios DG, et al. Efficacy of pedicle screw fixation in the treatment of spinal instability and failed back surgery: a 5-year review. J Neurosurg 1998;89:371–377
68. Deutsch H, Musacchio MJ. Minimally invasive transforaminal lumbar interbody fusion with unilateral pedicle screw fixation. Neurosurg Focus 2006;20:E10
69. Ozgur BM, Hughes SA, Baird LC, et al. Minimally disruptive decompression and transforaminal lumbar interbody fusion. Spine J 2006;6:27–33
70. Gibson JN, Waddell G, Grant IC. Surgery for degenerative lumbar spondylosis. Cochrane Database Syst Rev 2000;3:CD001352
71. Gibson JN, Waddell G. Surgery for degenerative lumbar spondylosis. Cochrane Database Syst Rev 2000;2:CD001352

8 Facet-Mediated versus Discogenic Pain: Differences in Presentation and Treatment

Jason M. Highsmith and Gerald Rodts Jr.

Understanding spinal anatomy is essential to understanding potential sources of pain. Pain is the result of mechanical or chemical irritation of nociceptive fibers in the bone, cartilage, and ligamentous capsules. Some cases of low back pain can be attributed to the complex interaction of these structures at articulating surfaces. Although the disk space is traditionally considered more complex, the paired facet joints posteriorly should not be underestimated.

Accurate diagnosis of pain generators in the spine is vital to achieving a good surgical outcome. Although a solid bony fusion can reduce motion at both the disk space and the facet joints, it is important that therapies target the specific source of pain. Many surgeons choose interbody fusion as an adjunct to conventional onlay or intertransverse process fusion, particularly in patients with a suspected discogenic source of their low back pain. Likewise, posterior decompression with medical facetectomies (with associated denervation of the facet) has been directed at patients suffering from facet-based pain. An accurate understanding of these competing modalities is increasingly important as disk and facet arthroplasty options grow.

Anatomy and Pathology

Because the nucleus of the lumbar disk is avascular with no innervation, discogenic pain more accurately reflects pain originating from the annulus and end plates. Discogenic pain typically results from stimulation of nociceptors in the cartilaginous end plates, the outer anulus fibrosus as well as the periosteum of the vertebral bodies.[1] An extensive network of small nerve fibers and free endings has been demonstrated in the superficial annulus and surrounding longitudinal ligaments.[2] Annular tears, although causing pain of their own, can lead to pathologic loading of the disk space and resultant inflammation of the end plates. The chemical irritation caused by the release of prostaglandins and interleukins in the area of a disk herniation can heighten localized back pain in addition to causing radiculopathy.

The facets are sliding joints lined with synovial membrane. They do not have intervening cartilage. Inflammation in bone-on-bone contact or the surrounding cartilaginous capsule is considered the etiology of facet-based pain. Severe trauma can cause rupturing of the facet joint, but more typically chronic inflammatory changes lead to excessive bone growth with hypertrophy of the surrounding joint and impending autoarthrosis of the joint. Studies show an extensive distribution of small nerve fiber in the joint as well as nerve containing substance P.[2] High-threshold mechanoreceptors have also been visualized.[2] Physiologic studies have shown sensitization and excitation of these nerves as well as those in the surrounding muscle when exposed to inflammatory and nociceptive stimuli.

In reality, it is difficult to compartmentalize a patient's back pain into either discogenic or facet-based entirely. Pathology frequently involves both areas, which is one significant limitation of arthroplasty as a treatment option. In their review of 100 consecutive patients who proceeded to fusion, Wong et al[3] found that all patients had at least one contraindication to total disk arthroplasty. Facet arthrosis was a common complicating factor in patients with degenerative disk disease (DDD). Not surprisingly, the authors concluded that the average fusion patient does not have isolated discogenic pain.

A large population of patients with presenting low back pain was evaluated using medial branch block, provocative diskography, and sacroiliac (SI) injections.[4] The authors diagnosed facet joint pain in 40%, discogenic pain in 26%, and SI joint pain in 2%, with the remaining patients having no specific diagnosis. Another review of the literature[5] found disk disruption to be the source of low back pain in 40%, facet pain in 10 to 15%, and SI pain in 15 to 20%. This study stated that the prevalence of facet joint pain among patients with low back pain seems to be between 15% and 40%. However, only 7% of patients have pure facet pain.[5]

Presentation

Discogenic pain is characterized by chronic low back pain that radiates into the hip and buttocks diffusely. It is exacerbated by activities that increase intradiskal pressure such as sitting, bending forward, coughing, and sneezing.

Intolerance of prolonged sitting is a common hallmark. Exercises that load the axial spine such as jogging and running may increase pain. These patients often report pain when ascending stairs because they flex their spine and load the disk space. Discogenic low back pain may or may not be associated with a radiculopathy as the degenerated disk often causes neurologic compression from herniated fragments or narrowing of the foramen.

Pain that is generated by the facets is often more positional in nature and has a less insidious course. Patients often get relief with certain positions and find maneuvers to decrease their symptoms. Posture alone is an important factor in exacerbating or relieving this pain. Understandably, these patients often find their pain worse with extension, which loads the facets. Descending a staircase is often painful for these patients, as they hyperextend their back to maintain an upright posture. Twisting and lateral bending can shift pain as the ipsilateral facet is loaded and the contralateral is unloaded. Facet is exacerbated with extension and rotation to symptomatic side.

Diagnosis

The physical exam provides valuable insight into the differentiation of discogenic versus facet-based pain. Simple standing and ambulation can often demonstrate postural tendencies to overcome pain.

Although traditionally described in the evaluation of pregnancy-induced back pain, several tests of SI disease can be applied to the patient with low back pain. A symptomatic SI joint may elicit pain in a supine patient whose pelvis is manually pressed apart (ventral gaping test) or pressed together (dorsal gaping test).[6] The SI joint fixation test can also be applied. This test is based on the premise that the symptomatic SI joint remains fixed and consequently elevated when the patient moves from the standing to the forward flexed position.

Patrick test (also called FAbERE test: flexion, abduction, external rotation, and extension) is another test for hip arthritis or SI joint disease. The patient flexes one hip with abduction and external rotation of the joint while maintaining extension of the contralateral hip. When the examiner loads the knee of the ipsilateral hip and reproduces back pain, the test is considered positive. Although these tests may provide some additional diagnostic information, an extensive review of the literature could not find sufficient specificity in the physical exam to diagnose SI disease.[7]

Imaging

Plain film imaging can provide some direction as to the differentiation of discogenic versus facet-mediated back pain. Lateral x-rays often demonstrate significant osteophyte formation at the disk space, suggesting chronic changes. Anteroposterior (AP) and oblique views are more helpful in evaluating the facets for hypertrophy and spondylosis. Flexion-extension plain films may show focal kyphosis around the disk space in patients with severe DDD or gross splaying of the posterior elements in those with facet arthropathy. Computed tomography (CT) imaging can demonstrate similar findings as well as end-plate changes in the disk space. However, imaging studies alone cannot predict which patients will respond to controlled diagnostic blocks of the facet joint.[7]

Magnetic resonance imaging (MRI) has provided exceptional detail of the disk space and surrounding soft tissues. MRI can demonstrate annular tears, disk integrity and hydration, as well as inflammation in the surrounding bony end plates and vertebral bodies. However, as mentioned in Chapter 7, the "dark disk" phenomenon does not truly reflect an epidemic of DDD. Reliance on MRI findings alone is not sufficient to make the diagnosis. A recent study showed that up to 30% of healthy young adults with no back pain had disk degeneration on their MRI scans.

Diskography is considered by many to be the gold standard for diagnosing discogenic low back pain. Patients with grade 4 or 5 disk degeneration and presence of a high-intensity zone on MRI typically have concordant pain on provocative diskography.[8]

When diskography is combined with CT imaging, there are several advantages. First, the initial injection in the disk space and resultant pressure readings can yield critical information about disk compliance. Second, axial, sagittal, and coronal imaging of the disk during and after the procedure reflects disk integrity. Third, the presence of negative controls on either side of the affected level can localize the lesion to a specific level, thus simplifying the picture. Fourth, the administration of local anesthesia through the diskography needle can confirm a pathologic diagnosis. Finally, the ability to have a blinded examiner administer the test reduces bias by the surgeon. Tolerance of the procedure can also provide prognostic information as to how well a patient would tolerate surgical intervention. Typical CT diskography findings with concordant pain were fissured/ruptured disks and contrast extending into/beyond the outer annulus on CT.[8] The specificity and sensitivity of diskography are high for the diagnosis of disc degeneration.[7] However, the diagnosis of discogenic pain has been more elusive.

An extensive review of the literature on diskography[9] found technique to be a confounding factor, particularly with regard to the specificity of the test. Although false-positive rates have been quoted as high as 36%,[10] even when performed with low-pressure technique, more recent studies have suggested the rate to be less than 10%.[11] Although specificity is still debated, there is strong evidence for the sensitivity of lumbar diskography in the diagnosis of DDD.

Treatment

Although many interventional therapies exist, there is no "gold standard" with which to compare the results of interventional tests.[7] Epidural steroid injections can provide relief of radicular pain and pain from stenosis, but DDD and facet arthropathy do not typically respond.

Based on an extensive review of the literature, a medial branch block was found to be the most effective means to perform facet joint blocks.[7] However, the specificity of this modality is only 65%.[7] Also patients with previous lumbar surgery tend to have a higher false-positive rate than those who had not undergone previous surgery.[12]

Although several treatments have yielded conflicting results,[7] the evidence in favor of diagnostic facet joint blocks for the diagnosis of facet joint pain was considered strong in both the cervical and lumbar spine.[13,14] Interventional therapies are gaining credibility in the diagnosis and treatment of facet and discogenic back pain.

Conclusion

Facet and discogenic pain vary markedly in their presentation, diagnosis, and treatment. As new imaging modalities arise and clinical accuracy improves, we will continue to improve the foundation on which our therapeutic decisions are based.

References

1. Mayer HM. [Discogenic low back pain and degenerative lumbar spinal stenosis - how appropriate is surgical treatment?] Schmerz 2001;15:484–491
2. Cavanaugh JM, Ozaktay AC, Yamashita T, et al. Mechanisms of low back pain: a neurophysiologic and neuroanatomic study. Clin Orthop Relat Res 1997;166–180
3. Wong DA, Annesser B, Birney T, et al. Incidence of contraindications to total disc arthroplasty: a retrospective review of 100 consecutive fusion patients with a specific analysis of facet arthrosis. Spine J 2007;7:5–11
4. Manchikanti L, Singh V, Pampati V, et al. Evaluation of the relative contributions of various structures in chronic low back pain. Pain Physician 2001;4:308–316
5. Hildebrandt J. [Relevance of nerve blocks in treating and diagnosing low back pain–is the quality decisive?] Schmerz 2001;15:474–483
6. Colliton J. Managing back pain during pregnancy. Medscape Womens Health 1997;2:2
7. Saal JS. General principles of diagnostic testing as related to painful lumbar spine disorders: a critical appraisal of current diagnostic techniques. Spine 2002;27:2538–2545
8. Lim CH, Jee WH, Son BC, et al. Discogenic lumbar pain: association with MR imaging and CT discography. Eur J Radiol 2005;54:431–437
9. Resnick DK, Malone DG, Ryken TC. Guidelines for the use of discography for the diagnosis of painful degenerative lumbar disc disease. Neurosurg Focus 2002;13:E12
10. Carragee EJ, Alamin TF, Carragee JM. Low-pressure positive discography in subjects asymptomatic of significant low back pain illness. Spine 2006;31:505–509
11. Derby R, Lee SH, Kim BJ, et al. Pressure-controlled lumbar discography in volunteers without low back symptoms. Pain Med 2005;6:213–221
12. Cohen SP, Larkin TM, Chang AS, et al. The causes of false-positive medial branch (facet joint) blocks in soldiers and retirees. Mil Med 2004;169:781–786
13. Boswell MV, Trescot AM, Datta S, et al. Interventional techniques: evidence-based practice guidelines in the management of chronic spinal pain. Pain Physician 2007;10:7–111
14. Manchikanti L, Staats PS, Singh V, et al. Evidence-based practice guidelines for interventional techniques in the management of chronic spinal pain. Pain Physician 2003;6:3–81

9 Posterolateral Fusion with or without Pedicle Screws for Low Back Pain

Sharad Rajpal and Gregory R. Trost

Low back pain (LBP) is one of the most common reasons for chronic disability in adults and early retirement in Western societies.[1] Approximately 70 to 85% of adults experience at least one episode of LBP, whereas 15 to 20% of adult males suffer from disabling back conditions.[2,3] Spinal fusion (SF) has traditionally played a vital role in stabilization and healing of certain spinal conditions, including scoliotic deformities, infections, and traumatic spinal fractures. Although the volume of SF procedures has increased dramatically over the past two decades, the indications for SF in degenerative spinal diseases (DSDs) remains unclear and, at times, controversial. Among SF techniques, posterolateral fusion (PLF) with or without pedicle screw instrumentation is still used widely by spine surgeons.[4–6]

Historical Background

Early therapeutic indications for SF were primarily for managing spinal instability secondary to infections and pathologic or scoliotic deformities. Albee[7] performed the first posterior spinal fusion for the treatment of Pott disease in 1911, in which he implanted an interspinous tibial graft to provide internal fixation and promote spinal stabilization. In 1917, Hibbs[8] reported the role of SF in the prevention of progressive deformity in degenerative scoliosis. The role of SF quickly expanded to include the treatment of developmental deformities and spinal trauma. In 1929, Hibbs and Swift[9] popularized the concept of SF in the treatment of DSD for a series of degenerative spine conditions. Mixter and Barr[10] in 1934 and Howorth[11] in 1943 advocated SF for the treatment of ruptured lumbar disks. In the midst of the fusion era, Watkins[12] introduced the *posterolateral fusion technique* in 1953, which involved the fusion of the facet joints, pars interarticularis, and base of the transverse processes (TPs). Wiltse and Hutchinson[13] later modified this technique to include the lamina into the fusion bed.

The use of instrumentation to augment bony fusion dates back to 1891, when Hadra described the first interspinous wiring technique using silver wire.[5,6] In 1909 Lange reported achieving spinal stability using rigid steel celluloid rods affixed to either side of the spinous processes with silk thread and steel wires.[14] Early instrumentation hardware, however, was limited to interspinous wiring and sublaminar wiring and was mainly used to treat symptomatic scoliosis. Improvements in surgical techniques and instrumentation continued over the ensuing decades. Luque introduced the use of multiple sublaminar wires, and Cotrel and Dubousset used laminar hooks to achieve spinal stability. Introduction of the pedicle screw by Roy-Camille and Magerl marked a breakthrough in the field of complex spine surgery. Roy-Camille et al[15] popularized the semirigid screw and plate system, whereas Steffee et al[16] championed the rigid pedicle screw and plate interface model. Increasing interest in interbody fusion sparked the development of carbon-fiber interbody cages by Brantigan and Steffee[17] and titanium metal alloy cages by Bagby and Kuslich.[18]

Innovations and advancements in the field of bone graft materials and bone fusion biology have stimulated the field of SF research.[19–21] New surgical adjuncts, such as endoscopy for minimally invasive spine surgery (MISS) and stereotactic image-guided techniques, as well as technologic advancements in diagnostic tools and instrumentation hardware, have provided surgeons with a wide spectrum of surgical techniques.

Advantages and Disadvantages

With the exception of interbody fusion, PLF has biomechanical advantages over other types of posterior fusion techniques.[4–6,12,22,23] The intertransverse arthrodesis is positioned anatomically closer to the center of rotational and bending forces and, therefore, helps to minimize the added stress placed upon the fusion sites by spinal segmental motion. Also, locally exposed muscles provide a generous vascular supply to the fusion graft bed. These factors help increase the overall graft fusion success. The modified Wiltse technique, with sacrospinalis muscle splitting, enables access to the fusion site and safe pedicle screw placement.[13]

Major disadvantages of the midline PLF approach include the long incision and wide dissection required to gain adequate bony exposure of the involved TPs, laminae, and facet joints. The wide exposure can also result in muscular ischemia with a potentially diminished blood supply to the fusion bed. Furthermore, despite the solid fusion seen in patients who have undergone PLF, several patients continue to have persistent lumbar pain, a condition sometimes termed *fusion disease*. Because the bone grafts are lying free in the fusion bed, there is an increased risk of graft displacement and resultant migration of the fusion mass to a different level with an ensuing pseudarthrosis.

■ Indications

Despite its long tradition and popularity, SF for DSD remains controversial; there lacks a common consensus in the standards of care and indication criteria for surgical LBP management. Furthermore, the lack of a "gold standard" assessment for SF results has created difficulties in surgical outcome evaluation and in determining the therapeutic effectiveness of fusion procedures.[4–6]

Advances in instrumentation hardware, surgical techniques, and diagnostic imaging tools have resulted in a transition of fusion indications from well-established conditions such as scoliosis, infections, and trauma to the more controversial entities of spinal instability and DSD. Commonly encountered DSD conditions are degenerative disk disease (DDD), spinal stenosis, isthmic and degenerative spondylolisthesis, degenerative scoliosis, and pseudoarthrosis/failed back syndrome (FBS). PLF has been widely performed to treat all of these DSD conditions.

Disk Herniation/Herniated Nucleus Pulposus

There is no substantial evidence in the literature to support the routine use of spinal arthrodesis in the treatment of herniated nucleus pulposus (HNP). Several independent, retrospective studies have demonstrated the effectiveness of simple decompressive diskectomy in the treatment of herniated disk disease.[2,24,25] Clinical improvements, such as alleviation of pain and sensorimotor deficits, faster recovery, and early return to work, have been reported to be significantly higher in surgically treated groups compared with medically treated groups. Hakelius[6] reported that these clinical improvements, however, appear to equalize after 6 months and without statistical clinical difference at the 7-year follow-up. Nashold and Hrubec[26] reported that 50% of patients treated for HNP continued to have debilitating back symptoms regardless of the type of treatments used, and additional surgery was warranted (14.7% surgical group versus 13.9% nonsurgical group). They concluded that there was no difference in long-term outcome between conservative medical therapy and decompressive surgery.

Early authors advocated routine spinal arthrodesis in addition to diskectomy for the treatment of lumbar disk herniation. In 1934, Mixter and Barr[10] identified HNP as the etiology for back and radicular pain and treated patients surgically with satisfactory outcome. They subsequently recommended concomitant SF because they believed that surgical removal of the disk resulted in structural weakness in the intervertebral disk space with ensuing progressive disk space collapse and structural instability. Howorth[11] in 1943 also advocated spinal arthrodesis as an adjunct for the management of HNP.

Retrospective series have failed to show any clinical improvement when comparing diskectomy alone versus diskectomy and fusion. In fact, many authors have reported higher morbidity and significant complication rates with the added fusion. Lehmann et al,[27] in a 20-year follow-up study, reported a 40% incidence of spinal instability and spinal stenosis in patients treated with simultaneous fusion for HNP. Likewise, Knutsson[28] found 20% spinal instability after 13 years in patients who had undergone L4-S1 fusion surgery, with 5% of these patients clinically symptomatic.

The concept of using concomitant fusion with diskectomy has fallen out of favor because of a lack of support in the literature. Decompressive diskectomy has instead proven to be therapeutic for leg and back pain secondary to HNP. However, there is no evidence that routine spinal arthrodesis with diskectomy improves surgical outcome in the management of lumbar disk herniation, with the exception of multiple disk herniations.

Spinal Stenosis/Spondylosis

Spinal spondylosis represents a spectrum of nonspecific, generalized spinal degenerative conditions in which marked central, lateral recess, and foraminal stenosis are frequently observed. Because of the physical and mechanical constraints from the overall reduction in the diameter of the spinal canal, decompressive surgery is generally accepted as the treatment of choice.[5,6,23,29–31]

Indications for fusion in lumbar stenosis are often based on initial clinical or radiographic evidence, and less frequently on intraoperative findings, that suggest the presence of spinal instability at the time of spinal canal decompression. Extensive spinal decompression, such as generous or complete intraoperative facetectomy with or without pars resection, can often lead to structural instability. Decompressive laminectomy with concomitant SF has long been shown to improve back and radicular symptoms and to reduce the incidence of postoperative slippage, and thus has resulted in improved clinical outcomes.[6,23,30]

The applicability of SF for spinal stenosis has solely been empirical and based on retrospective studies. The incidence of increasing lumbar instability has been reported as ranging anywhere from 10 to 60% following extensive decompression for lumbar stenosis.[31–33] The risk of developing postoperative instability has been strongly associated with the presence of concomitant degenerative spondylolisthesis. White and Wiltse[33] reported a 60% chance of developing increased postoperative slip in patients with lumbar stenosis and degenerative spondylolisthesis. Two thirds of patients who underwent decompression with partial facetectomy were found to have increased postoperative slip, resulting in worse clinical outcome.[31]

Routine fusion with decompression for patients with concomitant degenerative spondylolisthesis resulted in 64 to 100% good or excellent results.[32] Feffer et al[29] treated

19 patients with lumbar stenosis and degenerative spondylolisthesis and found 100% good clinical outcome in patients who underwent fusion compared with 72% without fusion. Bolesta and Bohlman[34] reported 100% good clinical outcomes with decompression and fusion versus only 50% with decompression alone. Simultaneous spinal arthrodesis with decompression for lumbar stenosis thus improves radicular symptoms and back pain and decreases postoperative spondylolisthesis.

Johnson and Kirwan[22] recognized several potential risk factors for spinal instability development following decompression surgery: female gender, preoperative unstable flexion/extension study, preexisting degenerative spondylolisthesis, and complete facetectomy. Reynolds and Wiltse[23] advocated fusion in patients younger than 60 years of age with preexisting degenerative spondylolisthesis and in patients younger than 50 years of age with preexisting isthmic spondylolisthesis. Herkowitz and Kurtz[30] reported a reduced postoperative slip and 64% fusion rate with noninstrumented PLF. Fritzell et al[35,36] found that although functional outcomes are not influenced by the addition of pedicle screw fixation PLF in patients with LBP from degenerative spondylolisthesis, the addition of pedicle screws improved fusion success but at a risk of higher complication rates. When comparing patients undergoing PLF with or without supplementary pedicle screw fixation, Thomsen et al[37] found an increase in operative time, blood loss, and reoperation rate in those patients undergoing supplementary pedicle screw fixation, but with no significant difference in functional outcome or fusion rate between the two treatment groups. In their comparison of instrumented and noninstrumented PLF, Christensen et al[1] found a benefit to pedicle screw fixation on fusion success rates as well as functional improvement with pedicle screw fixation in patients with degenerative lumbar spinal disease requiring SF.

In general, patients with spinal stenosis typically respond well to decompressive surgery. However, in situations in which extensive disruption of facet joints, pars, or both is identified intraoperatively, fusion with or without instrumentation should be considered. Furthermore, PLF, with or without instrumentation, can improve clinical outcome in patients with spinal stenosis and concomitant degenerative spondylolisthesis.

Isthmic Spondylolisthesis

It is estimated that 5 to 8% of the general population may have bilateral pars interarticularis defects, but less than 50% of these individuals eventually progress to any clinically relevant spondylolisthesis.[6,38] Early treatment of symptomatic spondylolysis and spondylolisthesis has relied heavily on nonsurgical modalities such as external bracing devices, physical therapy for truncal strengthening, and nonsteroidal antiinflammatory drugs (NSAIDs). Steiner and Micheli[39] reported a 9% progression to symptomatic spondylolysis or low-grade slip that eventually required fusion. Turner and Bianco[40] found that 34% of their patients deteriorated with pain and debilitating musculoskeletal complaints to the point requiring surgical intervention.

Surgical treatments for isthmic spondylolisthesis have been discussed extensively in the literature, including simple repair of pars defects, decompression alone (Gill procedure), complex in situ fusion, decompression with in situ fusion, and combined reduction/fixation with simultaneous fusion. Review of the literature from retrospective fusion series has suggested that combined fusion with concomitant decompression is the preferred treatment for isthmic spondylolisthesis.[22,41–44] With the historical success of alleviation of symptoms, PLF has been shown to be effective in the treatment of isthmic spondylolisthesis; the reported fusion rate for ranges from 27 to 100% for various fusion techniques and from 66 to 89% for PLF.[5,6,41] Risk factors that may result in unsatisfactory outcomes include male gender, middle age, tobacco use, and preoperative radicular symptoms.[41]

Harrington introduced instrumentation with PLF in 1967 using distraction rods, sublaminar hooks, and a transiliac sacral bar. Following Harrington's initial attempt to use pedicle screw instrumentation for spinal stability, Harrington and Dickson[45] reported no advantage in reducing the listhesis. For isthmic spondylolisthesis, many have found PLF with or without anterior fixation to be more successful than other posterior fusions, such as posterior intralaminar fusions, and to provide better relief of symptoms.[42] To date, instrumentation with pedicle screw placement has been an integral part of the treatment of isthmic spondylolisthesis. Lenke et al[43] reported a discouragingly low 50% solid fusion with noninstrumented in situ fusion, but greater than 80% had a good clinical outcome. Reynolds and Wiltse[23] reported 90% of patients with high-grade LS-SI slips treated with in situ fusion to have resolved hamstring pain and, subsequently, 71% of patients remained free of symptoms. Compared with historical controls, Jacobs et al[46] reported a 90% fusion rate using transfacet screw fixation methods.

The incidence of postoperative slip for patients undergoing PLF for isthmic spondylolisthesis ranges from 11 to 72%. Possible causes include excessive bending stress or deformation of fusion mass leading to subsequent pseudarthrosis. Despite high fusion success rates reported in many series, it remains challenging to correctly diagnose solid fusion. Boxall et al[60] assessed 10 patients with isthmic spondylolisthesis who underwent bilateral PLF and diagnosed all patients with a solid fusion using radiographic evidence. Following surgical exploration due to persistent symptoms, however, 70% of these patients were found to have pseudarthrosis. McGuire and Amundson,[44] in their study of 27 patients, failed to see any statistically significant improvement in fusion rate with the addition of instrumentation. They reported a 72% versus 78% fusion rate with noninstrumented versus rigid pedicle screw fixation, respectively, and concluded that instrumentation did not enhance the bony fusion rate (at least when fusion was determined radiographically).

Despite the controversy in fusion surgery, there is convincing evidence that PLF results in the improvement of clinical symptoms due to isthmic spondylolisthesis. The addition of pedicle screws or other instrumentation techniques, such as transfacet screw fixation, may improve fusion rates.[46,47]

Discogenic Pain

Crock[48] was the first to examine the mechanism of pain of discogenic origin. He subsequently coined the term *internal disk derangement* to describe unremitting lumbar spinal pain that (1) persisted longer than 4 months, (2) was not responsive to conservative care, and (3) was reproduced with diskography. In a sense, *discogenic pain syndrome* (DPS) represents a continuum of pathologies that mainly involve the diseased intervertebral disk. It is also known as DDD, internal disk derangement, annular tear, and dark disk disease. In many instances, these pain entities can be diagnosed by magnetic resonance imaging (MRI) or diskography.[49–52]

Early nonfusion treatments for pain of discogenic origin included diskectomy, percutaneous diskectomy, and chymopapain injection. These treatment modalities, however, were found to be ineffective. Contemporary SF techniques have included PLF with or without instrumentation, posterior lumbar interbody fusion (PLIF), anterior lumbar interbody fusion (ALIF), and combined anterior/posterior fusion.

Because the presumed pain generator in DDD is the disk itself, posterolateral fusion may be inadequate for eliminating pain of discogenic origin. Despite excellent fusion rates of higher than 80% reported in several fusion series, clinical correlation, which ranged from 57 to 67%, has been disappointing. According to Zucherman et al,[53] the addition of pedicle screw fixation has resulted in 89% successful fusion rate but with only 60% clinical success. Weatherley et al[54] documented five patients with continued LBP despite satisfactory solid PLF who went on to have complete resolution of symptoms following ALIF.

The goal of management is to eliminate the pain that appears to originate from within the disk space. This may require complete disk ablation and elimination of disk motion. Biomechanical studies have demonstrated that the most effective method for eliminating motion between two vertebral bodies is through interbody fusion. In fact, the mechanical strength in ALIF has been found to be twice as strong compared with that of PLF.[55,56]

Colhoun et al[49] found an 88% satisfactory result in his nonconsecutive series of patients who underwent fusion following positive diskography. Other authors have reported clinical outcome and fusion success rates ranging from 73 to 89% for the anterior approach. In the case of combined anterior and posterior fusion, several clinical series have reported overall clinical success rates as high as 60 to 80%.

In a prospective randomized study of patients with single-level L5-Sl degenerative disk disease, Nachemson et al[57] compared the fusion outcome of different surgical techniques in the management of DDD and reported 80% fusion rate with PLF, 91% with PLIF, and 100% with ALIF using interbody fusion cages. Kuslich et al[18] had a 91% fusion rate and a 92% clinical success rate in their series using an interbody cage.

■ American Association of Neurosurgeons/CNS Guidelines

In 2005, the American Association of Neurological Surgeons and Congress of Neurological Surgeons (AANS/CNS) Joint Section on Disorders of the Spine and Peripheral Nerves produced a set of evidence-based guidelines regarding the performance of lumbar fusion for degenerative disease.[58] Their review focused on the surgical treatment of LBP in patients with DDD or low-grade degenerative spondylolisthesis that was treated with PLF with or without pedicle screw fixation. Although they concluded that there was insufficient evidence to recommend a treatment standard or guideline, they offered the following options:

1 Pedicle screw fixation is recommended as a treatment option for patients with LBP treated with PLF who are at high risk of fusion failure because fusion success rates are improved with the use of pedicle screw fixation.
2 Pedicle screw fixation should not be used routinely as an adjunct to PLF in treating patients with chronic LBP secondary to DDD because the evidence is conflicting regarding the benefit of pedicle screw fixation on functional outcomes.
3 The use of pedicle screw fixation is associated with higher costs and complications.

■ Technique

The objective of lumbar surgical fusion is to obtain a solid arthrosis and reduce pain and disability, all with the least amount of risk to the patient. Without bony fusion, instrumentation will eventually fail. Adequate quantity and quality of bone graft, as well as meticulous preparation of the recipient bed, enhances the likelihood of a bony fusion. In addition, the use of instrumentation has been associated with an increased probability of a successful fusion; instrumentation is not, however, required in all cases (as previously discussed).

The patient is first placed in the prone position on the Jackson operating table (the table that we prefer). The basic principle of patient positioning is to achieve abdominal decompression while maintaining lumbar lordosis. With the

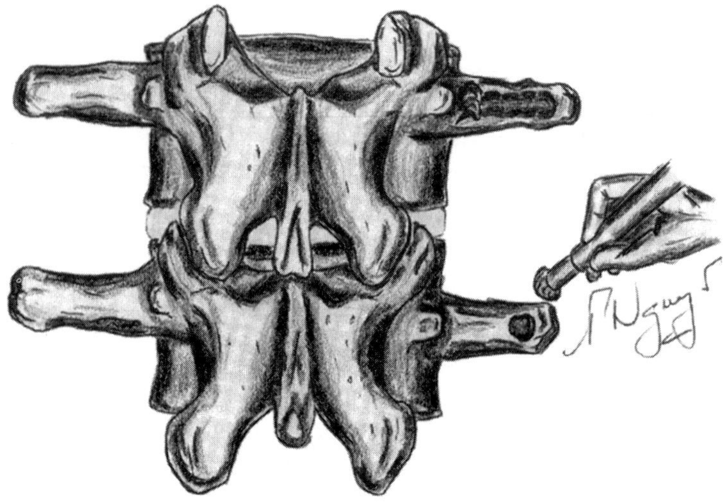

Fig. 9.1 The dorsal lumbar spine. The fusion bed is first prepared by creating a hole in the lateral aspect of the transverse process with a cutting burr drill bit.

patient's legs extended at the hip, the posture is maintained with the correct lordosis and sacral inclination. Tribus et al[59] discussed the importance of proper surgical positioning during lumbosacral fusion, and found the kneeling position to be suboptimal for posterior fusion techniques, especially in multiple-level fusions.

Surgical exposure initially requires visualization of the spinous processes and facet complex. Electrocautery is used to define the lateral aspect of the facet joint in a subperiosteal plane. Deep retractors are used to retract the paraspinal muscles laterally. The TPs are best exposed with cauterization of the attachments of the paraspinous muscles to the TPs while retracting back any overlying fatty tissue. Dissection is performed to the lateral tip of the TPs via a subperiosteal dissection with the electrocautery but with care not to plunge ventrally where the nerve roots are traveling obliquely.

The fusion bed must be thoroughly prepared prior to placement of the bone graft. Decortication of the dorsal bony surfaces should include exposure down to the underlying cancellous core of the TP, facet joint, and pars interarticularis. Decortication of the TP is achieved with a variety of instruments, such as a cutting burr, osteotome, or curette. We prefer creating a curl of bone in the TP using a large curette. This doubles the surface area for engraftment and, at the same time, creates a vascularized pedicle of bone. This is accomplished initially by drilling a hole in the distal portion of the TP (**Fig. 9.1**). A large curette or cutting burr is then placed in the hole and gently wiggled medially to create a corticocancellous strip that remains attached medially (**Fig. 9.2**). Equally important, the lateral surface of the facet joint must also be prepared with a cutting burr or curette. The adjacent surfaces of the facet joints can be removed with a narrow-tipped rongeur and then packed with bone graft to enhance fusion. Although any exposed bony surface should be decorticated prior to bone grafting, decortication should not be so aggressive that it compromises the integrity of the spine or instrumentation.

To optimize fusion, a generous quantity and quality of bone graft must be used. Autograft should be used whenever possible, whereas allograft may be sufficient for interbody fusions. Autograft can be harvested from the iliac crest or from the bony decompression. The use of bone fusion enhancers, such as bone morphogenetic protein-2 (BMP-2), may lower the rate of pseudarthrosis and accelerate the

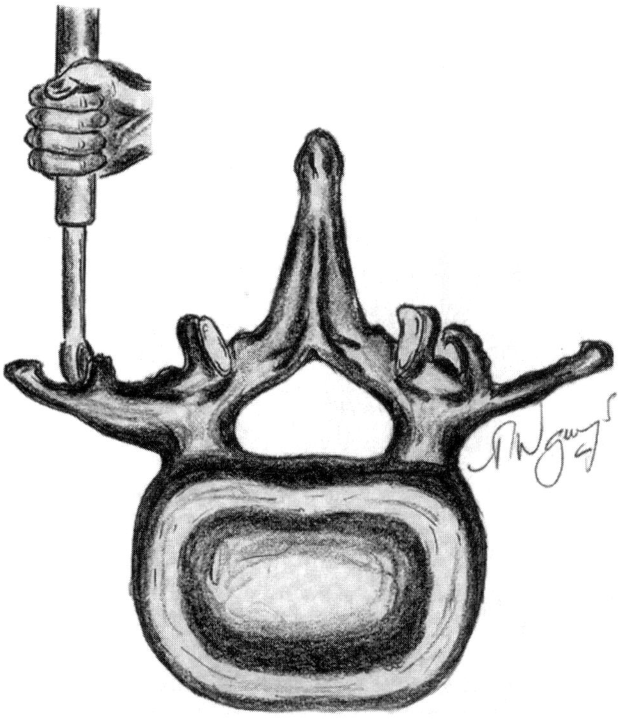

Fig. 9.2 Axial view of the lumbar spine. Once the initial hole is drilled in the lateral aspect of the transverse process, a large curette or cutting burr drill bit is moved with a gentle wiggle motion (left transverse process in image) medially to create a well-vascularized corticocancellous bony strip. A bony curl on the right transverse process in this image has previously been created and is ready for graft placement.

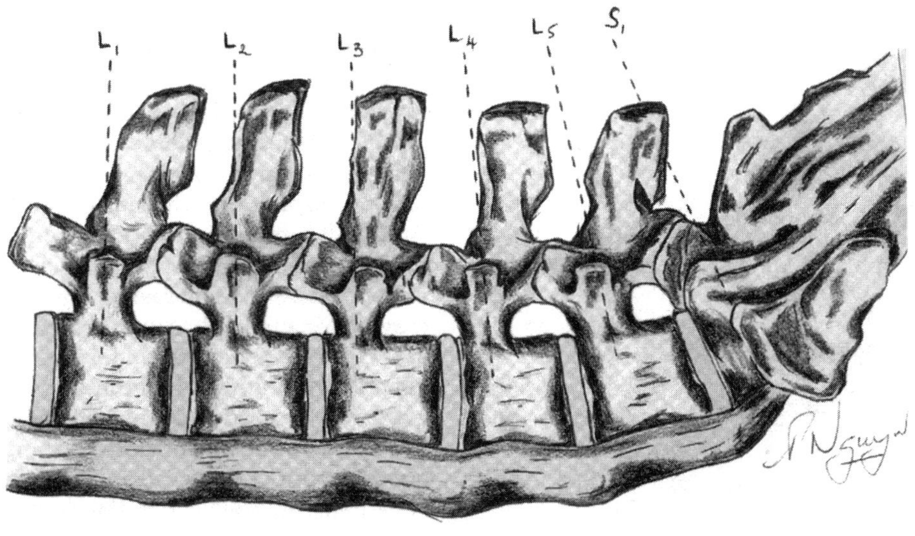

Fig. 9.3 Lateral view of the lumbosacral spine. Demonstration of the rostrocaudal angle of each pedicle from L1 to S1. This should serve as the trajectory for intraoperative pedicle screw placement.

development of fusion. For short segment fusions, unilateral posterior iliac crest harvesting provides adequate bone for grafting. For longer, more complex fusions, bilateral iliac crest bone harvesting may be necessary. Also, autograft may be used either alone or in combination with allograft or demineralized bone matrix if an adequate supply of autograft is unobtainable. Any extra bone obtained from the initial decompression should be cleaned of soft tissue and cut into small match-head–size pieces. The importance of adequate bone grafting cannot be overemphasized as this has been shown to be one of the factors that can influence fusion outcome.[20,60] The bone graft is carefully applied to the decorticated surfaces in a continuous fashion, forming a bridge from one segment to the next.

For instrumented fusions, a thorough knowledge of the anatomy of the lumbosacral spine is mandatory if safe and accurate placement of pedicle screws is to be accomplished. Because pedicle screws are used as the primary anchoring device in lumbosacral fusions, preoperative assessment of the anatomy on imaging studies and a familiarity with the pertinent instrumentation system ensures a smooth operation and increases the likelihood of a good outcome.

Because of possible complications with pedicle screw placement, one must familiarize oneself with each individual lumbar and sacral pedicle size, as well as the potential variations. The width of each pedicle varies and is slightly increased in size rostrocaudally. In addition, there is a more caudal trajectory through the pedicles of lower lumbar and sacral levels **(Fig. 9.3)**. The appropriate screw trajectory through a pedicle must be precise to avoid any compromise of the spinal canal or neural foramen. The angle of pedicle placement also varies from one level to another. A general rule of thumb is that there is an increasing angle of screw trajectory for lower lumbar and sacral pedicles. For each level descending along the lumbosacral spine, the angle of screw placement is 5 degrees more medial **(Fig. 9.4)**.

A variety of methods have been described for placing pedicle screws. We prefer first determining the intersection between the midpoint of the base of the TP and the superior articular facet as the entry point for screw placement. The bony surface is then decorticated with a cutting burr until the cancellous appearance of the pedicular core is encountered. A pilot hole is then created with the drill or sharp awl. The pedicle is then probed with firm advancing pressure and a gentle twisting motion in the planned trajectory until the anterior vertebral cortical surface is felt. The distinctive resistance of the cortical surface to the probe is unique and better appreciated with experience.

The ultimate control of any probing device must be maintained at all times to prevent plunging the instrument beyond the anterior cortex of the vertebral body. In osteoporotic and arthritic patients, great caution is needed because of the poor bone quality, making a through-and-through probing a heightened risk. We recommend repeatedly assessing the pedicle with a probe between instrument changes for inadvertent penetration of the cortical wall in all directions. Once all of the pedicles pilot holes have been drilled and probed, radiographs are obtained with markers placed in each hole to document correct location and appropriate trajectories. Any additional adjustments of the trajectories are performed prior to screw placement. Final screw placement is confirmed with a final lateral radiograph **(Fig. 9.5)**.

Frameless stereotactic image guidance can be used as an adjunct to safe and accurate pedicle screw placement. This technology is safe and effective, albeit with increased radiation exposure to the surgeon and patient. Preoperative imaging data can be used prior to surgery to help in planning screw trajectory and to determine screw diameter and length. All of this information can be mated to the actual intraoperative anatomy through registration and the image-guided tools used to locate and create the pedicle screws pilot holes.

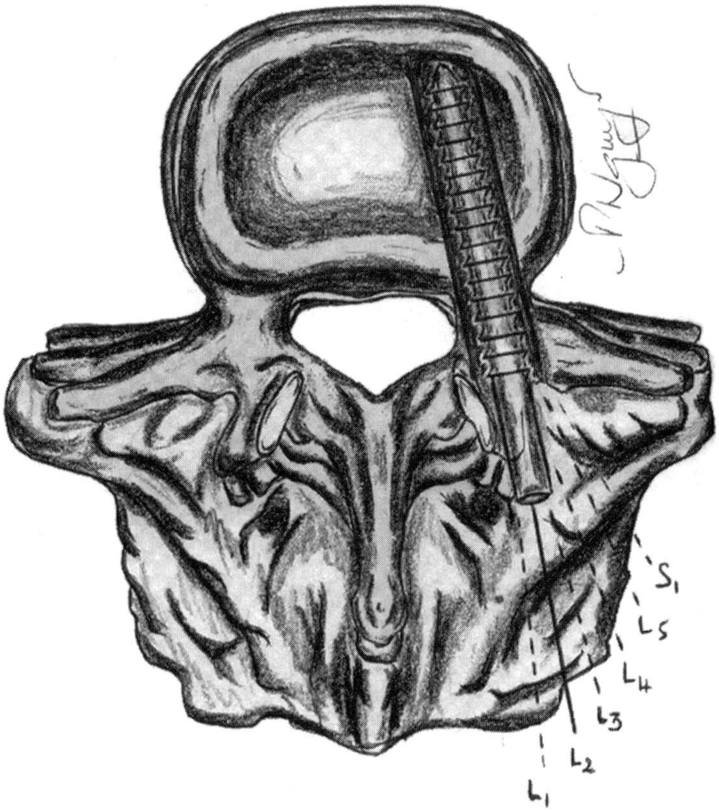

Fig. 9.4 Axial view demonstrating the angle and trajectory of pedicle screw placement. Entry site is at the junction between the midpoint of the base of the transverse process and superior articular facet. The angle of the trajectory becomes more medial as one travels more caudally down the lumbosacral spine.

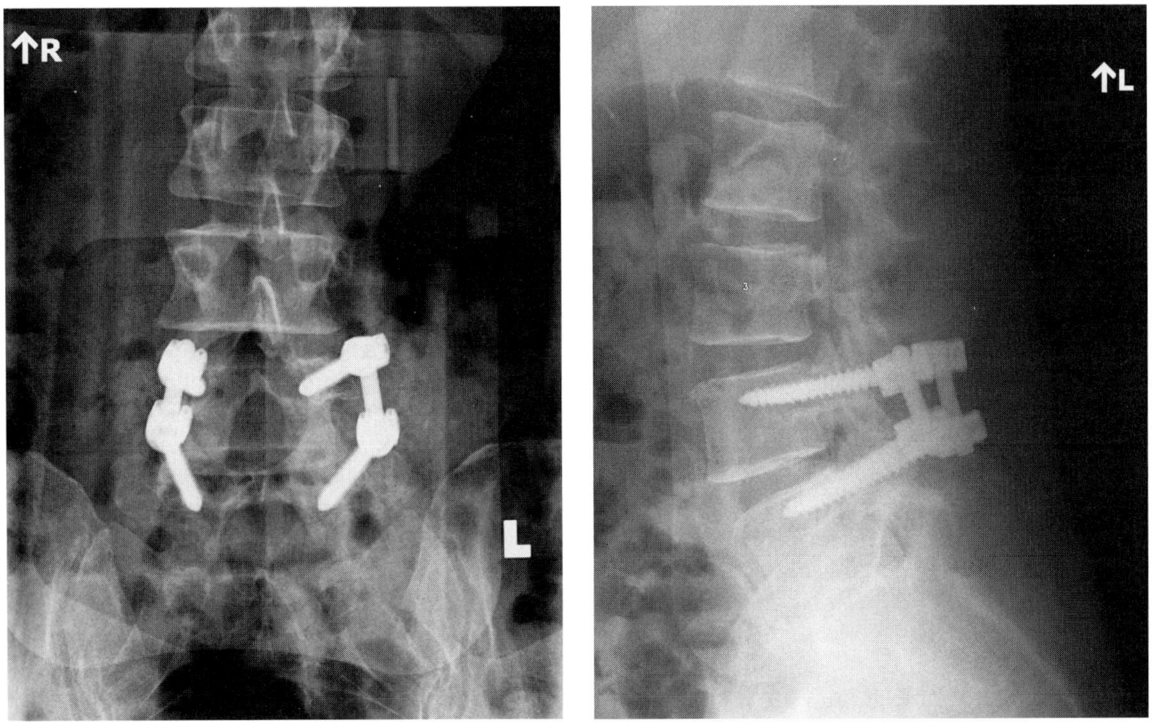

A B

Fig. 9.5 Anteroposterior **(A)** and lateral lumbosacral **(B)** spine x-rays. Instrumented posterolateral fusion (PLF) with L4-L5 pedicle screws (Legacy; Medtronic Sofamor Danek, Memphis, TN) in a 49-year-old patient with history of LBP and mild spondylolisthesis. Symptoms improved following fusion surgery.

The surgeon must be familiar with the instrumentation system to be implanted. Most commercially available systems come with standard screws ranging in diameter from 5.0 or 5.5 mm to as wide as 7.5 to 8.5 mm. Custom-made screws with a smaller diameter of 4.5 mm are also available. Standard screw lengths typically range from 30 to 75 mm. Furthermore, pedicle screws are available with fixed or multiaxial heads, and coupling devices can vary from system to system. The intricacies of each particular system are beyond the scope of this chapter.

■ Complication Avoidance and Management

Posterolateral fusion of the lumbosacral spine can be a formidable undertaking associated with a variety of complications. The surgeon must be aware of the pitfalls at each stage of the procedure. Thus there must be careful planning and meticulous execution of the procedure to minimize such complications.

Blood Loss Posterolateral fusions require extensive exposure of musculoskeletal components and can lead to considerable blood loss. Meticulous hemostatic control throughout the operation greatly reduces blood loss; bleeding should be controlled at the time of discovery with monopolar or bipolar electrocautery. Although liberal utilization of electrocautery decreases blood loss, thermal injury to areas where bone grafting will take place can impede fusion; therefore, care must be taken to avoid excessive injury to exposed bone. In addition to hemostatic techniques, various strategies are available to limit the use of blood transfusion, including the use of either autologous blood donation or cell-saver suction systems.

Infections The avoidance of infection is best accomplished by strict adherence to sterile technique throughout the procedure, appropriate preoperative antibiotics dosing (and intraoperative re-dosing if necessary), and meticulous technique during wound closure. A consistent operative team can also help shorten the operating time to reduce the risk of infection. If an infection does occur, removal of hardware is not always necessary because there are a variety of strategies available for treatment. We recommend wound reexploration with infected tissue debridement and copious irrigation with pulsatile lavage containing antibiotics. Appropriate cultures should be obtained intraoperatively to confirm the preoperative diagnosis and guide the antibiotic choice. The wound can be closed with drains to allow for wound drainage; drain removal occurs once output has decreased. We find that occasional consultation with the infectious disease specialists may also be of benefit. Discontinuation of antibiotics can be determined by clinical findings and by laboratory indicators, such as white blood cell count, sedimentation rate, and C-reactive protein. If the patient fails to respond to the treatment, wound reexploration with removal of the hardware is inevitable. In the event that hardware removal is necessary, it is recommended that removal be delayed until after fusion has occurred if possible.

Incorrect Surgical Level Incorrect identification of the fusion level can occur in patients who have had previous surgery or in those who may require simultaneous decompressive surgery. Despite the familiarity of spinal anatomy, direct observation and palpation can sometimes be unreliable, and therefore an intraoperative lateral radiograph should be obtained routinely.[61]

Hardware Malpositioning Malpositioned hardware can often lead to complications involving the neural structures. Placement of bone graft ventrally between the transverse processes can inadvertently contact and compress the nerve root. Direct compromise of nerve roots can result in symptoms ranging from mild paresthesias to significant sensorimotor deficits. The appropriate treatment for such complications depends solely on signs and symptoms presented. Treatment plans may vary from no immediate treatment to possible urgent removal of the offending device.

Pseudarthrosis/Nonunion It is important to realize that instrumentation serves as an adjunct to fusion, is used to provide spinal rigidity, allows bony fusion to occur, and has been shown to enhance fusion rates.[4,62–65] Without good solid bony fusion, all hardware will eventually fail. Treatment of hardware failure is usually dictated by symptoms. Nonunion has been reported in the range of 35 to 59% in noninstrumented fusions and in the range of 0 to 14% of instrumented fusions.[63,64] Physiologic properties of fusion have been studied thoroughly, and several factors have been shown to enhance or retard fusion via a variety of mechanisms.[20,66,67] Cigarette smoking has been implicated in an increased risk of nonunion or pseudarthrosis, as well as in risk of other systemic problems such as stroke, hypertension, cardiorespiratory-related problems, and cancers. Brown et al[68] reported a 40% incidence of pseudarthrosis in smokers versus 8% in nonsmokers. Deguchi et al[69] found the fusion rate in smokers to be lower regardless of whether or not instrumentation was used. McGuire and Amundson[44] reported 100% fusion rates in nonsmokers and 56% in smokers. Smoking cessation is therefore highly recommended in preparation for fusion procedure; the patient should be advised to cease smoking for at least 1 month preceding a fusion and for 6 months afterward. In addition, because the initial phase of fusion is an inflammatory response and because the use of NSAIDs has been shown to decrease fusion rates in animal models, NSAIDs cannot be used for at least 6 weeks postoperatively.[69,70]

Within the fusion bed there are several factors that must be considered to optimize the fusion environment. The fusion mass receives its blood supply from the surrounding musculature. Necrotic or nonviable tissues should be debrided from the area surrounding the fusion bed prior to closure. As mentioned earlier, thermal injury to the transverse processes through overzealous use of cauterization can impede fusion growth and should be avoided. Because nutrition plays a major role in the recuperation and healing process following fusion surgery, the patient's nutritional status should also be optimized.

Dural Tear Dural tear is not an uncommon occurrence in lumbar spine surgery. If feasible, primary closure is usually effective. Any one of the currently available commercial glue products can be used as an adjunctive measure for security. We routinely use 48 hours of flat bedrest following the repair of a dural tear to prevent the development of posture-related headaches. In a few instances, spinal fluid leaks may not be reparable by primary closure and may require more complex treatment options. Patching with muscle, fascia lata, or bovine pericardium has been used by many with reasonably good outcome. In these cases, however, cerebrospinal fluid (CSF) diversion and glue, in addition to patching, can be greatly beneficial.

Injury to Surrounding Structures Vascular and visceral injuries rarely occur during placement of posterior instrumentation, but their occurrence has been well documented in the literature. Again, these complications can be avoided if the surgeon pays meticulous attention to detail. Preoperative planning with imaging studies or information provided from frameless stereotactic systems helps reduce these risks by providing adequate information regarding pedicle dimensions, trajectory, and screw length. Complications to structures adjacent to the graft site must also be considered. Because the cluneal nerve is located approximately 8 cm lateral to the posterior superior iliac spine, injury to these nerves can occur and can lead to pain at the harvest site. The sciatic nerve and superior gluteal vessels are positioned in the proximity of the sciatic notch and therefore are vulnerable to injury during bone harvesting. Stress fractures of the hip can occasionally occur following the removal of bone or in patients with severe osteoporosis.

Fusion operations are physiologically stressful operations. Thus medical complications are not uncommon and can be minimized with vigilant treatment of the patient in the postoperative period. Ileus, deep venous thrombosis, fluid overload, and atelectasis are but a few of these complications.

■ Conclusion

Spinal arthrodesis continues to claim an important position in the treatment of DSD and is routinely performed for the treatment of many spinal degenerative conditions, including spinal stenosis with concomitant degenerative spondylolisthesis, isthmic spondylolisthesis, and other degenerative conditions. Instrumentation has also been shown to improve both fusion outcome and postoperative clinical outcome. However, difficulties remain in developing universal criteria for making a correct diagnosis of successful fusion versus failed fusion. The addition of instrumentation hardware must be carefully considered, with a good understanding of both the potential risks and benefits.

References

1. Christensen FB, Hansen ES, Laursen M, Thomsen K, Bunger CE. Long-term functional outcome of pedicle screw instrumentation as a support for posterolateral spinal fusion. Spine 2002;27:1267–1277
2. Swanson JA, Hoecker JL. Concise review for primary-care physicians. Mayo Clin Proc 1996;71:179–183
3. Loeser JD, Volinn E. Epidemiology of low back pain. Neurosurg Clin North Am 1991;2:713–718
4. Fraser RD. Interbody, posterior, and combined lumbar fusion. Spine 1995;20(suppl):167S–177S
5. Hanley EN. The indications for lumbar spinal fusion with and without instrumentation. Spine 1995;20(suppl):143S–153S
6. Zdeblick TA. The treatment of degenerative lumbar disorders. A critical review of the literature. Spine 1995;20(suppl):126S–137S
7. Albee FH. Transplantation of a portion of the tibia into the spine for Pott's disease. JAMA 1911;57:885–886
8. Hibbs RA. Treatment of deformities of the spine caused by poliomyelitis. JAMA 1917;69:787–796
9. Hibbs RA, Swift WE. Developmental abnormalities at the lumbosacral juncture causing pain and disability. Surg Gynecol Obstet 1929;48:604–612
10. Mixter WJ, Barr JS. Rupture of the intervertebral disc with involvement of the spinal canal. N Engl J Med 1934;211:210–215
11. Howorth MB. Evolution of spinal fusion. Ann Surg 1943;117:278–289
12. Watkins MB. Posterior fusion of the lumbar and lumbosacral spine. J Bone Joint Surg Am 1953;35A:1014–1018
13. Wiltse LL, Hutchinson RH. Surgical treatment of spondylolisthesis. Clin Orthop Relat Res 1964;35:116–135
14. Lange F. Support for the spondylitic spine by means of buried steel bars attached to the vertebra. Clin Orthop Relat Res 1986;203:3–6
15. Roy-Camille R, Saillant G, Mazel C. Plating of thoracic, thoracolumbar and lumbar injuries with pedicle plates. Orthop Clin North Am 1986;17:147–159
16. Steffee AD, Biscup RS, Sitkowski DJ. Segmental spine plates with pedicle screw fixation. A new internal fixation device for disorders of the lumbar and thoracolumbar spine. Clin Orthop Relat Res 1986;203:45–53
17. Brantigan JW, Steffee AD. A carbon fiber implant to aid interbody lumbar fusion: two-year clinical results in the first 26 patients. Spine 1993;18:2106–2107
18. Kuslich SD, Ulstrom CL, Griffith SL, et al. The Bagby and Kuslich method of lumbar interbody fusion: history, techniques, and

2-year follow-up results of a United States prospective, multicenter trial. Spine 1998;23:1267–1278
19. Boden SD, Schimandle JH. Biologic enhancement of spinal fusion. Spine 1995;20(suppl):113S–123S
20. Boden SD, Martin GJ, Barone M, et al. The use of coralline hydroxyapatite with bone marrow, autogenous bone graft, or osteoinductive bone protein extract for posterolateral lumbar spine fusion. Spine 1999;24:320–327
21. Martin GJ, Boden SD, Titus L, et al. New formulations of demineralized bone matrix as a more effective graft alternative in experimental posterolateral lumbar spine arthrodesis. Spine 1999;24:637–645
22. Johnson JR, Kirwan EO. The long-term results of fusion in situ for severe spondylolisthesis. J Bone Joint Surg Br 1983;65:43–46
23. Reynolds JB, Wiltse LL. Surgical treatment of degenerative spondylolisthesis. Spine 1979;4:148–152
24. Davis RA. A long-term outcome analysis of 984 surgically treated herniated lumbar discs. J Neurosurg 1994;80:415–421
25. Pappas CT, Harrington T, Sonntag VK. Outcome analysis in 654 surgically treated lumbar disc herniations. Neurosurgery 1992;30:862–866
26. Nashold BS, Hrubec Z. Lumbar Disc Disease: A Twenty-Year Clinical Follow-Up Study. St. Louis: Mosby, 1971
27. Lehmann TR, Spratt KF, Tozzi JE, et al. Long-term follow-up of lower lumbar fusion patients. Spine 1987;12:97–104
28. Knutsson F. The instability associated with disc degeneration in the lumbar spine. Acta Radiol 1944;25:593–609
29. Feffer HL, Wiesel SW, Cuckler JM, et al. Degenerative spondylolisthesis: to fuse or not to fuse. Spine 1985;10:287–289
30. Herkowitz HN, Kurz LT. Degenerative lumbar spondylolisthesis with spinal stenosis. A prospective study comparing decompression with decompression and intertransverse process arthrodesis. J Bone Joint Surg Am 1991;73:802–808
31. Lombardi JS, Wiltse LL, Reynolds J, et al. Treatment of degenerative spondylolisthesis. Spine 1985;10:821–827
32. Rosenberg NJ. Degenerative spondylolisthesis: predisposing factors. J Bone Joint Surg Am 1975;57:467–474
33. White AH, Wiltse LL. Spondylolisthesis after extensive lumbar laminectomy. J Bone Joint Surg Am 1976;58:727–728
34. Bolesta MJ, Bohlman HH. Degenerative spondylolisthesis. Instr Course Lect 1989;38:157–165 Review
35. Fritzell P, Hagg O, Wessberg P, et al Swedish Lumbar Spine Study Group. Chronic low back pain and fusion: a comparison of three surgical techniques: a prospective multicenter randomized study from the Swedish lumbar spine study group. Spine 2002;27:1131–1141
36. Fritzell P, Hagg O, Wessberg P, et al. Swedish Lumbar Spine Study Group. 2001 Volvo Award Winner in Clinical Studies: Lumbar fusion versus nonsurgical treatment for chronic low back pain: a multicenter randomized controlled trial from the Swedish Lumbar Spine Study Group. Spine 2001;26:2521–2532
37. Thomsen K, Christensen FB, Eiskjaer SP, et al. The effect of pedicle screw instrumentation on functional outcome and fusion rates in posterolateral spinal fusion: a prospective randomized clinical trial. Spine 1997;22:2813–2822
38. Hanley EN, Levy JA. Surgical treatment of isthmic lumbosacral spondylolisthesis: analysis of variables influencing results. Spine 1989;14:48–50
39. Steiner ME, Micheli LJ. Treatment of symptomatic spondylolysis and spondylolisthesis with the modified Boston brace. Spine 1985;10:937–943
40. Turner RH, Bianco AJ. Spondylosis and spondylolisthesis in children and teen-agers. J Bone Joint Surg Am 1971;53:1298–1306
41. Hanley EN, Levy JA. Surgical treatment of isthmic lumbosacral spondylolisthesis: analysis of variables influencing results. Spine 1989;14:48–50
42. Harris IE, Weinstein SL. Long-term follow-up of patients with and without grade III and IV spondylolisthesis. Treatment with and without posterior fusion. J Bone Joint Surg Am 1987;69:960–969
43. Lenke LG, Bridwell KH, Bullis D, et al. Results of in-situ fusion for isthmic spondylolisthesis. J Spinal Disord 1992;5:433–442
44. McGuire RA, Amundson GM. The use of primary internal fixation in spondylolisthesis. Spine 1993;18:1662–1672
45. Harrington PR, Dickson JH. Spinal instrumentation in treatment of severe progressive spondylolisthesis. Clin Orthop Relat Res 1976;117:157–163
46. Jacobs RR, Montesano PX, Jackson RP. Enhancement of lumbar spine fusion by use of translaminar facet joint screws. Spine 1989;14:12–15
47. Reich SM, Kuflik P, Neuwirth M. Translaminar facet screw fixation in lumbar spine fusion. Spine 1993;18:444–449
48. Crock HV. Internal disc disruption: a challenge to disc prolapse fifty years on. Spine 1986;11:650–653
49. Colhoun E, McCall IW, Williams L, et al. Provocative discography as a guide to planning operations of the spine. J Bone Joint Surg Br 1988;70:267–271
50. Modic MT, Pavliced W, Weinstein MA. Magnetic resonance imaging of the intervertebral disc disease. Radiology 1984;152:103–111
51. Modic MT, Steinberg PM, Ross JS, et al. Degenerative disc disease: assessment of changes in vertebral body marrow with MR imaging. Radiology 1988;166:193–199
52. Wetzel FT, LaRocca SH, Lowery GL, et al. The treatment of lumbar spinal pain syndromes diagnosed by discography. Lumbar arthrodesis. Spine 1994;19:792–800
53. Zucherman J, Hsu K, Picetti G, et al. Clinical efficacy of spinal instrumentation in lumbar degenerative disc disease. Spine 1992;17:834–837
54. Weatherley CR, Prickett CF, O'Brien JP. Discogenic pain persisting despite solid posterior fusion. J Bone Joint Surg Br 1986;68:142–143
55. Lee CK, Vessa P, Lee JK. Chronic disabling low back pain syndrome caused by internal disc derangements. Spine 1995;20:356–361
56. Zdeblick TA, Smith GR, Warden KE, Eng MB, McAfee PC. Two-point fixation of the lumbar spine. Differential stability in rotation. Spine 1991;16(suppl):S298–S301
57. Nachemson A, Zdeblick TA, O'Brien JP. Controversy: lumbar disc disease with discogenic pain. What surgical treatment is most effective? Spine 1996;21:1835–1838
58. Resnick DK, Choudhri TF, Dailey AT, et al. Guidelines for the performance of fusion procedures for degenerative disease of the lumbar spine. Part 12: pedicle screw fixation as an adjunct to posterolateral fusion for low-back pain. J Neurosurg Spine 2005;2:700–706
59. Tribus CB, Belanger TA, Zdeblick TA. The effect of operative position and short-segment fusion on maintenance of sagittal alignment of the lumber spine. Spine 1999;24:58–61
60. Boxall D, Bradford DS, Winter RB, et al. Management of severe spondylolisthesis in children and adolescents. J Bone Joint Surg Am 1979;61:479–495
61. Ebraheim NA, Inzerillo C, Xu R. Are anatomic landmarks reliable in determination of fusion level in posterolateral lumbar fusion. Spine 1999;24:973–974

62. Kaneda K, Kazama H, Satoh S. Follow-up study of medial facetectomies and PLF with instrumentation in unstable degenerative spondylolisthesis. Clin Orthop Relat Res 1986;203:159–167
63. Lorenz M, Zendrick M, Schwaegler P, et al. A comparison of single-level fusions with and without hardware. Spine 1991;16(suppl):S455–S458
64. Zdeblick TA. A prospective, randomized study of lumbar fusion. Preliminary results. Spine 1993;18:983–991
65. Zdeblick TA. Introduction of discogenic back pain. 13th Annual Meeting of the North American Spine Society, October 1998
66. Glazer PA, Heilmann MR, Lotz JC, et al. Use of electromagnetic fields in a spinal fusion. A rabbit model. Spine 1997;22:2351–2356
67. Goodwin CB, Brighton CT, Guyer RD, et al. A double blind study of capacitively coupled electrical stimulation as an adjunct to lumbar spinal fusions. Spine 1999;24:1349–1356
68. Brown CW, Orme TJ, Richardson HD. The rate of pseudoarthrosis (surgical nonunion) in patients who are smokers and patients who are nonsmokers: a comparison study. Spine 1986;11:942–943
69. Deguchi M, Rapoff AJ, Zdeblick TA. Posterolateral fusion for isthmic spondylolisthesis in adults: analysis of fusion rate and clinical results. J Spinal Disord 1998;11:459–464
70. Glassman SD, Rose SM, Dimar JR, et al. The effect of postoperative nonsteriodal anti-inflammatory drug administration on spinal fusion. Spine 1998;23:834–838

10 Anterior Lumbar Interbody Fusion

Rick C. Sasso, A. Kirk Reichard, and Shenil Shah

■ Historical Background

Anterior lumbar interbody fusion (ALIF) was first used in the treatment of tuberculosis and lumbar spondylolisthesis.[1–3] Although described by Capener[4] in 1932 as the "ideal" operation for spondylolisthesis, he further elaborated that "the technical difficulties of such procedure, however, preclude their trial." This statement was soon to be proven wrong by numerous technical advances in ALIF. When initially developed, the transperitoneal approach for lumbar arthrodesis was the norm, but was later replaced by the retroperitoneal approach. The first description of the transperitoneal approach was published in 1906 by Muller,[5] and Iwahara[6] first reported the later approach in 1944. Further broadening the scope of ALIF, Lane and Moore[7] in 1948 reported ALIF as a treatment for lumbar degenerative disk disease. Here they used the transperitoneal approach with an allogenic bone graft in 97 patients, reporting a 54% fusion rate after 8 months and a clinical success rate of 94%.

Further developing Iwahara's retroperitoneal approach, Hodgson and Stock[8,9] established the foundation for the modern era of ALIF while treating Pott disease with different bone grafting materials. Debridement of the necrotic tissue, followed by decompression of the spinal canal, allowed them to place corticocancellous blocks of autogenous bone into the defect to obtain arthrodesis. The dowel technique, developed by Ralph Cloward in 1953, involved the use of cylindrical shaped corticocancellous dowels. Although Cloward[10–12] used a posterior approach, his methods for disk removal, end-plate preparation, and grafting were widely used. Following Cloward's dowel technique, four individuals adapted this to make their own innovations in bone grafting methods. Two of them, Harmon[13] in 1963 and Sacks[14] in 1965, were the first to utilize the dowel technique for an anterior lumbar fusion. The third, Crock, developed a cylindrical allograft for the anterior approach to the lumbar spine. Finally, the fourth, O'Brien et al,[15] modified a technique of using trapezoidal bone blocks for the treatment of lumbar discogenic pain through ALIF. They later developed a hybrid interbody graft using a biologic fusion cage (femoral cortical allograft ring) packed with autogenous cancellous bone graft. By using autogenous iliac crest bone graft, rapid incorporation and vascularization of the graft are achieved, as well as long-term stability.[16] Furthermore, the femoral allograft ring allows for acute stability of the construct and a compatible framework for host bone ingrowth.[15]

Despite the success in safely exposing the anterior lumbar spine, in the 1970s and 1980s stand-alone ALIF was not a reliable procedure due to low fusion rates. Early in the development of the procedure, there was great discrepancy among success rates. The reported numbers were incredibly inconsistent, with some reporting huge success and others complete failure. For example, Lane and Moore,[7] as stated previously, reported a 94% clinical success rate. In contrast, though, Adkins[17] in 1955 had a fusion rate of 1%. Early reports encompassing numerous surgical techniques and a heterogeneous group of patients demonstrated a fusion rate of 95% by Harmon,[13] 70% by Hoover,[18] 90% by Crock,[19] and 96% by Fujimaki et al.[20] However, other reports cited fusion rates of 19%, 40%, 45%, and 56% by Calandruccio and Benton,[21] Nisbet and James,[22] Raney and Adams,[23] and Flynn and Hoque,[24] respectively. A 1972 study conducted from the Mayo Clinic and authored by Stauffer and Conventry[25] concluded definitively that the stand-alone ALIF had a low success rate. After reporting on 83 patients who underwent ALIF without instrumentation between 1959 and 1967, they found an extremely low success rate, with pseudarthrosis occurring in 44%. The Mayo Clinic study resulted in a review of the ALIF as a stand-alone procedure, and it soon after fell out of favor, particularly for the indication of lumbar degenerative disk disease and lumbar axial back pain.

In response to these low fusion rates, a technique combining an ALIF with posterior fusion became very common.[26] Although the anterior approach continued to be utilized for the diskectomy, lordosis restoration, and fusion block insertion, a posterior approach was used to access the posterior elements for instrumentation and stabilization **(Fig. 10.1)**. The addition of posterior instrumentation increases stability across the segment and decreases motion while the fusion solidifies. Despite having a very high fusion rate, the magnitude of the circumferential fusion increased morbidity. Although the ALIF usage had been revitalized with posterior instrumentation, the search for a better construct continued.

These new innovations included anterior lumbar instrumentation, first reported by Humphries et al[27] in 1961. They developed a slotted, contoured plate that was placed over the anterior lumbar spine in an attempt to enhance arthrodesis. Another advance in anterior hardware was the cylindrical cage. The first cylindrical cages were modified from a smooth, stainless steel, fenestrated cylinder (Bagby

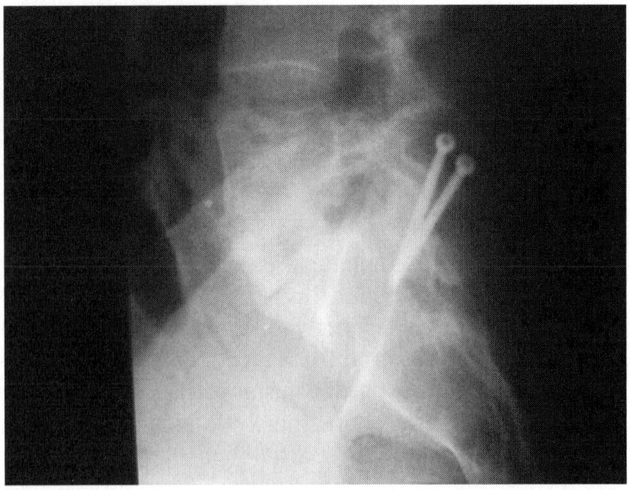

Fig. 10.1 Lateral radiograph of circumferential fusion using a femoral ring allograft for the anterior lumbar interbody fusion (ALIF) and translaminar facet screws for posterior stability.

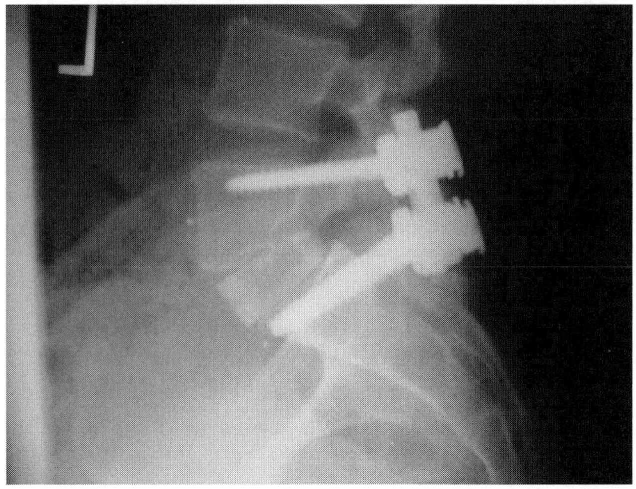

Fig. 10.2 Lateral radiograph of circumferential fusion using a femoral ring allograft for the ALIF and pedicle screws and rods for posterior stability.

basket) used by Bagby and colleagues in the mid-1970s and early 1980s to treat Wobbler syndrome, which is a chronic cervical instability causing myelopathy in thoroughbred horses.[28] In Bagby's procedure, he packed the cage with cancellous bone chips obtained from the reaming of the cervical decompression, thus eliminating the need for an autograft harvest. Further, the cage was developed with perforations in its walls to allow for bone ingrowth and to enhance fusion. This construct allowed for early stability and improved arthrodesis. Animals studies corroborated the success of this procedure with fusion rates as high as 88%.[28–31] Following the original cylindrical cage, more and more improvements in the design of the cages led to the Bagby and Kuslich design (BAK, Spine-Tech, Minneapolis, MN), which was first implanted in humans in 1992.[32] This BAK titanium cage was threaded and screwed into the end plates for stabilization and fusion of the segment. Another similar device developed by Ray[33] (Ray TFC, Surgical Dynamics, Norwalk, CT) was initially used in posterior lumbar interbody fusion (PLIF) but was later adapted to the ALIFs as well.

Although cylindrical cages were originally metal alloy, the development of machined bone dowels provided several advantages. Threaded bone dowels are similar in nature to a metal cage, but differ in that they are osteoconductive, incorporated over time, radiographically benign, and easier to revise.

Despite the rampant usage and initial success of the threaded cylindrical cage in the late 1990s, the next generation, the lumbar tapered (LT) cage, has several advantages over the cylindrical predecessor. It provides the same benefits of a cylindrical device, but allows the surgeon to symmetrically ream the end plate while restoring lordosis. Symmetric reaming prepares the end plate for fusion and preserves the strength.

In addition, LT cages packed with recombinant human bone morphogenetic protein (rhBMP-2) perform as well as those packed with autograft.

Other constructs include trapezoidal cages. Trapezoidal constructs can be made from various materials, but several features are shared, including a large footprint for maximum end-plate coverage and a large inner volume for bone graft and future fusion maturation.

Although cages continue to be widely used, femoral ring allografts (FRAs), as well as other trapezoidal implants are growing in popularity. The rhBMP-2 is also commonly used during all spinal fusions. Using rhBMP-2 decreases donor-site morbidity, as well as operating room time, and has proven to be as effective as autologous bone. Not surprisingly, the surgical approach has again been revisited, and recent research has shied away from laparoscopic approaches in favor of a retroperitoneal "mini" open approach. Although the ALIF was conceived over 100 years ago, it continues to be updated and improved with each new generation of implant and surgeon.

The ALIF has developed over decades, and specific attributes have been identified as primary contributors to a successful outcome. With the disk as the pain generator, removal of the pain source with a total diskectomy addresses the patient's presenting complaint. Also, restoration of disk height can alleviate foraminal stenosis. Re-creation of native lordosis may decrease juxtalevel stress. And lastly, posterior stabilization maximizes the likelihood of fusion **(Fig. 10.2).**

■ Biomechanics

The greatest strength of the vertebral body is present in the peripheral subchondral bone of the cortical end plate.

When threaded cages are used, the preparation process violates this peripheral ring of subchondral bone. Although this process compromises the strong ring of subchondral bone and theoretically raises the risk of subsidence, it also exposes vascular cancellous bone that may facilitate healing.

In contrast, to prepare the intervertebral space for a nonthreaded, trapezoidal implant, such as an FRA, the strong peripheral ring of subchondral bone is preserved and directly supports the graft while fusion occurs. In the past when FRAs were fashioned by the surgeon on the back table, the size and shape were difficult to match, and this strong ring of subchondral bone may not have been maximally utilized. Now, FRAs are more frequently manufactured, and thus size and shape are more predictable. This enables the surgeon to match the implant to the patient and build the most stable construct. In addition, manufactured FRAs have the benefit of insertion instruments that distract the adjacent vertebral bodies and ensure proper alignment and placement.

The spine endures a wide range of biomechanical forces, from 400 N while standing, to greater than 7000 N during heavy lifting,[34,35] with an maximum compression strength of 10,000 N.[36] The selected implant should not fail under these loads. When tested, modern-day implants usually sustain the maximum loads, with failure occurring at the end plate or the sacroiliac joint.[37] With implants infrequently failing, every effort must be made to utilize the intrinsic strength and healing potential of the end plate to promote rapid fusion. Considering that the implants usually do not fail, when constructs do fail, it generally results in subsidence of the implant into the vertebral body, or cavitation. As the end plate fails, either due to violation during preparation or after excessive loading, the implant migrates into the vertebral body and the segment collapses. Cavitation is addressed by choosing an implant with a large contact area, or footprint. A larger footprint provides a bigger foundation for the implant, decreasing the load per square inch **(Fig. 10.3)**.

Subsequently, a successful implant should be mechanically strong to withstand compressive loads while providing an osteogenic, osteoinductive, and osteoconductive matrix. Many metal alloy implants provide strength and stability but are unable to incorporate these other attributes. To compensate, metal implants provide an environment that allows the surgeon to place an autogenous cancellous bone graft, which does accomplish these later goals. Although metal implants can provide an environment that is fusion friendly, it is limited by the specific design and subsequent volume available for the fusion to traverse through the implant. To maximize the area available for fusion, the surgeon should expose the entire end plate with a total diskectomy,[38] as well as choose an implant that provides the most volume for the biologic substrate and future fusion block.

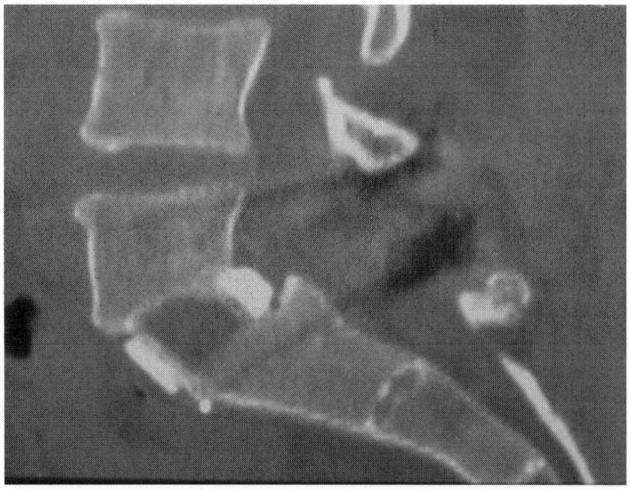

Fig. 10.3 Sagittal reconstruction of a computed tomography (CT) scan with a femoral allograft at L5-S1 demonstrating a large footprint and support on the peripheral endplate.

Implant design affects how the load is transmitted to the adjacent vertebra and may contribute to juxtalevel discogenic pain.[39] A recent biomechanical analysis revealed that greater implant contact area transmits loads to the adjacent segment in a more physiologic manner and could decrease adjacent level pain, as Kumar et al[39] found in 2005 that implants with smaller surface areas transmit loads in a similar manner to a degenerative disk that causes discogenic pain. In addition, physiologic stress patterns are better recreated when the patient's lordotic curve is restored. Consequently, when choosing a device, the largest appropriate implant should be carefully implanted after a total diskectomy. This would theoretically prepare the end plate in the correct fashion, load the adjacent vertebra more physiologically, and, when fused, minimize the risk of juxtalevel disease and pain.

Rh-BMP-2 is now routinely used for spinal fusions. The decrease in donor-site morbidity and operating room (OR) time are inviting; however, a recent study found a concerning trend. This prospective cohort study found a lower fusion rate with rhBMP in FRAs. Although, the ALIFs studied were stand-alone, the fusion rate was decreased with the use of rhBMP. The authors believe that the drop in fusion rate, although insignificant, may be secondary to rhBMP-induced resorption of the FRA **(Fig. 10.4)**. If the ring is absorbed more quickly, the graft may weaken or fragment, which allows motion at the segment before fusion occurs, resulting in an unsatisfactory outcome.[40] This stand-alone study reinforces the significance of stabilizing the fusion segment. Although FRA implants are stable at the time of implantation, rhBMP may accelerate the resorption process and destabilize the segment before fusion can occur. Posterior stabilization with pedicle screws or translaminar facet screws provides the needed stability necessary for fusion.

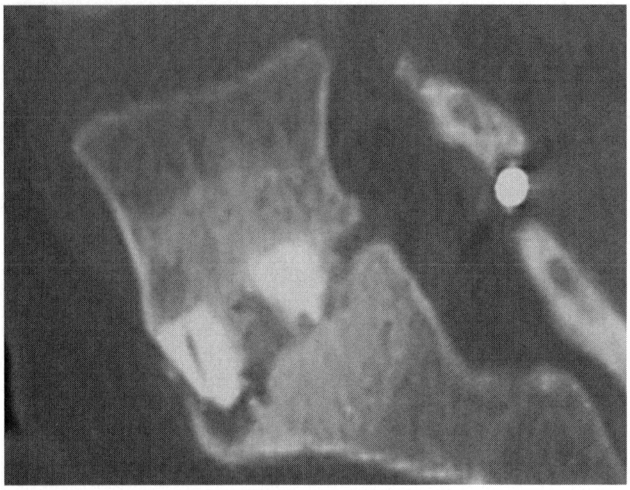

Fig. 10.4 Sagittal reconstruction of CT scan with a femoral allograft packed with recombinant human bone morphogenetic protein (rhBMP-2) demonstrating early resorption of bone at the caudal graft–host junction.

Although the ALIF was conceived as a stand-alone device, posterior instrumentation has proven to be optimal for reliable fusion. Even though the stand-alone ALIF does have intrinsic stability, posterior stabilization is recommended because posterior instrumentation provides stability in the range the cage does not.[41] Several implant options have been used, two of which are pedicle screws and translaminar facet screws. Ferrara et al[42] performed a biomechanical comparison of these two constructs and found both to be reliable constructs, with similar properties. After 180,000 cycles, both constructs were equivalent with regard to stiffness and motion. With similar biomechanical properties, implant choice can be determined by other factors, including surgeon preference, and patient-specific characteristics.

Although both constructs have similar integrity, multiple factors should be considered. Best and Sasso[43] recently reviewed 105 ALIF patients receiving translaminar screws or pedicle screws, and they found that the OR time was greatly reduced with translaminar screws, and the blood loss was significantly less.[43] Translaminar screw placement combines a midline incision and percutaneous screw placement, thus decreasing the overall incision length. To place translaminar facet screws, less muscle stripping is required, the cephalad facet joint is not disrupted, and instrumentation prominence is not an issue.[44] Despite the benefits of translaminar facet screws, patients with a prior complete laminectomy and removal of the spinous process or those with spondylolysis are not candidates.

Understanding the biomechanics of the spine is critical to interpreting the principles with the latest implants and techniques. Despite the ever-changing approach to lumbar disk disease, the ALIF relies on removal of the entire degenerative disk, preserving end-plate strength, re-creating physiologic lordosis, eliminating motion across the segment, and most importantly, achieving a stable fusion.

■ Patient Selection

Most low back pain is transient and self-limiting; however, 5% does not respond to nonoperative treatment.[45,46] Although this small percentage of patients does not improve with the most conservative measures, the surgeon must be confident that all conventional alternatives have been exhausted. Leaving options behind and moving ahead too quickly places risks on patients who would have improved without surgery and puts the surgeon at risk of an unacceptable outcome. Utilizing conservative methods and screening tests with high predictive value improves practice outcomes.

The ALIF is a commonly used surgical intervention to treat discogenic low back pain not controlled by nonoperative measures. Indications for an interbody fusion include degenerative disk disease of one or two adjacent levels of the lumbar spine, with severe, chronic, disabling, low back pain lasting longer than 6 months and unresponsive to adequate nonoperative therapy.[33,47] Less than three levels should be addressed at a time because the risk of pseudarthrosis increases with each additional level fused and clinical success decreases.[48–50]

The pathophysiology of discogenic pain is poorly understood; however, we do know that other factors, such as compensation and pending litigation, affect outcomes.[51] These confounding variables must be accounted for prior to determination of the definitive therapy. The importance of the history and physical examination cannot be overstated; the interaction with the patient is an opportunity for the surgeon to assess the patient's expectations and determine if the patient is motivated by secondary gain.

Magnetic resonance imaging (MRI) is a sensitive and specific tool for diagnosing disk pathology;[52] however, asymptomatic disk pathology or herniation can be as high as 34%.[53] Boden et al[53] studied 20- to 39-year-olds, and found that more than one third had asymptomatic disk degeneration and more than one fifth had asymptomatic disk herniations. MRI should not be used as a screening tool and should be ordered only when clinical suspicion is high for spinal pathology.

Although controversial, diskography can provide the surgeon additional information prior to surgical intervention. Diskography is a diagnostic tool that many feel correlates pathoanatomy and symptomatology in patients with primary discogenic pain. Several studies suggest improved outcomes in interbody fusion patients after supportive preoperative diskography.[54–56] Re-creation of concordant pain with diskography especially under low pressures can verify the pain source or help rule out pathology at a specific level **(Fig. 10.5)**.

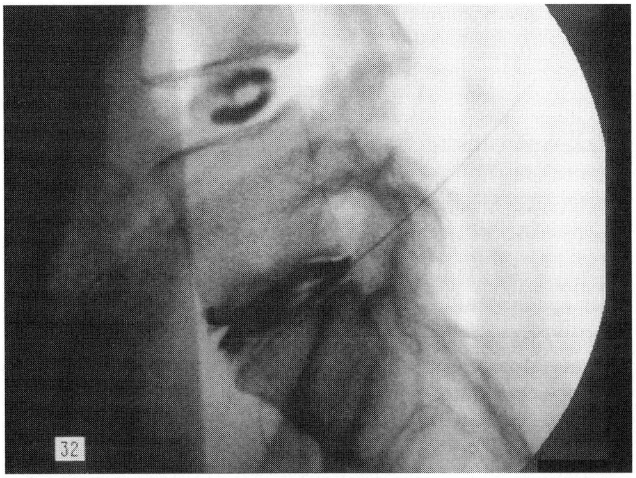

Fig. 10.5 Lateral radiograph during diskography with a morphologically abnormal L5-S1 disk and a normal L4-L5 disk.

Another provocative test with predictive value is the selective nerve root injection (SNRI), which can elucidate the pathophysiology of the pain generator in patients with complex disk disease or nontraditional radiculopathy. A positive result, meaning the patient has 100% relief of symptoms following the injection of anesthetic, correlates with the benefits achieved following surgical intervention of simply decompressing the offending nerve.[57] This procedure is easily performed by an experienced anesthesiologist and gives the surgeon an added layer of confidence before surgical intervention (**Fig. 10.6**).

Operative intervention for spinal pathology places the patient at risk. Utilizing available diagnostic tools improves patient outcome and avoids low-yield surgical intervention. The least expensive and most easily used tools likely are the history and physical examination of the patient.

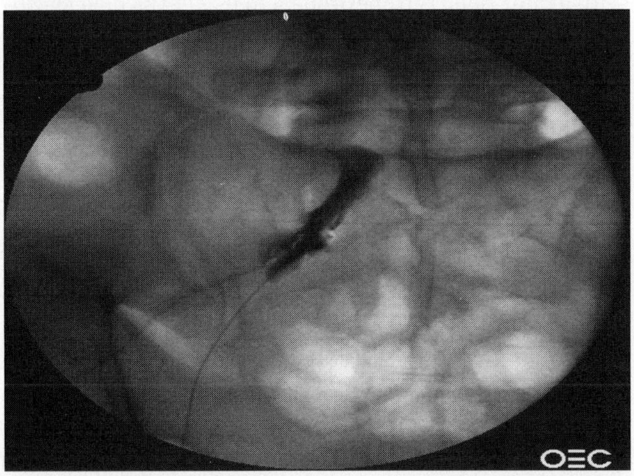

Fig. 10.6 Anteroposterior radiograph during selective nerve root injection (SNRI) of the left S1 nerve.

Clinical Studies

The ALIF has evolved over several decades through constant reevaluation and technique revision. To date, the most reliable constructs employ an anterior fusion that is stabilized posteriorly with instrumentation. Several attempts have been made to optimize an anterior-only, stand-alone technique; however, fusion rates have been less reliable. Posterior instrumentation provides the additional stability needed for rapid fusion, and now with the addition of rh-BMP, donor-site morbidity can be eliminated.

Despite the wide usage of cylindrical cages throughout the 1990s, no prospective fusion data was available until 2004. Starting in 2000, 140 patients were enrolled in a prospective, randomized, controlled, clinical trial comparing fusion rates of stand-alone threaded cages and stand-alone FRAs.[58] The 13 surgeons who took part in the trial implanted either a pair of cylindrical threaded titanium cages or an FRA. Both implants were packed with autograft, and fusion was evaluated at 6-month intervals by a board-certified radiologist. At 6 months, 95% of the threaded cages were fused as compared with only 10.9% of the FRAs, and the superior fusion rate remained in favor of threaded cages throughout the study. The highest fusion rate obtained by the FRA control group was 51.9% at 2 years, in contrast to the lowest fusion rate seen with the threaded cages was 95% at 6 months. Regardless of the outstanding fusion capacity of threaded cages, clinical outcomes remained equal between groups.[58] These surprising clinical findings may be explained by Fraser's[59] analysis in 1995, which attributes the clinical success of the ALIF to the surgical approach to the pathologic disk and not the fusion status.

The more recent emergence of LT cages enables surgeons to restore lumbar lordosis while achieving the similarly high fusion rates seen with cages. Burkus et al[60] compared LT cages implanted with rh-BMP-2 and FRA with autologous bone graft, and found no difference in outcomes, supporting the use of rh-BMP-2.[60] Having an off-the-shelf substitute for autologous bone graft allows surgeons to spare their patients the morbidity associated with donor sites, without sacrificing the osteoinductive properties needed for a fusion (**Fig. 10.7**).

Although donor-site morbidity has overshadowed autologous bone grafting, a prospective analysis was lacking. The senior author of this chapter participated in the first prospective analysis of over 200 spinal fusion patients randomized to an autologous donor arm and an rh-BMP arm comparing postoperative pain. Nearly one third of the autologous donors had persistent donor-site pain 2 years postoperatively compared with zero pain in the rh-BMP randomized group.[61] The ability to eliminate donor-site pain is an appealing option for the spine surgeon, despite appearing to be an added expense.

A comparison of an off-the-shelf osteoinductive growth factor reveals that they are in fact a cost-effective way of

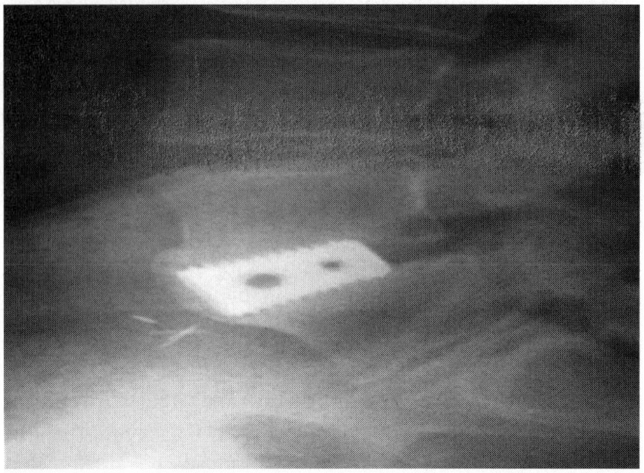

Fig. 10.7 Lateral radiograph of ALIF with an lumbar tapered (LT) cylindrical cage and BMP.

decreasing patient morbidity and maximizing patient outcomes. This 2003 evaluation found that the cost of BMP is offset by reductions in other care expenses. For example, valuable OR time is reduced with the use of a protein substitute, the postoperative period is less painful, and less nursing staff wound care is required for the patient.[62]

Reduction of OR time is beneficial for patients as well as for surgeons. Similar to using rhBMP, performing a 270-degree fusion (posterior instrumentation without fusion after an ALIF) versus a 360-degree fusion may be another effective way to trim OR time. A 2001 prospective randomized trial failed to reveal any clinical difference with the addition of the posterior instrumentation. The Oswestry Low Back Disability Index (ODI) and the Numerical Rating Scale (NRS) were used to evaluate outcomes following ALIF with or without posterior stabilization, and there were no statistical clinical differences.[63] Without clinical support of the posterior fusion, surgeons could choose to decrease operative supply cost (i.e., supplies needed for posterior fusion), shorten OR time, and decrease intra/postoperative complications.

Evaluation of patient success can be addressed from many perspectives. A clinical evaluation may reveal a pain-free patient with total resolution of symptoms despite a radiographic result that may be discordant, or vice versa. Using interval plain radiographs and computed tomography (CT) scans, a recent study shows that LT cages plus rhBMP compared favorably with LT cages plus autograft, and those supplemented with rhBMP achieved more bone formation outside the cage. Both constructs formed bone similarly through the implant, but rhBMP improved bony fusion outside the cage. This confirms that rhBMP is not only comparable to autologous bone graft as an osteoinductive agent, but may be superior when specifically evaluating bone formation outside the stabilizing construct.[64]

Multiple papers support the stability of threaded cages and the clinical success;[33,65,66] however, a recent retrospective review revealed an increased complication rate with threaded devices compared with nonthreaded trapezoidal block-type constructs. This retrospective review identified a significantly higher number of intraoperative complications with threaded devices and the tools used to prepare the site and insert the devices. The study also found more postoperative complications; however, this was not statistically significant. The greatest numbers of complications seen were vascular in nature, including both intraoperative and postoperative. Most of these complications can be linked to the added steps required to prepare the level for the threaded device and the insertion instrumentation.[58]

The surgical techniques employed to expose the anterior lumbar spine focus on the preservation of adjacent structures to minimize long-term complications. The anterior lumbar spine can be approached via a transperitoneal or extraperitoneal approach using various incisions. As with other surgical disciplines, minimally invasive techniques have been pioneered with varying results. The laparoscopic anterior lumbar interbody fusion (LALIF) first appeared in the late 1990s,[67,68] with positive results presented by the early users. Initial LALIF reports indicated that the procedure was a safe, less invasive procedure, with less blood loss and faster patient recovery. However, follow-up reports found LALIF to be more time-consuming, and the touted benefits similar to those achieved with a "mini" open retroperitoneal approach.[69,70] In 2003, Chung et al[71] performed a 47-patient side-by-side comparison of the LALIF and the mini-ALIF and reported similar clinical and radiographic outcomes, with no identifiable advantages to the LALIF, despite the added technical challenge. Not only have the proclaimed benefits of the laparoscopic approach been challenged, but also specific complications are higher with the LALIF.

Two studies in 2003 reported a higher risk of retrograde ejaculation following a transperitoneal LALIF as compared with a mini-open retroperitoneal ALIF.[72,73] The delicate superior hypogastric plexus lies on top of the L4–S1 anterior spine and innervates the internal vesical sphincter. Damage to the plexus can cause retrograde ejaculation in men. The transperitoneal approach, either laparoscopic or open, dissects through this fragile web of nerves, whereas an open retroperitoneal approach, mini or traditional, sweeps the plexus from left to right. Retraction of the plexus as a whole versus dissection through it appears to decrease the risk of internal vesical sphincter denervation.

Imaging

Evaluation of interbody arthrodesis is difficult and controversial secondary to various fusion criteria.[50,59,74,75] Varying criteria include bridging bone and no motion on flexion and extension films, whereas others allow limited motion.

Radiographic assessment is also limited by the materials implanted.

Computed tomography and plain x-ray are traditionally used to assess fusion. Utilizing these tools, pseudarthrosis is identified by lucency around the cage, motion across the segment, or lack of bridging bone extending through the cage. Unfortunately, no study, other than histologic, is 100% reliable. Even with the improved quality of reconstructed, thin-segment, high-resolution CT, it is also unreliable in evaluation of fusion status.[38,74,76,77]

Post-ALIF pain is often attributed to pseudarthrosis. A follow-up study of patients with persistent back pain following ALIFs with radiographically confirmed fusions found a high rate of pseudarthrosis upon reoperation. Six of seven patients had pre-revision CT scans that failed to show peri-implant lucency. Seven of eight patients had pre-revision plain films showing no signs of loosening. The CT scan and plain films were both hindered with the use of a metal implant as compared with a bone allograft, making the predictive value of these screening tools low when metal implants were used.[74,77]

In addition, Cizek and Boyd[74] performed a cadaveric study on three different implant materials to determine the predictive value of CT scan versus plain radiographs for identification of a fusion. They compared bone cages, titanium cages, and carbon fiber cages, and found that neither CT scan nor plain radiograph was reliable. Fusions identified on CT were often refuted with plain films and vice versa.

Another study on pig-tailed macaques *(Macaca nemestrina)* reexamined this controversy, finding thin section helical CT better than plain films at identifying the presence of fusion; however, the extent of fusion was overestimated on CT when compared with histology. The predictive values of the CT results were greater in this nonhuman study with 83% concordance between the CT and the histology, versus 45% concordance with plain radiographs.

In summary, radiographic assessment of interbody fusions is suboptimal secondary to interpretation and implant artifact. Although these tools may be beneficial for identification of the grossly positive or negative result, the more difficult cases may require additional studies and possibly surgical exploration for definitive diagnosis.

Conclusion

Low back pain is generally treated with nonoperative measures, including nonsteroidal antiinflammatory drugs (NSAIDs), physical therapy, lifestyle modification, and time. Unfortunately, not all patients with discogenic pain respond to nonoperative treatment. A thorough preoperative evaluation should be able to determine patients with primary discogenic pain who may respond to operative arthrodesis.

The mini-open retroperitoneal ALIF approach allows the surgeon to maximize exposure without compromising the superior hypogastric plexus or the rectus muscles. The mini-ALIF approach is retroperitoneal and minimally invasive in nature with a low complication rate.

Choosing an implant is a personal decision and should be founded in clinical success. FRA has proven to be successful, especially with posterior instrumentation, and has unique benefits with regard to postoperative imaging. When an FRA is used in conjunction with posterior instrumentation and an off-the-shelf osteogenic biologic, an ideal construct for a 360-degree fusion has been created. Additionally, using translaminar facet screws to minimize soft tissue insult will optimize clinical success.

Our current assessment of spinal pathology will continue to change and our treatment options will too. Although spine surgery is an ever-changing world, the patient interactions and clinical success that motivate those involved is a constant.

References

1. Mercer W. Spondylolisthesis with a description of a new method of operative treatment and notes of ten cases. Edinburgh Med J 1936;43:545–572
2. Burns B. An operation for spondylolisthesis. Lancet 1933;224:1233–1239
3. Ito H, Tsuchiya J, Asami G. A new radical operation for Pott's disease. J Bone Joint Surg Br 1934;16:499–515
4. Capener N. Spondylolisthesis. Br J Surg 1932;19:374–386
5. Muller W. Transperitoneale freilegung der wirbelsaule bei tuberkuloser spondylitis. Dtsch Z Chirop 1906;85:128–137
6. Iwahara T. A new method of vertebral body fusion. Surgery 1944;8:271–287
7. Lane JD, Moore E. Transperitoneal approach to the intervertebral disc in the lumbar area. Ann Surg 1948;127:537–551
8. Hodgson A, Stock F. Anterior spinal fusion. Br J Surg 1956;44:226–275
9. Hodgson AR, Stock FE. Anterior spine fusion for the treatment of tuberculosis of the spine. J Bone Joint Surg Br 1960;42:295–310
10. Cloward RB. Spondylolisthesis: treatment by laminectomy and posterior interbody fusion. Clin Orthop Relat Res 1981;154:74–82
11. Cloward RB. The treatment of ruptured lumbar intervertebral discs by vertebral body fusion. J Neurosurg 1953;10:154–168
12. Cloward RB. Lesions of the intervertebral disks and their treatment by interbody fusion methods. Clin Orthop Relat Res 1963;27:51–77
13. Harmon PH. Anterior excision and vertebral body fusion operation for intervertebral disc syndromes of the lower lumbar spine. Clin Orthop Relat Res 1963;26:107–127
14. Sacks S. Anterior interbody fusion of the lumbar spine. J Bone Joint Surg Br 1965;47:211–223
15. O'Brien JP, Dawson MH, Heard CW. Simultaneous combined anterior and posterior fusion. Clin Orthop Relat Res 1986;203:51–77
16. Holte DC, O'Brien JP, Renton P. Anterior lumbar fusion using a hybrid interbody graft. A preliminary radiographic report. Eur Spine J 1994;3:32–38

17. Adkins EWO. Lumbosacral arthrodesis after laminectomy. J Bone Joint Surg Br 1955;37:208–223
18. Hoover NW. Methods of lumbar spine fusion. J Bone Joint Surg Am 1968;50:194–210
19. Crock HV. Anterior lumbar interbody fusion: Indications for its use and notes on surgical technique. Clin Orthop Relat Res 1982;165:157–163
20. Fujimaki A, Crock H, Bedbrook G. The results of 150 anterior lumbar interbody fusion operations performed by two surgeons in Australia. Clin Orthop Relat Res 1982;165:164–167
21. Calandruccio RA, Benton BF. Anterior lumbar fusion. Clin Orthop Relat Res 1964;35:63–68
22. Nisbet NW, James A. Results of intervertebral bony fusions. J Bone Joint Surg Br 1956;38:952–953
23. Raney FL, Adams JE. Anterior lumbar disc excision and interbody fusion used as a salvage procedure. J Bone Joint Surg Am 1963;45:667–668
24. Flynn JC, Hoque MA. Anterior fusion of the lumbar spine. End-result study with long-term follow-up. J Bone Joint Surg Am 1979;61:1143–1150
25. Stauffer RN, Coventry M. Anterior interbody lumbar spine fusion: Analysis of Mayo Clinic studies. J Bone Joint Surg Am 1972;54:756–768
26. Kozak JA, O'Brien JP. Simultaneous combined anterior posterior fusion: An independent analysis of a treatment for the disabled low back pain patient. Spine 1990;15:322–328
27. Humphries AW, Hawk WA, Berndt AL. Anterior interbody fusion of lumbar vertebrae. Surg Clin North Am 1961;41:1685–1700
28. DeBowes RM, Grant BD, Bagby GW. Cervical vertebral interbody fusion in the horse: a comparative study of bovine xenografts and autografts supported by stainless steel baskets. Am J Vet Res 1984;45:191–199
29. Bagby GW. Arthrodesis by the distraction-compression method using a stainless steel implant. Orthopedics 1988;11:931–934
30. Crawley GR, Grant BD, White KK. A modified Cloward's technique for arthrodesis of the normal metacarpophalangeal joint in the horse. Vet Surg 1988;17:117–127
31. Wagner PC, Grant BD, Bagby GW, et al. Evaluation of spine fusion as treatment in the equine wobbler syndrome. Vet Surg 1979;8:84–88
32. Kuslich SD, Ulstrom CI, Griffith SL, et al. The Bagby and Kuslich method of lumbar interbody fusion. History, technique, and 2-year follow-up results of a United States prospective, multicenter trial. Spine 1998;23:1267–1278
33. Ray CD. Threaded fusion cages for lumbar interbody fusions. An economic comparison with 360 fusions. Spine 1997;22:681–685
34. Nachemson AL, Schultz AB, Berkson MH. Mechanical properties of human lumbar spine motion segments: influence of age, sex, disc level and degeneration. Spine 1979;4:1–8
35. White AA, Panjabi MM. Clinical Biomechanics of the Spine, 2nd ed. Philadelphia: Lippincott, 1990
36. Dolan P, Earley M, Adams MA. Bending and compressive stresses acting on the lumbar spine during lifting activities. J Biomech 1994;27:1237–1248
37. Haher TR, Yeung AW, Merola AA, et al. An in vitro biomechanical investigation of spinal interbody fusion devices. 14th Annual Meeting of the North American Spine Society, 1999, Chicago
38. McAfee PC, Lee GA, Fedder IL, et al. A prospective randomized study of 100 anterior interbody cage arthrodeses: complete versus partial discectomy. 14th Annual Meeting of North American Spine Society, 1999, Chicago
39. Kumar N, Judith MR, Kumar A, et al. Analysis of stress distribution in lumbar interbody fusion. Spine 2005;30:1731–1735
40. Pradhan BB, Bae HW, Dawson EG, et al. Graft resorption with the use of bone morphogenetic protein: lessons from anterior lumbar interbody fusion using femoral ring allografts and recombinant human bone morphogenetic protein-2. Spine 2006;31:E277–E284
41. Phillips FM, Cunningham B, Carandang G, et al. Effect of supplemental translaminar facet screw fixation on the stability of stand-alone anterior lumbar interbody fusion cages under physiologic compressive loads. Spine 2004;29:1731–1736
42. Ferrara LA, Secor JL, Jin BH, et al. A biomechanical comparison of facet screw fixation and pedicle screw fixation: effects of short-term and long-term repetitive cycling. Spine 2003;28:1226–1234
43. Best NM, Sasso RC. Efficacy of translaminar facet screw fixation in circumferential interbody fusions as compared to pedicle screw fixation. J Spinal Disord Tech 2006;19:98–103
44. Beaubien BP, Mehbod AA, Kallemeier PM, et al. Posterior augmentation of an anterior lumbar interbody fusion. Spine 2004;29:E406–E412
45. Deyo RA, Cherkin D, Conrad D, Volinn E. Cost, controversy, crisis: low back pain and the health of the public. Annu Rev Public Health 1991;12:141–156
46. Frymoyer JW, Pope MH, Clements JH, et al. Risk factors in low back pain. An epidemiological survey. J Bone Joint Surg Am 1983;65:213–218
47. Kuslich SD, Ulstrom CL, Griffith SL, et al. The Bagby and Kuslich method of lumbar interbody fusion. History, technique, and 2-year follow-up results of a United States prospective, multicenter trial. Spine 1998;23:1267–1278
48. Kozak JA, O'Brien JP. Simultaneous combined anterior and posterior fusion: an independent analysis of a treatment for the disabled low-back pain patient. Spine 1990;15:322–328
49. Goldner JL, Urbaniak JR, McCollum DE. Anterior disc excision and interbody spinal fusion for chronic low back pain. Orthop Clin North Am 1971;(2):543–568
50. Chow SP, Leong JC, Ma A, Yau AC. Anterior spinal fusion for deranged lumbar intervertebral disc. Spine 1980;5:452–458
51.
52. Forristall RM, Marsh HO, Pay NT. MRI and contrast CT of the lumbar spine: comparison of diagnostic methods and correlation with surgical findings. Spine 1988;13:1049–1054
53. Boden SD, Davis DO, Dina TS, et al. Abnormal magnetic resonance scans of the lumbar spine in asymptomatic subjects: a prospective investigation. J Bone Joint Surg Am 1990;72:403–408
54. Gill K, Blumenthal S. Functional results after anterior lumbar fusions at L5–S1 in patients with normal and abnormal MRI scans. Spine 1992;17:940–942
55. Colhoun E, McCall IW, Williams L, et al. Provocation discography as a guide to planning operation on the spine. J Bone Joint Surg Br 1988;70B:267–271
56. Schwarzer AC, Aprill CN, Derby R, et al. The prevalence and clinical features of internal disc disruption in patients with chronic low back pain. Spine 1995;20:1878–1883
57. Sasso RC, Macadaeg K, Nordmann D, Smith M. Selective nerve root injections can predict surgical outcome for lumbar and cervical radiculopathy: comparison to magnetic resonance imaging. J Spinal Disord Tech 2005;18:471–478
58. Sasso RC, Kitchel SH, Dawson EG. A prospective, randomized controlled clinical trial of anterior lumbar interbody fusion using a titanium cylindrical threaded fusion device. Spine 2004;29:113–122

59. Fraser RD. Interbody, posterior and combined lumbar fusions. Spine 1995;20:S167–S177
60. Burkus JK, Gornet MF, Dickman CA, et al. Anterior lumbar interbody fusion using rhBMP-2 with tapered interbody cages. J Spinal Disord Tech 2002;15:337–349
61. Sasso RC, LeHuec JC, Shaffrey C, et al. Iliac crest bone graft donor site pain after anterior lumbar interbody fusion. J Spinal Disord Tech 2005;18:S77–S81
62. Polly DW, Ackerman SJ, Shaffrey CI, et al. A cost analysis of bone morphogenetic protein versus autologous iliac crest bone graft in single-level anterior lumbar fusion. Orthopedics 2003;26:1027–1037
63. Schofferman J, Slosar P, Reynolds J, et al. A prospective randomized comparison of 270 degree fusions to 360 degree fusions (circumferential fusions). Spine 2001;26:E207–E212
64. Burkus JK, Dorchak JD, Sanders DL. Radiographic assessment of interbody fusion using recombinant human bone morphogenetic protein type 2. Spine 2003;28:372–377
65. Rajaraman V, Vingan R, Roth P, et al. Visceral and vascular complications resulting from anterior lumbar interbody fusion. J Neurosurg 1999;91:60–64
66. O'Brien JP, Dawson MH, Heard CW, et al. Simultaneous combined anterior and posterior fusion. A surgical solution for failed spinal surgery with a brief review of the first 150 patients. Clin Orthop Relat Res 1986;203:191–195
67. Regan JJ, Aronoff RJ, Ohnmeiss DD, Sengupta DK. Laparoscopic approach to L4–L5 for interbody fusion using BAK cages: experience in the first 58 cases. Spine 1999;24:2171–2174
68. Lieberman IH, Willsher PC, Litwin DE, et al. Transperitoneal laparoscopic exposure for lumbar interbody fusion. Spine 2000;25:509–514
69. Liu JC, Ondra SL, Angelos P, et al. Is laparoscopic anterior lumbar interbody fusion a useful minimally invasive procedure? Neurosurgery 2002;51:S155–S158
70. Zdeblick TA, David SM. Laparoscopic versus mini anterior lumbar interbody fusion. Spine 2000;25:2682–2687
71. Chung SK, Lee SH, Lim SR, et al. Comparative study of laparoscopic L5–S1 fusion versus open mini-ALIF, with a minimum 2-year follow-up. Eur Spine J 2003;12:613–617
72. Escobar E, Transfeldt E, Garvey T, et al. Video-assisted versus open anterior lumbar spine fusion surgery: a comparison of four techniques and complications in 135 patients. Spine 2003;28:729–732
73. Sasso RC, Burkus JK, LeHuec JC. Retrograde ejaculation after anterior lumbar interbody fusion. Spine 2003;28:1023–1026
74. Cizek GR, Boyd LM. Imaging pitfalls of interbody spinal implants. 14th Annual Meeting of North American Spine Society, 1999, Chicago
75. McAfee PC. Interbody fusion cages in reconstructive operations on the spine. J Bone Joint Surg Am 1999;81:859–880
76. Heithoff KB, Mullin JW, Holte D, et al. Failure of radiographic detection of pseudoarthrosis in patients with titanium anterior lumbar interbody fusion cages. 14th Annual Meeting of North American Spine Society, 1999, Chicago
77. Weiner BK, Fraser RD. Spine update: lumbar interbody cages. Spine 1998;23:634–640

11 Posterior Lumbar Interbody Fusion

Nirav K. Shah, Mark R. McLaughlin, and Prithvi Narayan

The technique of posterior lumbar interbody fusion (PLIF) was first introduced in 1936, and later successfully adopted by Cloward in 1943. Iliac crest grafts were placed within an excised disk space after an extensive laminectomy and medial facetectomy. PLIF was found to have an overall 75% clinical success rate and 95% fusion rate.[1–3] The addition of pedicle screw fixation to augment interbody fusion did not gain wide acceptance in the past, and was employed largely based on surgeon's preference. We believe there is significant evidence to support the use of posterior segmental fixation to increase the rate of spinal fusion.[4–8] The addition of posterior segmental fixation places the interbody graft under compression and enhances the fusion rate, based on Wolff's law. More importantly, segmental fixation reconstructs the dorsal tension bond. This results in a highly rigid construct, and consequently a shorter time course for improvement of mechanical low back pain, especially in patients with demonstrated segmental instability. Although some surgeons advocate the routine addition of posterolateral intertransverse fusion, the PLIF technique obviates the need for the extra muscle dissection, thus minimizing postoperative pain.

Rarely, intertransverse arthrodesis in addition to PLIF may be indicated in an attempt to increase the likelihood of a successful fusion.

■ Goals

The goals of PLIF are as follows:

1. Improve fusion rates
2. Treat pseudarthrosis
3. Minimize postoperative pain related to intertransverse fusion
4. Serve as a radical diskectomy for recurrent disk herniation
5. Distract the neural foramina
6. Restore spinal alignment related to postlaminectomy kyphosis
7. Minimize postoperative external bracing time

■ The Interbody Device

Numerous interbody devices ranging from carbon fiber to titanium to machined allograft have been described. The shapes and sizes are also variable ranging from large cylindrical dowels to smaller impacted rectangular wedges. We prefer to use rectangular allograft wedges as interbody implants. In our experience, the decreased width of the rectangular wedge makes it is easier to navigate between the exiting and traversing nerve roots compared with the titanium cage or threaded bone dowel. Despite this decreased width, the rectangular implant preserves distraction of the disk space and foramina. By minimizing nerve root retraction through a generous facetectomy, the risk of motor and sensory deficits may be reduced. Furthermore, the rectangular allograft's modulus of elasticity is similar to that of the adjacent vertebral body, giving it extensive structural stability under axial compression. This bony allograft undergoes osseous integration without producing a metallic artifact on postoperative imaging.

The allograft bone products are available in various dimensions allowing customization for different disk spaces.

■ Advantages of Posterior Lumbar Interbody Fusion Over Anterior Lumbar Interbody Fusion

1. Uses a single incision to restore three-column stabilization when supplemented with pedicle screw fixation
2. Minimizes the risk of injury to the great vessels
3. Avoids retrograde ejaculation
4. Avoids gastrointestinal complications

■ Contraindications of Posterior Lumbar Interbody Fusion

1. Back pain in levels above L3, where retraction may cause spinal cord injury
2. Severe osteoporosis
3. Severe epidural fibrosis secondary to prior surgery, which increases the risk of bleeding and dural tears

■ Open Posterior Lumbar Interbody Fusion Technique

Step 1: Positioning the Patient and Preparation

We prefer to use the Jackson operating table with the patient's pressure points appropriately padded to achieve good abdominal decompression as well as to re-create the patient's normal lumbar lordosis and sagittal balance in the prone position. Once the patient is appropriately positioned, prepped, and draped, an appropriate-length midline incision is made. The subcutaneous tissues are divided down to the level of the lumbodorsal fascia. Once the fascia is identified a separate facial plane is dissected laterally to expose the posterior superior iliac spine (PSIS) if autograft harvest is employed.

Step 2: Autologous Iliac Crest Bone Graft Harvest

Harvesting of autologous iliac crest graft is losing popularity as other options such as bone morphogenetic protein (BMP) and other biologic devices are gaining greater acceptance. In patients with severe osteoporosis or smoking history who are at high risk for pseudarthrosis, autograft may still be the preferred option.

The fascia is opened over the PSIS, and the roof of the PSIS is exposed using subperiosteal dissection. A cortical window is opened in the PSIS using osteotomes, taking care to expose the cancellous bone but not to violate the anterior surface of the crest. The quantity of graft harvested is based on the number of levels for arthrodesis. The graft site is then irrigated and the bleeding is controlled with bone wax or other hemostatic agents. The fascia is then closed in a watertight fashion.

Step 3: Bony Exposure

The midline incision is extended deeper and the spinous processes of the appropriate spinal levels are exposed. Using subperiosteal dissection, the paraspinous muscles are dissected laterally to the base of the transverse processes bilaterally. The pars interarticularis (pars) is identified and dissected free. The pars is an important extra canalicular landmark for localizing the pedicle entry site and for identifying the exiting nerve root. It is useful to mark the preliminary pedicle entry sites prior to decompression while the normal anatomic bony landmarks are preserved. The entry sites can be reconfirmed with fluoroscopy and by direct palpation of the pedicle within the canal at the time of screw placement. (The technique of pedicle screw placement has been described elsewhere and is beyond the scope of this chapter.) It is vital to expose the base of the transverse processes and the pars of the superior and inferior vertebra before proceeding with the decompression.

Step 4: Decompression

The spinous processes and lamina are removed using rongeurs. A high-speed drill can be used to thin the entire posterior elements and the bone overlying the lateral recesses. This minimizes blood loss during this portion of the procedure and makes bone removal with a Kerrison

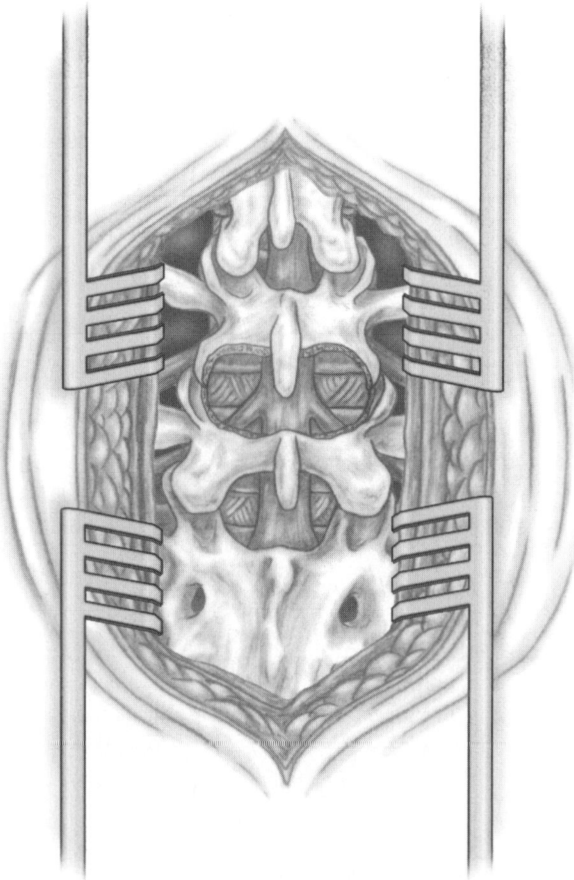

Fig. 11.1 A laminectomy, foraminotomy, and medial facetectomy are performed to expose the exiting and traversing nerve roots. The dissection and bony removal must be adequate enough to allow for minimal retraction of the nerve root while the interbody graft is being placed. (With permission from Medtronic Sofamor Danek.)

rongeur easier. After the decompression is performed, a bone chisel or osteotome is used to remove the medial aspect of the facet joint **(Fig. 11.1)**. Alternatively, in some patients, the spinous process and interspinous ligaments may be preserved. The decompression and access to the disk are accomplished through extensive bilateral laminoforaminotomies.

Step 5: Nerve Root Decompression

After the decompression of the spinal canal is completed, the pedicles of the superior and inferior vertebrae may be clearly visualized. A Woodson dissector is used to follow the course of the nerve laterally into the foramen, ensuring adequate decompression. A foraminotomy may be performed to complete the decompression.

Step 6: Prepare Graft Entry Portal

After the foraminotomy is performed and the remaining lateral recess exposure is completed, the epidural venous

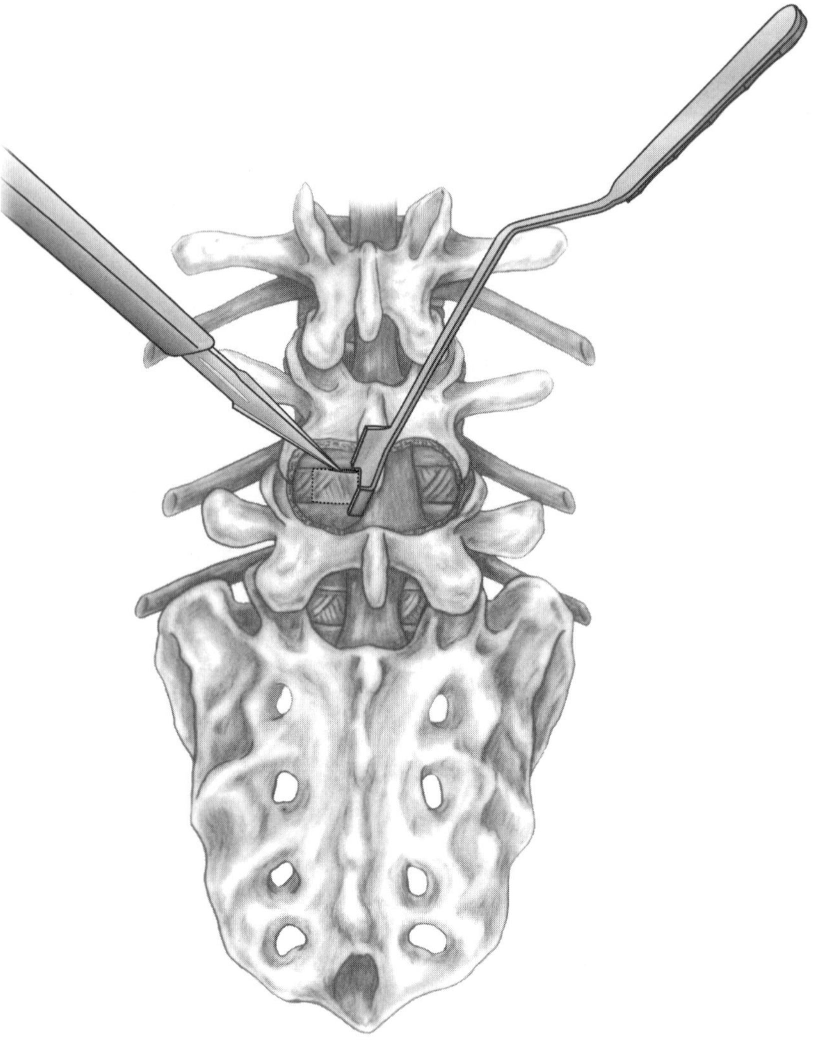

Fig. 11.2 An annulotomy and diskectomy are performed bilaterally, and soft tissue fragments are removed from the intradiskal space. This facilitates the removal of extruded fragments, and decompresses the canal. (With permission from Medtronic Sofamor Danek.)

plexus is identified and coagulated. The superior and inferior nerve roots must be identified, and the venous plexus of the superior nerve root must be carefully coagulated as well. It is important to release the tethering venous plexus to expose the true axilla of the exiting nerve root. This allows for a larger portal of entry for the interbody device and provides greater relaxation of the superior (exiting) nerve root. The combination of medial facetectomy and superior nerve root release minimizes the nerve root traction injury and the risk of durotomy and cerebrospinal fluid (CSF) leakage.

Step 7: Diskectomy

A radical diskectomy is performed after the incision of the annulus **(Fig. 11.2)**. It is performed bilaterally so that the soft fragments within the interspace and any extruded fragments are removed. It should be noted that pedicle screws may be inserted prior to this step to provide distraction of the disk space and foramen. This aggressive decompression allows for treatment of any symptomatic nerve root compression, as well as entry into the disk space for sequential distraction. A complete diskectomy may not be possible if there is a significant disk space collapse.

Step 8: End-Plate Preparation and Graft Placement

The disk space is sequentially dilated/distracted using fluoroscopy until the optimal disk space height is achieved, providing additional foraminal decompression. Distraction is completed by starting with the smallest distractor available **(Fig. 11.3)**. The sizes of the distractors vary from 7 to 14 mm. Once the distractor is tamped into place within the disk space, it is rotated 90 degrees to allow for distraction of the space. The T-handle is removed, attached to the next larger sized distractor, and placed in the contralateral disk space. This is repeated using progressively larger distractors on alternating sides until the optimal disk height is achieved. The final distractor or the largest one is left within the disk space in the distracted position.

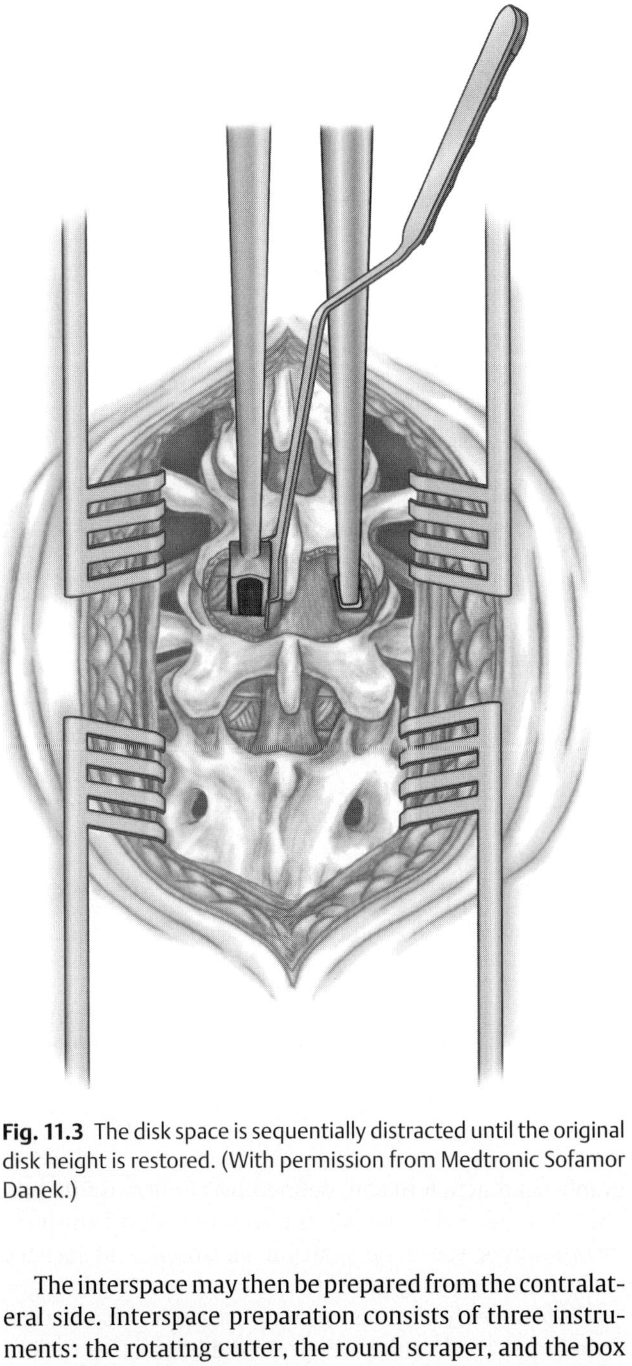

Fig. 11.3 The disk space is sequentially distracted until the original disk height is restored. (With permission from Medtronic Sofamor Danek.)

The interspace may then be prepared from the contralateral side. Interspace preparation consists of three instruments: the rotating cutter, the round scraper, and the box chisel. They are designed to sequentially remove the disk material and to create a channel that exposes the cancellous bone. While placing the rotating cutter, a nerve root retractor is used to gently retract and protect the nerve root. The depth markings on the instrument are used to assess the depth of insertion. The rotating cutter is inserted into the disk space with the cutting blades parallel to the dural sac. The optimal depth is verified by fluoroscopy. The cutter is rotated once or twice to remove osteophytes from the end plate. Removal of the osteophytes facilitates placement of the guides and free-hand chisel. The cutter is then rotated and carefully lifted out. This removes the soft tissue from the disk space. The rotation is continued with sweeping motions with sequentially larger cutters for the safe removal of the disk. This initial end-plate preparation is accomplished from the lateral annulus to the midline.

The remaining soft tissue and cartilaginous end plate are removed using the round scraper **(Fig. 11.4)**. Gentle scraping of the soft tissue with small repetitive motions in an anterior to posterior direction prepares the end plate. This step removes any residual soft tissue on the end plate and optimizes the contact between the bleeding end plate and the bone graft to enhance graft incorporation.

The cutting chisel ensures that the end plates are parallel and essentially creates the optimal channel to receive the impacted allograft wedge. The size of the cutting chisel for end-plate preparation may be determined prior to the surgery. A template overlay can be placed on the radiographic image at the adjacent level to determine the size. Alternatively, the size can be determined by comparison to the distractor size. The cutting chisel size should be ~1 to 2 mm larger than the distractor size. With the dura gently retracted, the guiding tongs of the cutting chisel is seated into the disk space **(Fig. 11.5)**. Under fluoroscopic guidance, the chisel is impacted into the interspace to a maximum depth of 30 mm. This depth may vary among patients. After impacting the cutting chisel to the desired depth, the slap hammer is attached to the chisel handle and rotated 90 degrees. The chisel is removed with a gentle upward stroke.

After the cutting chisel is removed, a distractor 1 mm larger than the expected wedge size is placed into the prepared disk space and rotated 90 degrees to maintain the disk space height. The distractor from the contralateral side is then removed, and the contralateral disk space is prepared as described above. Insertion of the interbody graft is not recommended until preparation of the entire disk space has been completed.

Once the end-plate preparation is complete, the wedge height and length is determined and appropriate grafts are chosen and prepared. The wedge height is determined by the preoperative template provided or based on the cutting chisel size (8, 10, or 12 mm). The length of the allograft wedge is determined by evaluation of the preoperative radiographs and the templating process as well as by intraoperative fluoroscopy. The appropriate-sized wedge is firmly attached to the inserter with a threaded trocar **(Fig. 11.6)**. The wedge is then gently impacted into the disk space at the appropriate angle until the implant is countersunk ~3 to 4 mm.

Step 9: Autograft Placement

Once the allograft wedge has been inserted on the contralateral side, the disk distractor is removed from the ipsilateral side, and morcellized autograft is packed into the prepared disk space between the midline structures. A second allograft wedge may then be inserted into the disk space along the previously prepared channel. Once it is

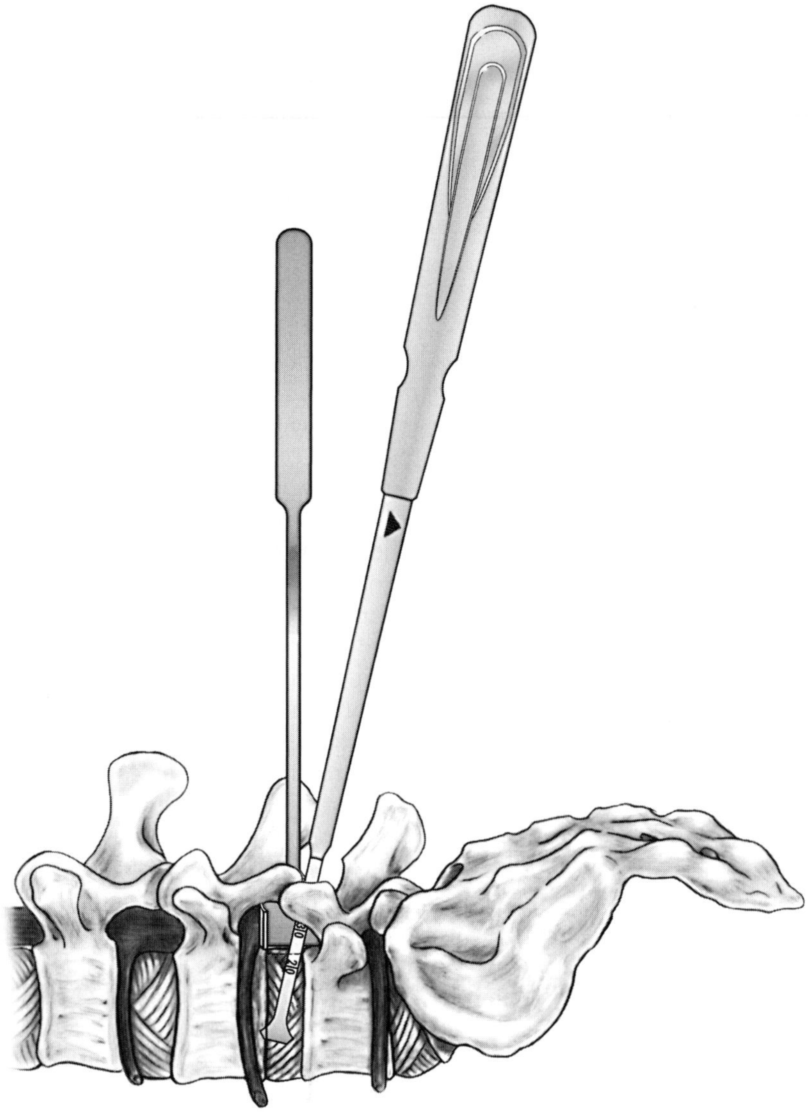

Fig. 11.4 The remaining soft tissue and cartilaginous end-plate coverings are removed from the end plate using the round scraper. (With permission from Medtronic Sofamor Danek.)

seated and the inserter is removed, any residual space between the wedge and the annulus may be filled with the remaining autograft **(Fig. 11.7)**.

■ Discussion

The overall assessment of PLIF results is extremely variable.[9] Limitations of some published reports in the past include concentration on the technique and relatively sparse short-term clinical follow-up.[10] More recent studies concentrate on outcome measures including radiographic and clinical outcomes. Radiographic measures allow very reliable comparisons of fusion rates and hardware complications among different studies.

Radiographic outcome measures of the various interbody options (titanium cages, threaded cortical bone dowel, rectangular bone wedges) include stability, defined by the absence of movement on flexion/extension radiographs, and actual fusion, defined by an increase in subchondral end-plate sclerosis, the presence of bridging bone incorporating the bone graft, or an absence of lucency around the interbody graft.[11]

Unfortunately, there is no consensus as to what the criterion for a good clinical result should be, such as the absence of residual pain, the absence of pain by relying on medication, good pain management on a continuing basis, or the ability to return to work.[10] Furthermore, clinical outcomes may be influenced by intraoperative complications including CSF leak or nerve traction injury. Recent studies not only demonstrate comprehensive radiographic data but also include more clinical outcome variables, such as the Prolo outcome measures, to demonstrate the overall efficacy of PLIF.

Review of recent PLIF results show that titanium cages without pedicle screw supplementation had a 91% stability rate.[12,13] Fusion rates could not be adequately assessed due to radiographic artifact created by the cages despite

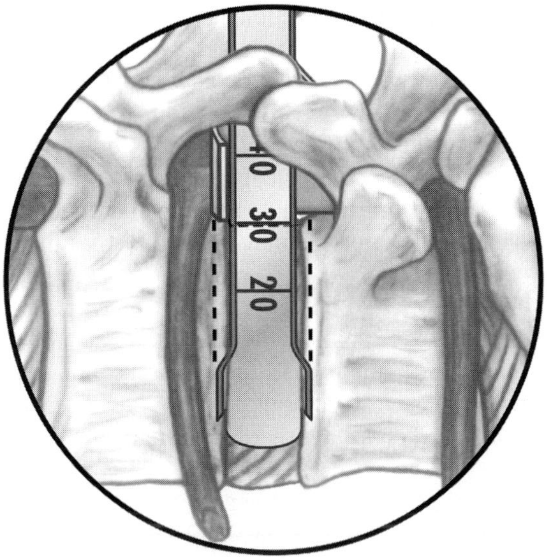

Fig. 11.5 Final end-plate preparation is performed with the use of the cutting chisel. The chisel is impacted into the disk space to a maximum depth of 30 mm. The dura is gently retracted. (With permission from Medtronic Sofamor Danek.)

computed tomography (CT) reconstructions. A 100% stability rate was noted on titanium cages supplemented with pedicle screw fixation along with a 95% fusion rate at the 1-year follow-up. Studies show consistent stability and fusion rates using rectangular bone wedges when supplemented with pedicle screw fixation. Overall, it appears that the various interbody devices may provide similar stability

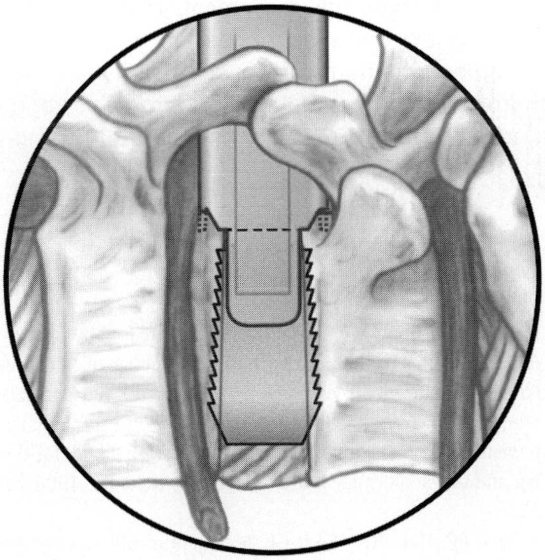

Fig. 11.6 The Tangent wedge is attached to the inserter with a threaded trocar. The wedge is then gently impacted into the interspace until it is 3 to 4 mm below the posterior margin of the vertebral body. (With permission from Medtronic Sofamor Danek. The Tangent® Impacted Posterior Instrument Set incorporates technology developed by Gary K. Michelson, MD.)

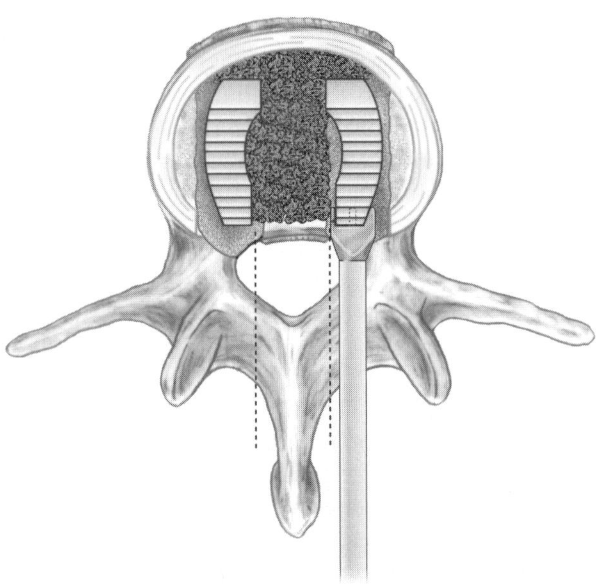

Fig. 11.7 Once the grafts are properly seated, segmental fixation may be applied using a standard technique. (With permission from Medtronic Sofamor Danek.)

whether they are stand-alone or augmented with pedicle screws, but the fusion rates are consistently improved with the latter.

Although the radiographic outcomes remained consistent among the various interbody grafts, clinical outcome measures did vary. Studies that combined both the stand-alone and pedicle screw augmented PLIF metallic/titanium devices showed a 10% incidence of transient nerve root injury and a 5% incidence of permanent nerve injury. On the other hand, use of the smaller rectangular bone wedges showed less than 1% permanent nerve root injuries.[14] The decreased incidence of nerve root injury in patients implanted with rectangular bone wedges is likely due to the decreased nerve root retraction compared with cylindrical dowels/cages. The incidence of CSF leak was 9% with titanium cages versus 1% with rectangular bone grafts.

In summary, good subjective clinical outcomes have been consistently demonstrated with the use of all types of interbody devices. In fact, multiple studies show overall satisfactory results, defined as excellent or good Prolo outcomes, to be 70% or greater.[14] Furthermore, there appears to be no significant statistical difference in clinical PLIF outcomes among various age groups.[15]

■ Minimally Invasive Posterior Lumbar Interbody Fusion Technique

The positioning of the patient is similar to that in the open technique. Using a biplanar or a two C-arm system, the surgeon must localize the superolateral aspects of the caudal and cranial pedicles bilaterally. Some systems advocate using a Kirschner wire (K-wire) overlying the pedicles to help this localization. This technique then employs incisions ~4 cm to the side of the midline bilaterally. An incision is made through the subcutaneous tissue and through the fascia to facilitate tissue dilation. Sequential dilators are used to split the muscle with the tubes centered between both pedicles. Retractors are then carefully placed over these dilators and the position confirmed by C-arm. The tubular retractor has the potential to expand once it is docked in place. The muscle splitting rather than subperiosteal dissection is the single most important advantage of this technique. Once the retractor is docked in position and expanded, it is held in place by ipsilateral fixation to the Jackson table. The retractor can be manipulated to various angulations to help visualize the anatomy clearly. Also, most retractors are expandable to allow for further anatomic detail. We prefer using the operative microscope to see through the tube, taking advantage of its light source. Bayoneted instruments including the drill, curets, and Kerrison rongeurs are quite useful to expand the surgeon's field of vision.

Once the appropriate level has been identified, ~50% of the caudal facet is drilled down along with its adjoining lamina and removed carefully. Once this is achieved, the traversing nerve root and axilla should be visible. With gentle retraction of the nerve root the interbody graft technique is completed as described above in the open procedure. Posterior instrumentation can then be placed through these incisions once the retractors are removed.

Early studies comparing minimally invasive approaches to traditional open surgeries show favorable results in terms of blood loss, less transfusion need, less postoperative back pain, quicker recovery, decreased muscle damage, and shorter hospital stay.[16] Minimally invasive PLIF also showed a similar surgical efficacy to the traditional open technique in the hands of experienced surgeons. However, the minimally invasive technique has a steep learning curve.[17]

Prospective studies with longer follow-ups are needed to determine the long-term benefits of minimally invasive PLIF. Intuitively, the major advantage of minimally invasive PLIF lies in the minimization of trauma to the muscles by using a muscle splitting technique rather than subperiosteal dissection, likely reducing the incidence of failed-back syndrome. In fact, postoperative atrophy of the paraspinal muscles may lead to further instability and persistent back pain. The level of serum creatine phosphokinase (CPK) has been shown to correlate with postoperative back pain. Studies have shown an increased serum CPK with open PLIF techniques compared with minimally invasive techniques.[16] This has given an impetus to the increased use of minimally invasive PLIF techniques.

■ Conclusion

Degenerative lumbar disk disease surgery has undergone tremendous changes over the past 30 to 40 years. Nevertheless, the idea that bone under compression leads to fusion is a time-tested axiom and remains the core principle of modern arthrodesis technique. The use of interbody devices has grown with our knowledge of lumbar anatomy and the use of pedicle screw instrumentation. The shape and size of this implant must allow for minimal disruption and injury to the existing structures. Furthermore, the placement of this interbody device should be familiar to most spinal surgeons. The modern era of spinal arthrodesis involves achieving better fusion rates through improved bone on bone contact. Interbody devices are successfully leading this movement. The future of spine surgery will expand and improve on interbody devices and techniques for minimally invasive placement not only to improve fusion rates but also to decrease postoperative pain and to improve recovery and surgical outcomes as well.

References

1. Branch CL. The case for posterior lumbar interbody fusion. Clin Neurosurg 1996;43:252–267
2. Cloward RB. The treatment of ruptured lumbar intervertebral discs by vertebral body fusion. J Neurosurg 1953;10:154–168
3. Dunsker SB. Lumbar spine stabilization: Indications. In: Black PM, ed. Clinical Neurosurgery, vol 36. Baltimore: Williams & Wilkins, 1998:147–158
4. Roy-Camille R, Saillant G, Mazel C. Internal fixation of the lumbar spine with pedicle screw plating. Clin Orthop Relat Res 1986;203:7–17
5. Zdeblick TA. A prospective, randomized study of lumbar fusion: Preliminary results. Spine 1993;18:983–991
6. Haid RW, Dickman CA. Instrumentation and fusion for discogenic disease of the lumbar spine. Neurosurg Clin N Am 1993;4:135–148
7. Haid RW, Morone MA. Spondylisthesis and spondylosis. In: Tindell GT, Cooper PR, Barrow DL, eds. The Practice of Neurosurgery. Baltimore: Lippincott Williams & Wilkins, 1996:2541–2560
8. Steffee AD, Biscup RS, Sitkowski DJ. Segmental spine plates with pedicle screw fixation: A new internal fixation device for the lumbar and thoracolumbar spine. Clin Orthop Relat Res 1986;203:45–53
9. Subach BR, Haid RW, Rodt GE, McLaughlin MR. Do current outcomes data support the technique of lumbar interbody fusion? Clin Neurosurg 2001;48:204–218
10. Simmons JW. Posterior lumbar interbody fusion. In: Frymoyer JW, ed. The Adult Spine. New York: Raven Press, 1991:1961–1987
11. McLaughlin MR, Haid RW, Rodts GE, Subach BR. Posterior lumbar interbody fusion: indications, techniques, and results. Clin Neurosurg 2000;47:514–527

12. Barnes B, McLaughlin MR, Birch B, et al. Threaded cortical bone dowels for lumbar fusion: Technique and short term results. Neurosurg Focus 1999;7:1–4
13. Barnes B, Rodts GE, McLaughlin MR, et al. Threaded cortical bone dowels for lumbar interbody fusion: Over 1-year mean follow-up in 28 patients. J Neurosurg 2001;95:1–4
14. McLaughlin MR, Barnes B, Rodts G. PLIF with allograft bone: Preliminary results comparing cylindrical dowels and impacted wedges. SpineUniverse.com.
15. Okuda S, Oda T, Miyauchi A, Haku T, Yamamoto T, Iwasaki M. Surgical outcomes of posterior lumbar interbody fusion in elderly patients. J Bone Joint Surg Am 2006;88:2714–2720
16. Suwa H, Hanakita J, Ohshita N, Gotoh K, Matsuoka N, Morizane A. Postoperative changes in paraspinal muscle thickness after various lumbar back surgery procedures. Neurol Med Chir (Tokyo) 2000;40:151–155
17. Salerni AA. A minimally invasive approach for posterior lumbar interbody fusion. Neurosurg Focus 2002;13:e6

12 Transforaminal Lumbar Interbody Fusion

David W. Polly Jr. and Edward Rainier G. Santos

Transforaminal lumbar interbody fusion (TLIF) has gained popularity in the treatment of various spinal disorders such as degenerative disk disease, spondylolisthesis, sagittal and coronal plane imbalance, and degenerative scoliosis.[1–10] This technique was originally described by Horst Blume[11] in 1985 and popularized by Harms and Jeszensky.[12] TLIF enables the performance of a circumferential arthrodesis with a single posterior approach through the foramen. Recent series have shown excellent fusion rates, correction of deformity, and clinical results with this technique.[1,2,4]

Transforaminal lumbar interbody fusion offers several advantages over other techniques of interbody fusion such as anterior lumbar interbody fusion (ALIF) and posterior lumbar interbody fusion (PLIF). ALIF is appealing because the exposure facilitates excellent clearance of the disk space, thereby increasing fusion rates. At the same time, the wide anterior annular release allows excellent restoration of disk space height and segmental lordosis. However, the anterior approach carries many possible complications, including retrograde ejaculation, vessel and ureteral injury, prolonged ileus, and lymphatic accumulation.[13]

The PLIF technique is similar to TLIF in that a separate anterior approach is not performed. However, TLIF eliminates many of the drawbacks seen with PLIF.[14] The ligamentum flavum and interspinous ligaments are preserved with TLIF. Furthermore, the more lateral approach makes dural retraction unnecessary, thereby decreasing the incidence of neural injury and dural tears.

Surgical Technique

The patient is placed under general anesthesia and positioned prone on either a Wilson frame or a four-poster frame. The abdomen must be free from any pressure to decrease intraoperative venous bleeding. The table must be radiolucent to allow intraoperative fluoroscopy if necessary.

After routine prepping and draping, a straight midline incision is made over the involved vertebrae. Dissection is carried through the subcutaneous tissues and onto the lumbodorsal fascia. At this point, there are two options for the fascial incision. If a concomitant decompression procedure is necessary, a midline fascial incision is made down to the spinous processes. Subperiosteal dissection is then performed to expose the lamina, facets, and transverse processes bilaterally. This facilitates performance of a decompressive procedure along with the TLIF.

If decompression is not necessary, the fascial incisions can be made bilaterally, approximately one and a half fingerbreadths lateral to the midline. Blunt dissection is then performed between the multifidus and longissimus muscles, to expose the pars interarticularis, facet joints, and transverse processes of the relevant segments.

The next crucial step is the induction of local kyphosis. This can be done in two ways. The first method is by pedicle screw instrumentation and distraction. If the patient has significant radicular symptoms, this is performed contralateral to the symptomatic side. After adequate exposure of the facet joint, pars, and transverse processes, the pedicle screws are inserted in a standard manner. A temporary distraction rod is then placed and locked in distraction. This facilitates exposure of the disk during the diskectomy. Alternatively, a distraction device that directly attaches to the pedicle screw heads may be used **(Fig. 12.1).** It must be noted that this distraction maneuver puts significant stress on the bone–screw interface, and pedicle fracture has occurred using this technique.

An alternative strategy is to use a crankable Wilson frame that allows the induction of kyphosis for the interbody work and then the restoration of lordosis at the end by cranking the frame down **(Fig. 12.2)**. When using the radiolucent crankable Wilson frame in conjunction with the Jackson table, excellent intraoperative anteroposterior (AP) and lateral fluoroscopy can still be achieved.

After adequate distraction is achieved, all soft tissues overlying the facet joint and pars interarticularis are removed. Excision of the facet joint is then is then performed. Using a ¼ inch straight osteotome, the inferior facet of the superior vertebra is resected. This osteotomy typically requires a vertical or oblique medial limb, and a transverse limb through the pars interarticularis **(Fig. 12.3).** Extreme care must be exercised so that the osteotomy does not extend into the pedicle superiorly. Angled curets are then used to remove the facet fragment, which is then cleaned of cartilage and soft tissues, milled, and saved.

The superior facet of the lower vertebra is then resected utilizing a ¼ inch osteotome or a high-speed drill **(Fig. 12.4)**. Resection is carried medially and inferiorly to the superior border of the pedicle. This may also require the use of Kerrison rongeurs so that the facet resection is

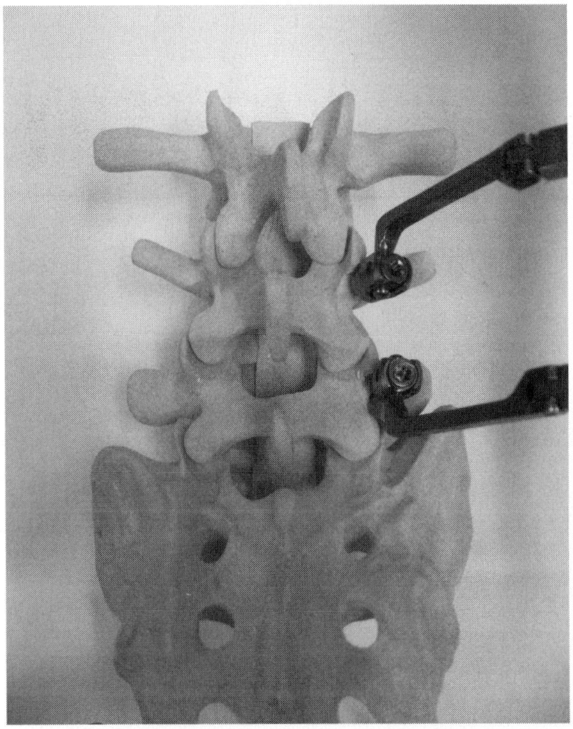

Fig. 12.1 Pedicle screw distraction device to induce local kyphosis.

flush to the superior pedicle wall. The lateral portion of the ligamentum flavum may be preserved because this protects the traversing nerve root. Blunt dissection is then performed with a Penfield dissector to expose the disk. There are usually capsular remnants and other soft tissues that need to be removed, as well as epidural veins that must be cauterized with a bipolar electrocautery. The exiting nerve and dorsal root ganglion (DRG), which are located in the superior portion of the foramen, should not be visualized. Placement of a cottonoid strip in the superior aspect of the foramen is helpful with retraction of soft tissues, as well as for protection of the exiting nerve and DRG.

Once there is adequate visualization of the disk space, an annulotomy is performed using a No. 15 blade **(Fig. 12.5).** This annular window typically measures 1.5 by 0.5 cm. The next step involves the use of a ¼ inch osteotome to remove the superior posterior lip of the inferior vertebra. This step is necessary because of the concave shape of the lumbar vertebral end plates. This step increases the working channel to the disk space by 2 to 4 mm and shifts the working area inferiorly and away from the exiting nerve.[1] Doing the same resection of the inferior posterior lip of the cephalad vertebra may also further increase the working channel. However, this vertebra often is just ventral to the DRG. Because of the sensitivity of the DRG, this step

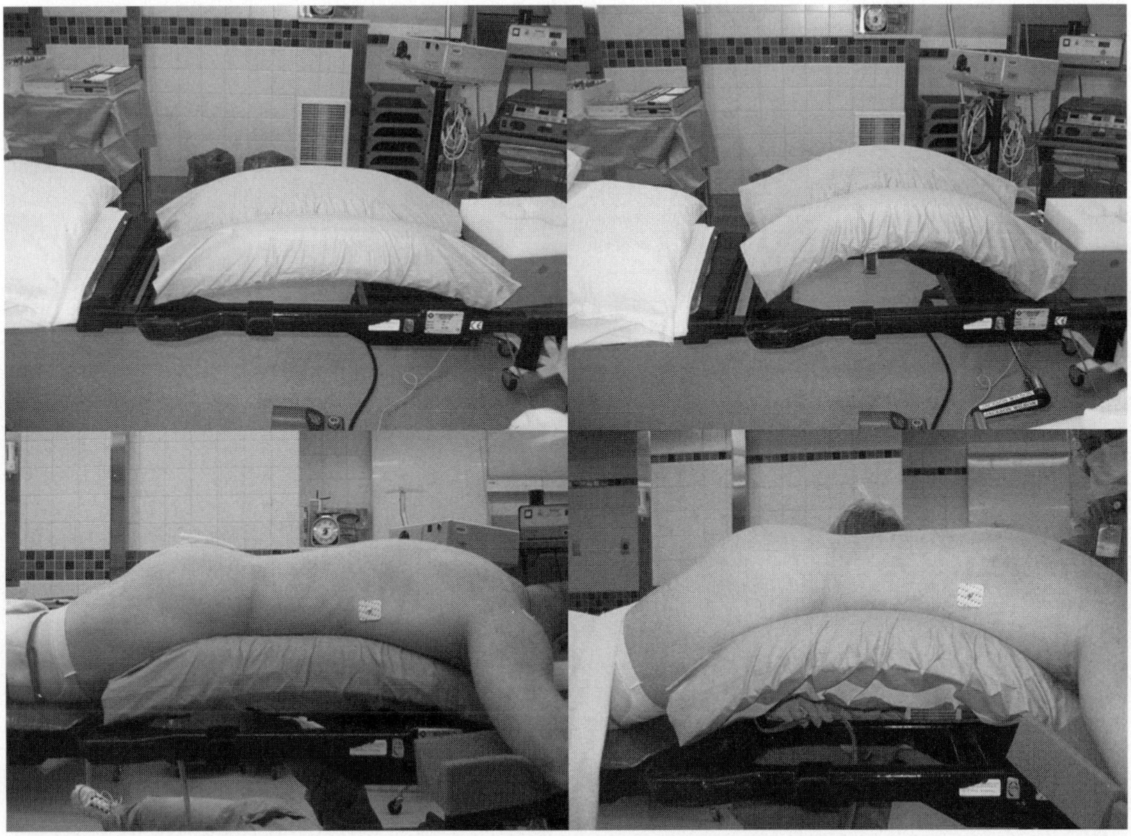

Fig. 12.2 The use of a crankable Wilson frame in TLIF facilitates local kyphosis induction.

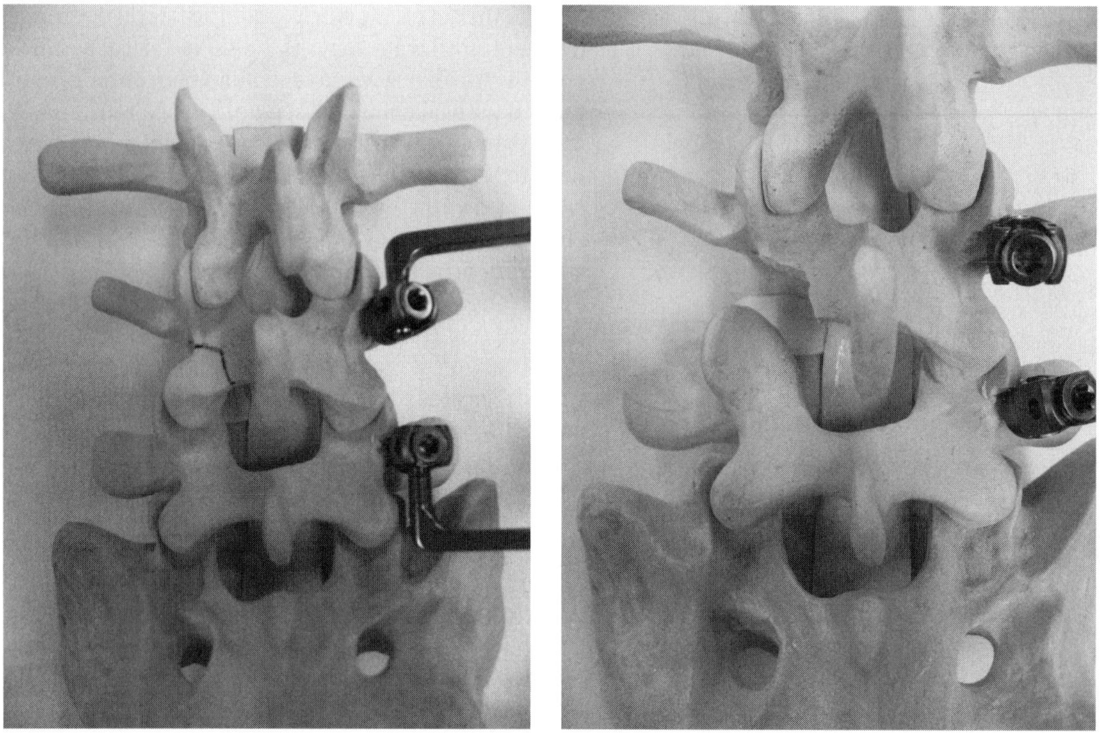

A B

Fig. 12.3 (A,B) Resection of the descending facet.

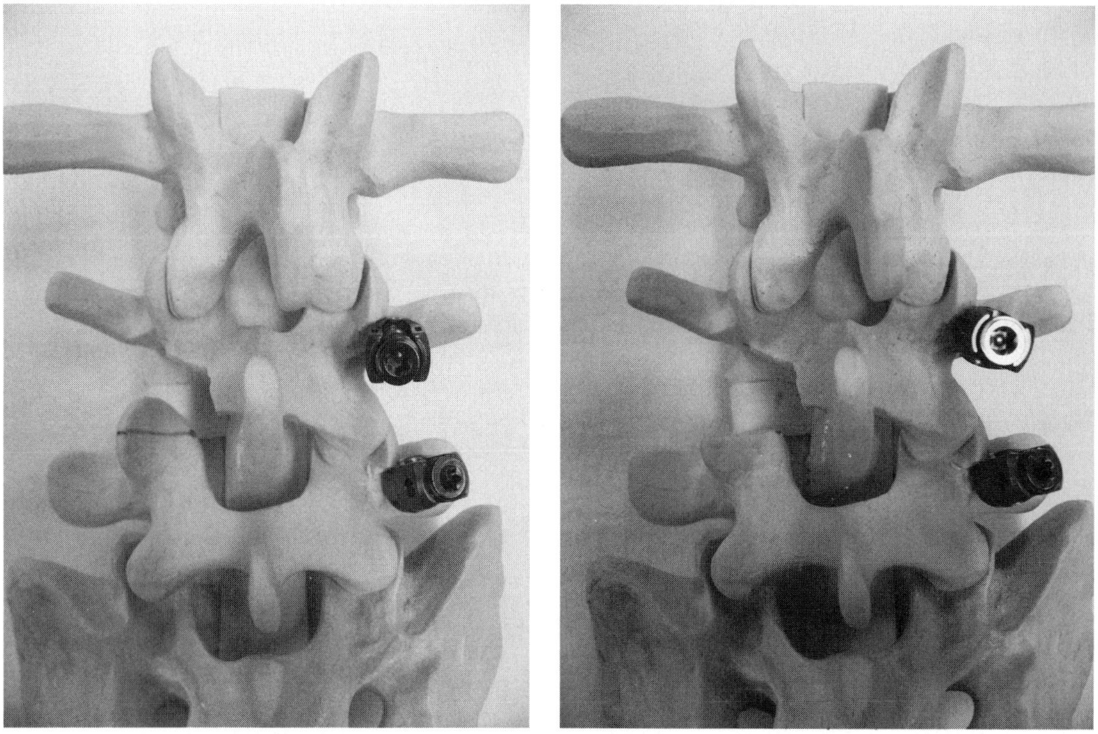

A B

Fig. 12.4 (A,B) Resection of the ascending facet.

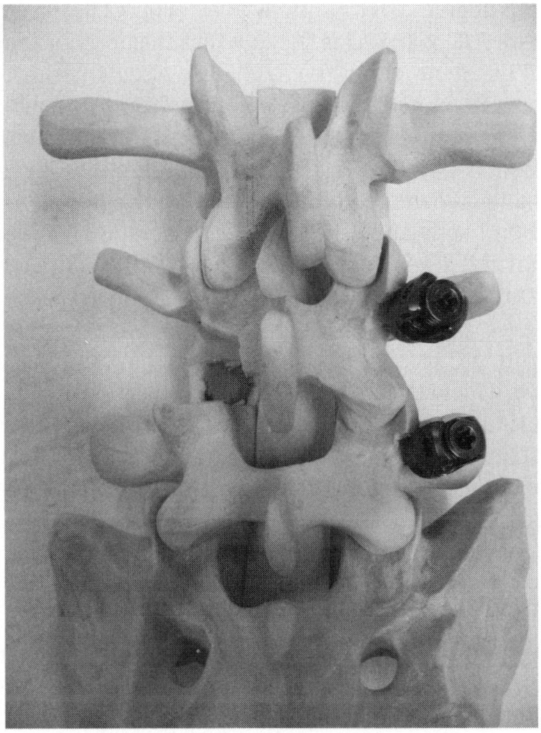

Fig. 12.5 Annulotomy to facilitate diskectomy.

carries significant risk. In general, it may be best to leave the DRG undisturbed. By identifying the caudal vertebra rostral pedicle margin at the disk space and sweeping the fat and nerve root cephalad with a cottonoid strip, the DRG is at less risk. In addition, the local kyphosis induction with the Wilson frame usually moves the DRG and exiting root out of the way.

The next key step is adequate removal of disk material. Specially designed curets and rongeurs are used to perform a near-total diskectomy. These instrumentation systems designed specifically for TLIF are widely available. Closkey et al[15] in 1993 demonstrated that fusion involving 30% of the cross-sectional area of the disk space was necessary for the trabecular bone to have adequate strength to carry physiologic loads. Studies have shown that a unilateral TLIF can remove approximately 55% or 11.8 cc of the disk material, and bilateral TLIF can remove 81% or 16.8 cc of the material.[16] This was in a setting where the operating surgeon was intentionally aggressive in removing the disk. Obviously, the amount of disk material removed is dependent on the disk volume so that significantly degenerated disks will have less volume available for removal. However, the percentages seem to be consistent. The disk not removed is typically the anterior and lateral annulus, which should not be removed with this technique because of the risk of vascular and visceral injury. In addition, the lateral and anterior annulus serves to contain the bone graft material within the disk space. The development of advanced bayoneted instruments may make unilateral TLIF more efficient.

Once the disk has been cleared out, adequate bone grafting is critical. A 3-cc syringe with its end cut off is probably the best way to deliver the bone graft into the disk space. Autologous iliac crest graft can be used. However, local bone from the facetectomies, as well as bone from any decompressive procedures usually suffices. The disk space should be able to handle a total volume of graft material of at least 12 cc. It is very common to be able to handle more.

The strategy of where to place the graft and where to place the structural implants has been a matter of some debate. The concept of placing graft material up against the anterior annulus allows for the development of a "sentinel sign" that can be seen on plain films. When present, confidence is high that there is a solid fusion. Placing a large volume of graft material anteriorly can preclude anterior cage placement, but up to 6 cc of graft can routinely be placed and not compromise anterior cage placement.

After placement of the bone graft, structural interbody support is placed. The choice of structural interbody support has also been a matter of debate. Two cylindrical titanium mesh cages were used early on because of availability and strength. The first one was inserted and rolled across to the contralateral side. Another cage was then placed next to it. Packing the vertically oriented cages with bone increased the volume of bone graft to achieve a fusion and probably increased the surface load-bearing area, thereby lessening the probability of settling. However, placement of two titanium cages can be technically challenging. Structural allograft bone is also being used in a variety of formats. Typically, this is either native cortical bone or processed allograft with the properties of solid cortical bone. Healing and remodeling of such a piece of allograft is not as reliable as autogenous cancellous bone. A variety of bioresorbable implants can also be used and have shown good radiologic and clinical results.[17] Further development of TLIF structural interbody support has progressed to a crescent-shaped one-piece implant. These implants are made of carbon fiber or polyether-ether-ketone (PEEK). The advantages include excellent structural support and radiolucency, allowing accurate assessment of fusion status. Furthermore, the crescent shape facilitates easier placement of the graft within the disk space.

There has been great debate about where the cages should be placed to minimize settling. Theoretically, the area where bone is most dense is in the ring apophysis. The end plate itself is less dense, and is really just condensed cancellous bone throughout the majority of its surface. However, the ring apophysis is only several millimeters wide, and placement of a structural interbody support on the ring apophysis, although optimal, requires very eccentric placement. Placement of cages anteriorly and in the midportion of the disk space has yielded good clinical and radiologic results. This location also allows placement of bone graft anteriorly on the disk space, which is desirable.

The availability of recombinant human bone morphogenetic protein (BMP) has changed many surgeons' approach to choice of bone graft. By using local bone (from the facet resection and products of decompression), supplemented with allograft bone and BMP, donor-site morbidity is avoided. The supplemental use of BMP in one series led to a 99% interbody fusion rate.[1]

■ Transforaminal Lumbar Interbody Fusion for Deformity Correction

Sagittal Plane Correction

Transforaminal lumbar interbody fusion can be a sagittal plane deformity correction strategy. When done in such a way as to place the implant in an anterior position, and then by applying posterior compression, lordosis restoration or even lordosis enhancement can be achieved. There is significant lordosis improvement compared with cylindrical screw in cages from a PLIF application.[18] Also, the vertically oriented mesh was better at restoring lordosis than even lordotic wedge-shaped structural allograft bone.[18]

When a bilateral TLIF approach is used, it functions similarly to a Smith-Petersen osteotomy (SPO). This allows substantial sagittal plane lordosis production of as much as 8 to 15 degrees over multiple levels **(Fig. 12.6)**. An advantage of TLIF over SPO is the fact that the anterior longitudinal ligament is preserved. The use of an anterior interbody graft in TLIF leads to pivoting mechanics, which is different from an SPO. In TLIF, the maximum achievable lordosis is based on the anterior annulus/anterior longitudinal ligament height and then posterior bone-on-bone vertebral body apposition. If this is attempted with a unilateral TLIF, then contralateral foraminal stenosis can result. In addition, if adequate height of the interspace is not achieved, there is the potential for central stenosis. But with appropriate facet resections, the foramen and lateral recess is widely decompressed. Bony apposition occurs centrally initially between the spinous processes (analogous to Baastrup phenomenon). Additional resection of the caudal edge of the suprajacent spinous process will allow further lordosation.

Coronal Plane Correction

Correction of coronal plane deformities can be achieved to a modest degree as well. TLIF can be done in an asymmetric function, resulting in correction of segmental coronal plane deformity. The primary strategy is to restore the disk space height in the concavity by inserting the biggest possible structural graft on that side. This concept of asymmetric cage placement to facilitate deformity correction has been espoused and initially adopted enthusiastically by many surgeons. However, only modest correction is achieved, and this application of TLIF has not been as

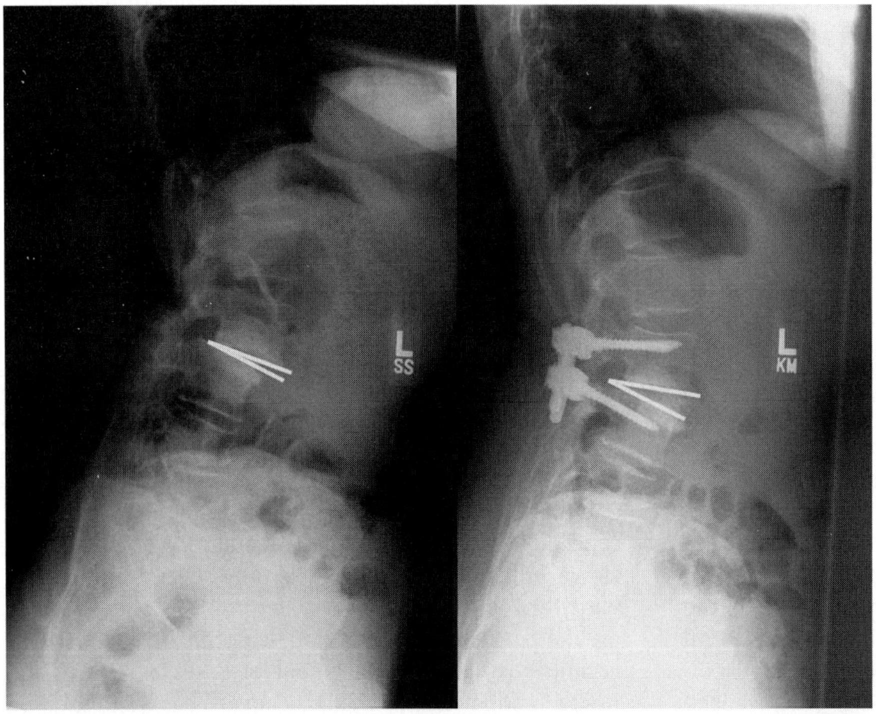

Fig. 12.6 Preoperative and postoperative x-rays showing correction of segmental kyphosis with bilateral TLIF.

widely practiced. A compression maneuver in the convexity of the scoliosis can also be helpful, but one must ensure that iatrogenic foraminal stenosis does not occur. Significant coronal deformity correction can be achieved through a wide facet resection bilaterally, a technique that is analogous to the wide posterior release described by Shufflebarger and Clark.[19]

■ Conclusion

We have described the basic techniques involved in TLIF for the treatment of degenerative lumbar conditions. Significant sagittal and coronal plane deformity correction can be achieved if necessary.

References

1. Anand N, Hamilton JF, Perri B, et al. Cantilever TLIF with structural allograft and RhBMP2 for correction and maintenance of segmental sagittal lordosis: long-term clinical, radiographic, and functional outcome. Spine 2006;31:E748–E753
2. Hackenberg L, Halm H, Bullmann V, et al. Transforaminal lumbar interbody fusion: a safe technique with satisfactory three to five year results. Eur Spine J 2005;14:551–558
3. Houten JK, Post NH, Dryer JW, et al. Clinical and radiographically/neuroimaging documented outcome in transforaminal lumbar interbody fusion. Neurosurg Focus 2006;20:E8
4. Lauber S, Schulte TL, Liljenqvist U, et al. Clinical and radiologic 2–4-year results of transforaminal lumbar interbody fusion in degenerative and isthmic spondylolisthesis grades 1 and 2. Spine 2006;31:1693–1698
5. Lowe TG, Tahernia AD, O'Brien MF, et al. Unilateral transforaminal posterior lumbar interbody fusion (TLIF): indications, technique, and 2-year results. J Spinal Disord Tech 2002;15:31–38
6. Moskowitz A. Transforaminal lumbar interbody fusion. Orthop Clin North Am 2002;33:359–366
7. Potter BK, Freedman BA, Verwiebe EG, et al. Transforaminal lumbar interbody fusion: clinical and radiographic results and complications in 100 consecutive patients. J Spinal Disord Tech 2005;18:337–346
8. Rosenberg WS, Mummaneni PV. Transforaminal lumbar interbody fusion: technique, complications, and early results. Neurosurgery 2001;48:569–574
9. Salehi SA, Tawk R, Ganju A, et al. Transforaminal lumbar interbody fusion: surgical technique and results in 24 patients. Neurosurgery 2004;54:368–374
10. Weiner BK, Nguyen HV, Hazard SW. Transforaminal lumbar interbody fusion: an independent assessment of outcomes in a difficult patient population. Med Sci Monit 2006;12:CR99–CR102
11. Blume HG. Unilateral posterior lumbar interbody fusion: simplified dowel technique. Clin Orthop Relat Res 1985;75–84
12. Harms JG, Jeszensky D. The unilateral, transforaminal approach for posterior lumbar interbody fusion. [in German] Oper Orthop Traumatol 1998;10:90–102
13. Villavicencio AT, Burneikiene S, Bulsara KR, et al. Perioperative complications in transforaminal lumbar interbody fusion versus anterior-posterior reconstruction for lumbar disc degeneration and instability. J Spinal Disord Tech 2006;19:92–97
14. Humphreys SC, Hodges SD, Patwardhan AG, et al. Comparison of posterior and transforaminal approaches to lumbar interbody fusion. Spine 2001;26:567–571
15. Closkey RF, Parsons JR, Lee CK, et al. Mechanics of interbody spinal fusion. Analysis of critical bone graft area. Spine 1993;18:1011–1015
16. Javernick MA, Kuklo TR, Polly DW. Transforaminal lumbar interbody fusion: unilateral versus bilateral disk removal–an in vivo study. Am J Orthop 2003;32:344–348
17. Coe JD, Vaccaro AR. Instrumented transforaminal lumbar interbody fusion with bioresorbable polymer implants and iliac crest autograft. Spine 2005;30:S76–S83
18. Groth AT, Kuklo TR, Klemme WR, et al. Comparison of sagittal contour and posterior disc height following interbody fusion: threaded cylindrical cages versus structural allograft versus vertical cages. J Spinal Disord Tech 2005;18:332–336
19. Shufflebarger HL, Clark CE. Effect of wide posterior release on correction in adolescent idiopathic scoliosis. J Pediatr Orthop B 1998;7:117–123

13 Minimally Incisional Transforaminal Lumbar Interbody Fusion

Praveen V. Mummaneni, Daniel C. Lu, and John H. Chi

In 1982, Harmsand Rolinger[1] described the transforaminal lumbar interbody fusion (TLIF) technique to create a 360-degree fusion via a single posterolateral approach. In the TLIF procedure, bone graft and an interbody spacer are placed via a posterolateral transforaminal route into a distracted disk space in conjunction with a supplemental pedicle screw construct. The safety and efficacy of TLIF has been demonstrated by several authors.[2–10]We have previously described the indications and contraindications for the TLIF (**Tables 13.1** and **13.2**).[5,6]

■ The Versa–Lumbar Interbody Fusion

The evolution of the TLIF procedure over the past 5 years has led to the development of a versatile approach to posterolateral lumbar interbody fusion that can be tailored to a patient's specific needs. We have named this versatile TLIF the versa–lumbar interbody fusion (VLIF).[5,6] For patients in whom a TLIF is indicated, the surgeon must choose which approach to use. An open approach may be selected as the best approach in cases involving multiple levels of surgery (e.g., deformity surgery). Conversely, a mini-open approach (using an expandable tubular retractor) or a minimally invasive approach (using a nonexpendable tubular retractor with percutaneous pedicle screws[11]) may be selected as the best-suited approach for patients who require a one- or two-level approach (**Table 13.3**). We avoid use of the minimally incisional TLIF in patients with scoliosis due to the difficulty with fluoroscopic imaging of the TLIF levels. We also avoid use of the minimally incisional TLIF in patients whose soft tissues are deeper than 8 cm from the skin to the bone due to difficulty positioning the retractors and the hardware at such depths. This chapter focuses on the single-level mini-open TLIF.

■ Operative Considerations

Patient Positioning

Optimal intraoperative positioning of the patient is critical to achieving success with the mini-open TLIF. We prefer to position patients prone on a standard operating table, using chest rolls to re-create physiologic lumbar lordosis. The operating table is placed in the reverse position with the base of the table under the patient's knees. This allows for intraoperative lateral fluoroscopy while avoiding the collision of the fluoroscope with the base of the operating table. The surgeon must avoid placing the patient in a flat-back or kyphotic position prior to performing the TLIF because the patient may be fused into that nonphysiologic position. For this reason, we do not perform lumbar fusions on a Wilson frame. Alternatively, if the surgeon positions the patient in lumbar hyperlordosis, then the procedure will become more difficult due to closure of the posterior disk space. In particular, obese patients with a large abdominal pannus who are positioned on an open bottom operating table are prone to being in hyperlordosis due to the effect of gravity on their pannus. For L4-L5 level fusions, we keep the operating table parallel to the floor. However, for L5-S1 fusions, we typically position the operating table in 20 to 30 degrees of reverse Trendelenburg to allow the surgeon to have a more convenient view of the inferiorly angled L5-S1 disk space. Once positioned, patients are given a perioperative dose of antibiotics.

■ Surgical Technique

Decompression

The location of the incision is planned utilizing biplanar fluoroscopy to identify and mark the skin overlying the appropriate facet complex. Specifically, on the anteroposterior fluoroscopy view, we mark the patient's skin with the superimposed position of the pedicles bordering the intended TLIF level. We then mark the intended incision by connecting a line between the outer portions of these two pedicles. Typically this incision is two fingerbreadths off the midline and allows for a paraspinal muscle splitting (Wiltse) approach to be performed. Following skin and fascial incision, a plane is developed on the lateral border of the paraspinal muscles by using progressively larger dilator tubes from the expandable retractor system (Pipeline, Depuy Spine, Raynham, MA, or METRX, Medtronic Sofamor Danek, Memphis, TN). For patients with unilateral nerve root compression, we perform the TLIF on the symptomatic side to ensure wide foraminal decompression and create a

Table 13.1 Indications for Lumbar Interbody Fusion

• Spondylolisthesis (usually grades I or II)
• Degenerative disk disease causing discogenic low back pain
• Recurrent lumbar disk herniation with significant mechanical back pain
• Postdiskectomy interbody space collapse with neuroforaminal stenosis and radiculopathy
• Third time or greater recurrent lumbar disk herniation with radiculopathy (with or without back pain)
• Treatment of pseudarthrosis
• Treatment of postlaminectomy kyphosis
• Treatment of lumbar deformity with coronal or sagittal plane imbalance

paramedian incision on the symptomatic side to access the facet complex overlying the compressed root.

An expandable tube retractor can then be docked on the facet complex after dilating the paraspinal lumbar musculature with sequential dilator tubes. Through this portal, we perform a radical facetectomy to decompress the nerve root. The retractor may be angled medially to also create a hemilaminectomy in patients who have coincidental canal stenosis. For patients with bilateral nerve root compression, bilateral expandable tube retractors may be utilized to attain bilateral access and perform bilateral decompression (**Fig. 13.1**).

Pedicle Screw Placement and Disk Distraction

To give the surgeon a visual landmark, the pedicle screw entry points (junction of the midpoint of the transverse process with the lateral facet) are identified and decorticated with a high-speed drill before the facetectomy is performed. The pedicles are then probed and tapped (**Fig. 13.2**) and covered with a small amount of bone wax to minimize bleeding. Subsequently, the pedicle screws placed on the side ipsilateral to the decompression are typically placed after the facetectomy and diskectomy and interbody graft

Table 13.2 Relative Contraindications for Lumbar Interbody Fusion

• Multilevel (more than three levels) degenerative disk disease (except in spinal deformity cases)
• Single-level disk disease causing radiculopathy without symptoms of mechanical low back pain or instability
• Severe osteoporosis (possible subsidence of interbody grafts through the end plates)

Table 13.3 When to Consider Use of the Mini-Open TLIF

One- or two-level TLIF in the following situations:
• Patients without scoliosis
• Patients with less than 8-cm depth of tissues between skin and spine
• Patients whose pelvis does not overlie the level of fusion

placement are complete because the hardware may limit an already small surgical field.

For the mini-open approach, the pedicle screws on the ipsilateral side of the decompression and interbody fusion are placed through the expandable tube retractor. The contralateral pedicle screws, however, can be placed either through a contralateral paramedian incision utilizing a second expandable tube retractor, or using a percutaneous pedicle screw system (Viper, Depuy Spine, or Sextant, Medtronic Sofamor Danek).

After the decompression is complete and the contralateral pedicle screws are in position, a diskectomy is performed. The pedicle screws contralateral to the interbody exposure are connected to a rod that is typically 4 to 5 cm in length. Sequential distraction of the interspace, which allows for tissue hysteresis, is gradually achieved using a combination of interspace wedges, intervertebral body spreaders, and serial distraction of the pedicle screws. An increase in disk height is accomplished and maintained by fixating the contralateral pedicle screws in the distracted position on the rod.

Endplate Preparation

If a non–bullet-shaped cage is to be used, then on the side of the planned cage placement the posterior "lip" of the superior and inferior end plate may be removed using an osteotome, an interbody box cutter, a Kerrison rongeur, or a small drill bit. Care is taken to protect the exiting nerve root and the lateral thecal sac during this maneuver. Removal of the posterior lip opens a wider "window" to the posterolateral disk space and facilitates more extensive disk excision. This step may not be needed if a bullet-shaped implant is used because it can self-distract the posterior lipping end plates. End plates are scraped with angled curets to debride cartilaginous surfaces until bleeding cancellous bone is exposed.

Interbody Fusion

Interbody arthrodesis is achieved with an osteoinductive and osteoconductive bone graft. Iliac crest autograft is an excellent option for bone graft because it has excellent osteoinductive and osteoconductive properties, but iliac crest autograft is associated with harvest-site morbidity in up to 25% of patients (donor-site pain, donor-site infection, and cosmetic issues).[12,13] Local autograft from the lamina

A

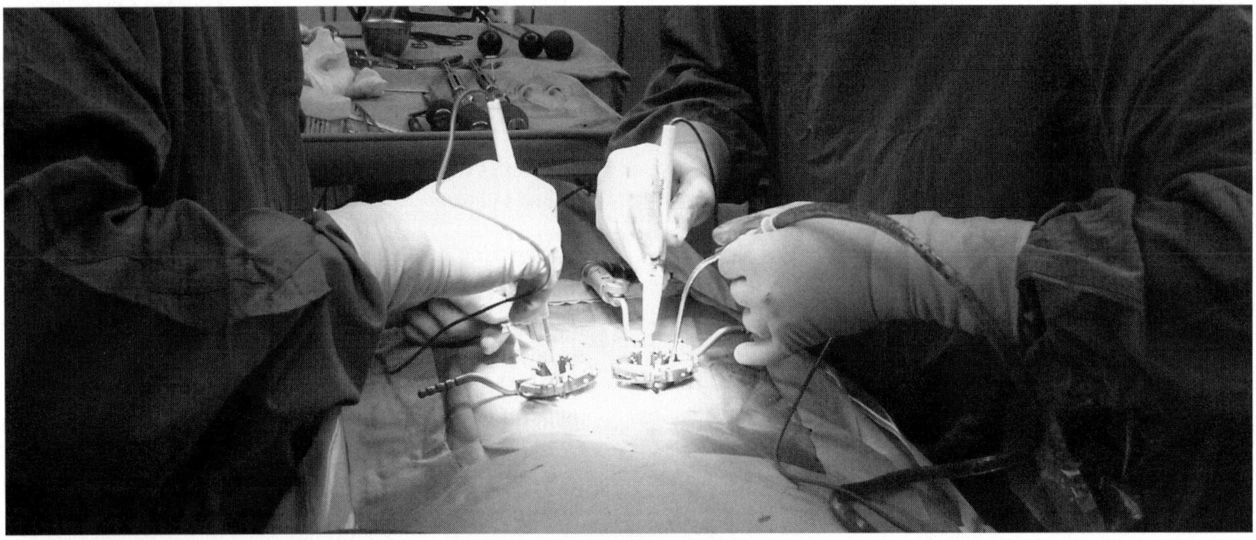

B

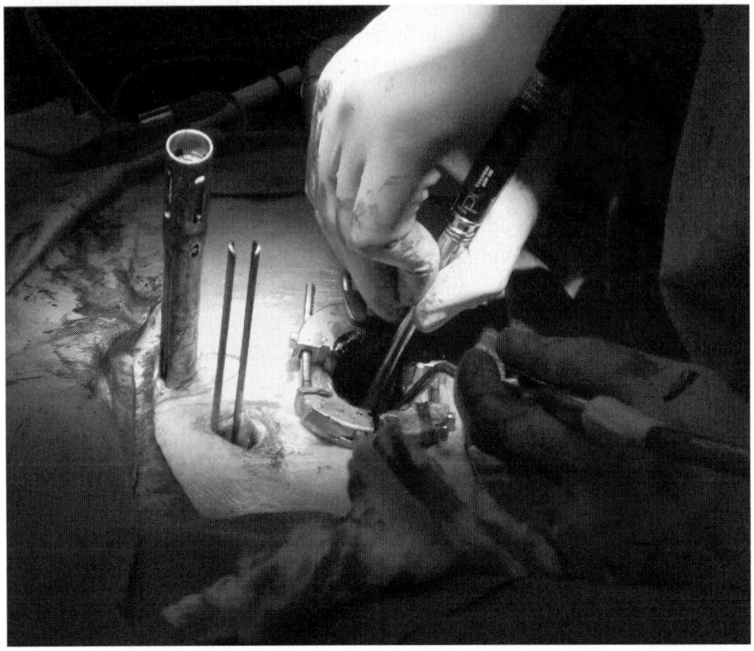

Fig. 13.1 (A) Intraoperative photograph of the placement of bilateral pipeline through which the pedicle screw placement and mini-open TLIF can be performed. **(B)** Photographs of interbody access via the pipeline with contralateral pedicle screw distraction in place.

or facet joint may not have the osteoinductive capability of iliac crest autograft and may not be sufficient to create a solid interbody fusion. Recently, the use of recombinant human bone morphogenetic protein-2 (rhBMP-2) in combination with local autograft has been reported to be an excellent alternative to iliac crest autograft to create interbody arthrodesis with a TLIF procedure. (The use of rhBMP-2 in the TLIF procedure is a Food and Drug Administration off-label use.) The use of rhBMP-2 eliminates the donor-site morbidity of iliac crest autograft. The rhBMP-2 sponge is typically placed anterior to and within the cage. To avoid foraminal bone formation, the rhBMP-2 sponge is not placed posterior to the cage.[7,14,15]

Following a complete interbody diskectomy, to maintain intervertebral body height, lumbar lordosis, and sagittal balance, a structural interbody spacer should be placed in the interbody space in addition to the osteoinductive graft material. Options for such spacers include titanium cages (circular, oval, rectangular, octagon, or boomerang shapes are available), polyether-ether-ketone (PEEK) cages, carbon fiber cages, structural machined allograft, or absorbable spacers such as the vacemic of polylactic acid (PL-DLA).

Historically, most TLIFs were performed with titanium cages in the interbody space. However, the modulus of elasticity of titanium is much greater than that of bone, and titanium cage subsidence through the vertebral body end plates may occur (especially in osteoporotic patients). Machined allograft dowels do not have the large modulus of elasticity that titanium has, but the supply of allograft bone is limited and nonuniform in shape. Allograft has the potential for viral disease transmission and rejection of donor allograft bone by the patient. The modulus of elasticity of bone is closely approximated by man-made nonresorbable polymers such as PEEK and carbon fiber cages, which have an unlimited supply and no risk of viral disease transmission or recipient rejection. Resorbable polymers, such as PL-DLA, initially also have a modulus of elasticity similar to bone. They can be packed with autograft, and once fusion takes place the PL-DLA is designed to resorb, leaving behind only the fused interbody bone. Like PEEK, PL-DLA is unlimited in supply and there is no risk of transmission of viral infection or recipient rejection.[5,16] The appropriate size of the spacer is selected using specifically designed trials. It has been our practice to use the Concorde Bullet spacer (Depuy Spine, Raynham, MA) for this purpose. Prior to placement of the spacer, we prefer to place an rh-BMP-2 sponge into the anterior disk space. When we utilize rh-BMP-2 for the interbody osteoinductive material, it is our preference to place the rhBMP-2 sponge into the anterior disk space and separate this sponge from the anterior thecal sac with the interbody spacer to avoid inducing heterotopic bone formation near the neural foramina. Local autograft from the facet joint (or from the iliac crest) is packed within the spacer itself (intracompartmental bone), and the spacer is positioned in the disk space **(Fig. 13.3).** Then autograft is packed posterior to the spacer (extracompartmental bone).[17] During interbody spacer placement, the lateral

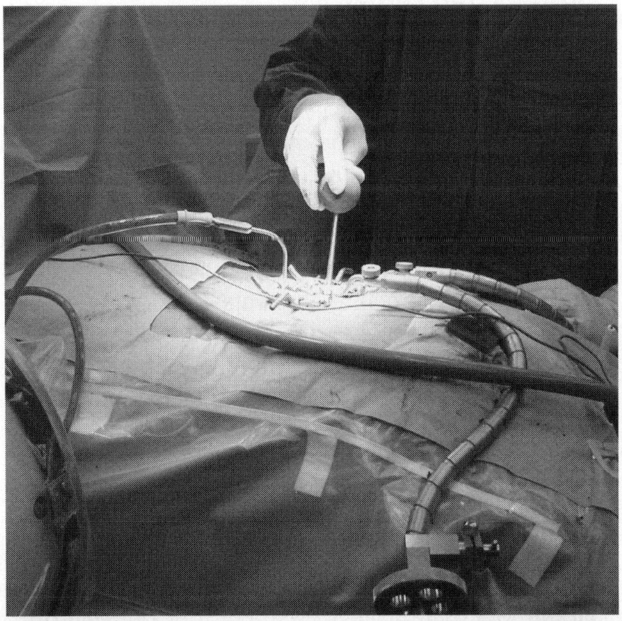
A

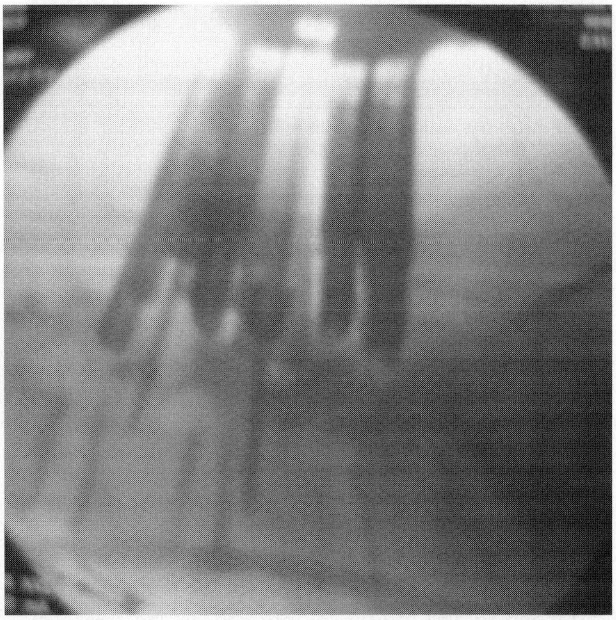
B

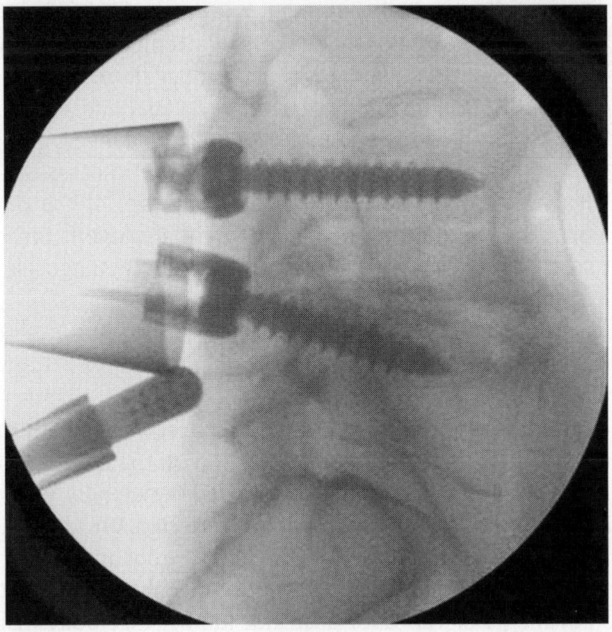
C

Fig. 13.2 Pedicle screws are placed in the standard fashion through the pipeline tube. **(A)** The pedicle is accessed with a pedicle finder. **(B)** The pedicle is tapped with an undersized tap. **(C)** The pedicle screws are placed on the side contralateral to the interbody spacer. Pedicle screws are placed on the side ipsilateral to the interbody spacer after the graft is in position.

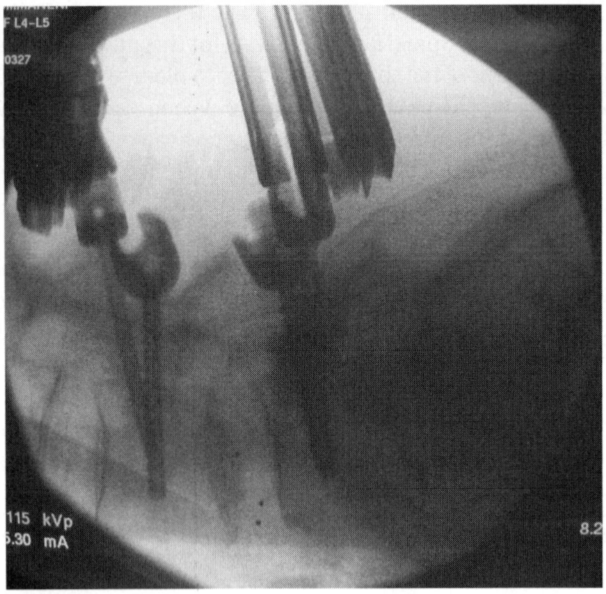

Fig. 13.3 After the diskectomy and interbody preparation is complete, a carbon fiber cage is inserted through the pipeline tube into the interspace.

dura may be protected with a small metal retractor. Usually, no retraction or minimal retraction of the thecal sac is needed during placement of the interbody spacer. The spacer is impacted until it is just under the posterior edge of the vertebral body and is then gradually rotated into position using an impactor.

Construct Compression and Posterolateral Fusion

After the interbody construct is placed, the pedicle screws are attached to and mildly compressed on the appropriate size rods **(Fig. 13.4),** thereby restoring lumbar lordosis while maintaining the restored disk height. It is important not to overcompress because it may create a contralateral foraminal stenosis in cases where no contralateral decompression has been performed. A posterior or posterolateral fusion may be added to increase the chances for solid arthrodesis; however, this is not mandatory. A standard closure in layers is performed. Following a mini-open TLIF, patients are encouraged to ambulate on the first postoperative day, and are typically discharged within 3 days.

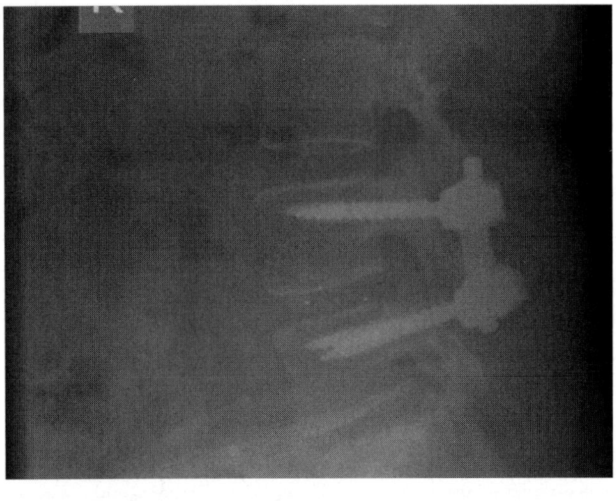

Fig. 13.4 Following cage placement, the pedicle screw and rod complex is mildly compressed and secured with locking cap screws.

■ Complication Avoidance and Management

Spinal Fluid Leaks

To avoid dural injury, we tend to delay dural exposure until later in the procedure. We prepare our pedicle screw entry points and tap the pedicles based on anatomic landmarks and fluoroscopy before we expose the exiting nerve root and lateral thecal sac. Furthermore, once the neural elements are exposed, we take care to protect them during hardware placement. For example, when we place the interbody spacer, we place a small Penfield dissector between it and the neural elements. In addition, when we place the pedicle screws and rods and compress the construct, we cover the exposed dural elements with a small cottonoid. Due to the limited exposure and reduced working space, cerebrospinal fluid (CSF) leaks encountered during the course of a mini-open TLIF can be difficult to repair. If a CSF leak occurs early in the procedure, we consider converting the operation into a posterolateral fusion to minimize tissue dissection. In cases where a CSF leakage is encountered during surgery, we attempt to sew the leak closed. We then place a small piece of Duragen (Integra NeuroSciences, Plainsboro, NJ) and inject fibrin glue Tisseal over the area of the leak in an attempt to seal it. We consider placing a subarachnoid lumbar drain in patients with CSF leaks if we do not achieve an adequate seal with our repair. It has not been our practice to convert a mini-open technique to a large open exposure in cases of CSF leakage. Rather, we feel it is an advantage of the mini-open technique that a smaller potential space is created so there is a smaller space for a pseudomeningocele to form.

Nerve Root Injury

During placement of the interbody spacer, we typically perform a minimal amount of retraction on the lateral thecal sac and, in patients with typical-sized nerve roots, we protect the exiting root with a small dissector. We usually do not have to retract the traversing nerve root at all, because we work in the axilla of the exiting nerve root. This is the advantage of TLIF over posterior lumbar interbody fusion

(PLIF); PLIF often requires significant thecal sac and traversing nerve root retraction.[6] However, a minority of patients have large exiting nerve roots or conjoined nerve roots that occupy almost the entire neural foramen. This can sometimes be appreciated on the preoperative magnetic resonance imaging (MRI) sagittal and coronal images, but on some occasions, it may not be appreciated until open operative exploration is undertaken. In these patients, it may be difficult to mobilize the nerve root to gain access to the posterolateral disk space. Because excessive nerve root retraction can result in radiculitis or nerve root injury, we avoid performing a TLIF on these patients. We prefer to perform a posterolateral fusion for these patients, and consider performing a subsequent mini-open anterior interbody fusion for them.[6]

Malpositioned Hardware

Placement of pedicle screws and interbody spacers through a small tubular corridor limits the surgeon's exposure and orientation. To compensate for this, the surgeon must have excellent working knowledge of the anatomy seen within the tubular retractor. To assist with orientation, we prefer to utilize fluoroscopy to identify and prepare the pedicle screw entry points early in the procedure to provide an anatomic reference point for the surgeon during the remainder of the procedure. The combination of anteroposterior and lateral fluoroscopy is an excellent method to check the position of the pedicles and to access them for subsequent pedicle screw placement. Another option is to use image-guided navigation. We have used FlouroNav and Stealth (Medtronic Sofamor Danek) successfully to place our hardware. However, use of image guidance requires a separate third midline incision to attach the arc for the navigation system to the spinous process. Once the pedicle screw entry holes are created, we utilize a small ball-tipped feeler probe to carefully palpate the inside of the pedicles to ensure there are no breaches in the pedicle walls. If a breach is palpated, an altered trajectory is chosen to avoid malpositioned pedicle screws. We prefer to position our interbody spacer in either the anterior or middle third of the interbody space **(Fig. 13.5).** If a spacer is positioned too far posteriorly, it may migrate back into the foramen through the aperture created by the surgeon. Fluoroscopy also assists with placement and positioning of the interbody spacer.

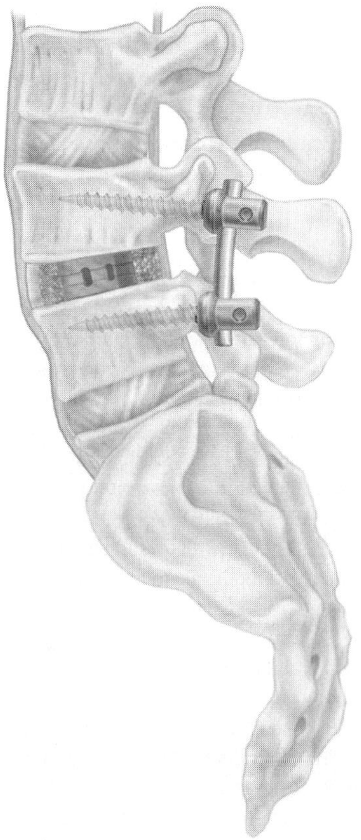

Fig. 13.5 Artist's illustration of the completed construct. Note the position of the cage in the middle of the disk space.

■ Discussion

Transforaminal lumbar interbody fusion is an excellent option to achieve a circumferential fusion by a single posterior approach. Recent advances in technique and instrumentation allow for the operation to be performed in a minimally invasive fashion that minimizes muscle dissection and scarring. There is a learning curve to this technique.

Transforaminal lumbar interbody fusion can be performed in a standard open fashion with a midline lumbar incision, in a mini-open fashion with expandable working tubes (as described here), or in a minimally invasive fashion using nonexpandable working tubes and percutaneous pedicle screws.[5] The open operation is associated with significant paraspinal muscle trauma, typical blood loss of 500 cc, and hospitalization averaging 5 days or more.[18] We prefer the open technique for cases with high-grade spondylolisthesis or cases with spinal deformity because it gives the best exposure of the three techniques and affords the greatest access for spinal realignment. The mini-open technique, on the other hand, minimizes paraspinal muscle trauma but has a moderate learning curve. It is our preferred technique in cases with low-grade (grade 1 or 2) spondylolisthesis or degenerative disk disease and is associated with an intraoperative blood loss of under 200 cc in our hands. It has been our experience that hospitalization following this procedure is reduced to about 3 days. The minimally invasive TLIF (through a nonexpendable tube on one side with percutaneous pedicle screws contralaterally as described by Foley et al[11])is associated with the least tissue trauma. The reported operative blood loss and hospital stay is similar to the mini-open technique, which we have described. The minimally invasive procedure, however, has a more difficult learning curve to master, in our experience. We have described the techniques that we use to obtain excellent exposure and to perform decompression while avoiding complications.

Acknowledgments

We are grateful to our colleagues Regis Haid and Jeff Pan for their insights.

References

1. Harms J, Rolinger H. [A one-stager procedure in operative treatment of spondylolistheses: dorsal traction-reposition and anterior fusion.] Z Orthop Ihre Grenzgeb 1982;120:343–347
2. Hee HT, Majd ME, Holt RT, Myers L. Do autologous growth factors enhance transforaminal lumbar interbody fusion? Eur Spine J 2003;12:400–407
3. Humphreys SC, Hodges SD, Patwardhan AG, Eck JC, Murphy RB, Covington LA. Comparison of posterior and transforaminal approaches to lumbar interbody fusion. Spine 2001;26:567–571
4. Kwon BK, Berta S, Daffner SD, et al. Radiographic analysis of transforaminal lumbar interbody fusion for the treatment of adult isthmic spondylolisthesis. J Spinal Disord Tech 2003;16:469–476
5. Lowe TG, Coe JD. Resorbable polymer implants in unilateral transforaminal lumbar interbody fusion. J Neurosurg 2002;97:464–467
6. Mummaneni PV, Haid RW, Rodts GE. Lumbar interbody fusion: state-of-the-art technical advances. Invited submission from the Joint Section Meeting on Disorders of the Spine and Peripheral Nerves, March 2004. J Neurosurg Spine 2004;1:24–30
7. Mummaneni PV, Pan J, Haid RW, Rodts GE. Contribution of recombinant human bone morphogenetic protein-2 to the rapid creation of interbody fusion when used in transforaminal lumbar interbody fusion: a preliminary report. Invited submission from the Joint Section Meeting on Disorders of the Spine and Peripheral Nerves, March 2004. J Neurosurg Spine 2004;1:19–23
8. Rosenberg WS, Mummaneni PV. Transforaminal lumbar interbody fusion: technique, complications, and early results. Neurosurgery 2001;48:569–574
9. Salehi SA, Tawk R, Ganju A, LaMarca F, Liu JC, Ondra SL. Transforaminal lumbar interbody fusion: surgical technique and results in 24 patients. Neurosurgery 2004;54:368–374
10. Whitecloud TS, Roesch WW, Ricciardi JE. Transforaminal interbody fusion versus anterior-posterior interbody fusion of the lumbar spine: a financial analysis. J Spinal Disord 2001;14:100–103
11. Foley KT, Holly LT, Schwender JD. Minimally invasive lumbar fusion. Spine 2003;28:S26–S35
12. Banwart JC, Asher MA, Hassanein RS. Iliac crest bone graft harvest donor site morbidity. A statistical evaluation. Spine 1995;20:1055–1060
13. Sawin PD, Traynelis VC, Menezes AH. A comparative analysis of fusion rates and donor-site morbidity for autogeneic rib and iliac crest bone grafts in posterior cervical fusions. J Neurosurg 1998;88:255–265
14. Burkus JK, Heim SE, Gornet MF, Zdeblick TA. Is INFUSE bone graft superior to autograft bone? An integrated analysis of clinical trials using the LT-CAGE lumbar tapered fusion device. J Spinal Disord Tech 2003;16:113–122
15. Lanman TH, Hopkins TJ. Lumbar interbody fusion after treatment with recombinant human bone morphogenetic protein-2 added to poly(L-lactide-co-D,L-lactide) bioresorbable implants. Neurosurg Focus 2004;16:E9
16. Alexander JT, Branch CL, Subach BR, Haid RW. Applications of a resorbable interbody spacer in posterior lumbar interbody fusion. J Neurosurg 2002;97:468–472
17. Mummaneni PV, Pan J, Haid RW, Rodts GE. Rh-BMP 2 contributes to the rapid creation of interbody fusion with utilized with the TLIF procedure. Presented at the Joint Section on Disorders of the Spine and Peripheral Nerves, San Diego, 2004
18. Mummaneni PV, Haid RW, Rodts GE. Lumbar interbody fusion: state of the art technical advances. In: Haid RW, Fessler R, eds. Lumbar Interbody Fusion: Cages, Dowels, and Grafts. St. Louis: Quality Medical Publishing, 2003:227–234

14 Bone Biology and Lumbar Fusion

Alex Hughes and Langston T. Holly

Lumbar fusion has become a widely accepted method in the management of a variety of disorders that require spinal stabilization, such as traumatic, degenerative, infectious, and neoplastic conditions. A variety of different fusion modalities exist, including interbody and posterolateral techniques. Irrespective of the exact modality performed, a thorough understanding of bone biology is essential to optimize the chances of a successful fusion. From the elegant macro- and micro-architecture of bone to the complexities of osteoconduction and cell signaling, the spine surgeon must be well versed in the factors associated with the reliable generation of bone. This chapter discusses the important aspects of bone biology with respect to lumbar fusion.

Architecture of Bone

The bone mass of the musculoskeletal system can be viewed simplistically as consisting of either cortical (compact) or cancellous (trabecular) bone. Overall, cortical bone comprises roughly 80% of the skeleton, whereas cancellous bone makes up the remainder. In practical terms, cortical bone (less than 20% porosity) is much denser than cancellous bone (50 to 90% porosity). The compact nature of cortical bone necessitates the very well organized haversian systems for vascular convection and support of cellular components within this largely acellular and avascular environment. Each osteon of haversian bone consists of concentric lamellae with osteocytes embedded in lacunae that surround a central high-pressure haversian canal. This architecture allows for a maximum density of structural matrix. Thus cortical bone is often defined as haversian bone. Relative to cancellous bone, cortical bone has a high Young's modulus and demonstrates more resistance to bending and torsion. The mechanical demands of the appendicular skeleton necessitate a high haversian bone content. Trabecular bone consists of arrays of stress-directed trabeculae surrounded by vast vascular channels. Individual trabeculae consist of parallel lamellae, or sheets of bone matrix with embedded osteocytes and surface osteoblasts and osteoclasts.[1] The peritrabecular tissues are composed of marrow contents that contain hematopoietic cell lines; angiogenic progenitor cells; vascular channels; lymphocytic cell lines and their progenitor cells; mesenchymal stem cells (MSCs); and bone, cartilage, and fibrous tissue progenitor cells.

Although the skeleton is 80% cortical bone, cancellous bone has five times the surface area due to its increased vascularity. Therefore, it lends itself to rapid remodeling and serves as the primary reservoir for calcium and phosphate homeostasis. Until the age of about 30 to 40 years, bone remodeling results in no net loss of bone mass because formation and absorption are roughly equal. About 10% of bone mass is remodeled each year in adults. Cancellous bone remodels by rapid osteoclast resorption followed by direct osteoblast generation of lamellae. Cortical bone, with a less cellular and vascular architecture, must form channels via osteoclastic tunneling or cutting cones. These new channels are then lined by osteoblasts and form concentric lamellae as a haversian canal system is regenerated with fresh matrix. Remodeling occurs within the paradigm suggested by Wolff's law. That is, compressive forces promote an electronegative environment (osteoblast stimulating), and tensile forces promote an electropositive environment (osteoclast stimulating) through conformational changes of collagen. The complexity of this piezoelectric effect has been expanded in recent years as more information has become available regarding the role of blood coagulation proteins (chiefly fibrin) in providing an osteoconductive scaffold during both remodeling and healing.[2]

Bone remodeling is performed by small packets of cells known as basic (or bone) multicellular units (BMUs). Each packet consists of osteoblasts, osteocytes, and osteoclasts that respond to systemic hormones and local cytokines. The osteoblasts, when stimulated, produce osteoid or organic bone matrix (40% dry weight of bone). Osteoid is 90% type I collagen and is responsible for the tensile strength of bone. The other 10% of osteoid consists of proteoglycans, noncollagenous matrix proteins (such as osteocalcin, osteonectin, osteopontin, and others), cytokines (such as interleukin-1 [IL-1], IL-6), and growth factors (e.g., transforming growth factor-β [TGF-β] superfamily, insulin-like growth factor [IGF]). Once osteoid has been introduced into the extracellular environment, mineral accretion begins usually within 10 days. Osteocalcin has an affinity for calcium and uncrystallized hydroxyapatite, whereas osteonectin binds hydroxyapatite crystals (calcium hydroxyapatite) to collagen. Osteoblasts also produce alkaline phosphatase, which releases phosphate groups from nucleotides, proteins, and alkaloids, thereby making it available for bone mineralization. The inorganic component of matrix contributes to the compressive strength of bone, thereby lending itself to the analogy of rebar (organic component) cement (inorganic/mineral component).[3–9]

Remodeling allows the skeleton to respond to stresses as well as replace aging bone matrix with new stock. The elderly suffer from not only an annual decrease of bone mass but also increasingly brittle bone matrix as collagen degrades with age faster than it can be remodeled (type I collagen is the largest organic component of bone matrix). This manifests itself in the axial skeleton, which is primarily cancellous bone, as increased compression fractures in the elderly population.[10,11] Women are significantly at risk because of a 25% smaller peak bone mass and an accelerated rate of loss during the first 5 years after menopause.

The architecture of the axial skeleton has implications not only for age-related change in bone morphology and clinical disease but also in surgical applications such as fusion. Specifically in the lumbar spine, the vertebral body consists almost entirely of trabecular bone surrounded circumferentially by a thin (around 1 mm) dense rind of compact trabecular bone **(Fig. 14.1).** Histologic analysis of this "cortex" of the lumbar vertebra demonstrates that in fact this is not true haversian bone. Rather, this layer is characterized by parallel sheets of lamellar bone that are loosely associated with vascular channels. The transverse processes and superior articular facets (lateral facets) can be thought of as extensions of the vertebral body and likewise are predominantly trabecular bone. In contrast, the posterior elements of the lumbar vertebral bodies are largely cortical-like and do not contain marrow-derived stem cells. This includes the spinous process, inferior articular facet, and the pars interarticularis.[1,10,12,13]

The arterial vascular supply to the spine is predominantly supplied by the bilateral segmental arteries that branch off the aorta. Of relevance for anterior approaches to the lumbar spine, the aorta bifurcates with some variability generally around L4-L5 in most people. The ventral branches of each bilateral segmental artery supply the vertebral bodies via ascending and descending branches. These branches travel underneath the posterior longitudinal ligament and enter the bodies in four separate ostia (two on each side). Perfusion studies have demonstrated maintenance of pulsatile flow to the vertebral bodies and spinal cord with unilateral occlusion of a single segmental artery.[14] The effect on fusion rates, however, remains unknown. The posterior elements and dura are supplied by smaller dorsal branches of the segmental arteries as well as by perforators from the paraspinal musculature. The vertebral body and its appendage structures (transverse process and superior articular facet) are supplied by a much higher flow arterial system than the posterior elements. Physiologically, this is expected given the increased cellularity and metabolic demands of trabecular bone. This anatomic architecture has important implications for lumbar spine fusion. Connectivity to the vertebral body or its appendages is essential for successful fusion (either interbody or intertransverse process posterolateral fusion). In simple terms, this connectivity is required for reliable fusion because it provides both access to a rich blood supply and an adequate stock of osteoprogenitor cells.[13,15,16]

Biology of Bone Healing

The human body demonstrates a consistent healing model in all tissues. Injury causes the release of tissue-specific growth factor and activates a platelet-mediated wound healing response. In bone, the most abundant growth factor is the TGF-β superfamily. This group, present in bone matrix at a concentration of 1 mg/kg contains the 15 recognized bone morphogenetic proteins (BMPs).[4] The released factors provide a chemotactic signal across their concentration gradient that serves to attract white blood cells and stem cells to the disrupted site. The white blood cells clear necrotic debris from the wound site as stem cells and progenitor cells begin to multiply to reach a critical mass that is tissue specific and required for the synthetic healing process. Under these conditions, MSCs demonstrate asymmetric division in which each cell produces a stem cell (to preserve that undifferentiated line) and progenitor cells. Depending on conditions, MSCs are capable of differentiating into osteoblast, chondroblast, adipocyte, fibroblast, and myoblast progenitor cells. Following this proliferative phase, the progenitor cell lines complete differentiation, undergo maturation, and begin depositing extracellular matrix.[17]

As in other tissues, the process of bone healing follows an orderly cascade. The initial event is followed by formation of a blood clot or hematoma and the initiation of an

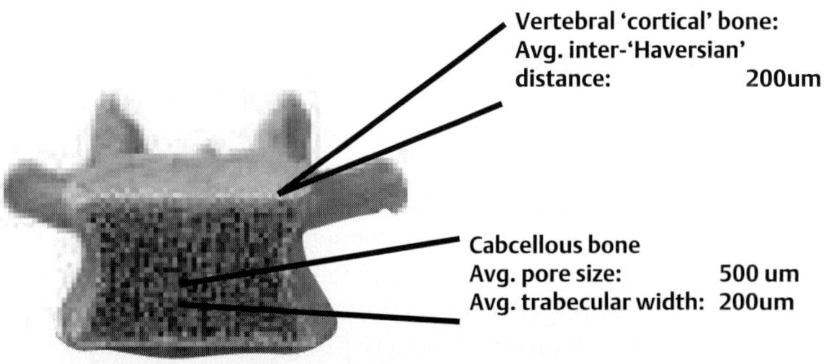

Fig. 14.1 Schematic demonstrating the macroarchitecture of a lumbar vertebral body.

inflammatory response. This initial hemorrhage phase exposes reactive plasma proteins to subendothelial tissue factors that activate the thrombin-clotting cascade. The end result is the formation of a three-dimensional latticework of fibrin threads that serves as a sticky matrix for platelet adhesion. This in turn releases platelet-derived growth factor (PDGF), vascular endothelial growth factor (VEGF), and TGF-β to attract macrophages, osteoprogenitors, and fibroblasts. Additionally, exposed local bone matrix, as previously discussed, also releases TGF-β (containing high amounts of the BMP family of proteins). Under these osteoinductive influences, the progenitor cells (derived from MSCs) start to proliferate to reach a critical mass and then undergo differentiation into chondrocytes or osteoblasts under the influence of local stimuli. These stimuli include biochemical signals released from bone, oxygen tension, inflammatory mediators, and mechanical conditions at the fracture site. Simultaneous with this proliferative phase begins a phase of neovascularization under the influence of VEGF. Under bone-inductive signal conditions when oxygen tension is relatively high and microstrain low (500 to 2000 microstrain), osteoblasts directly produce bone matrix in intramembranous bone formation. When bone-inductive signals are present but oxygen tension is low and microstrain is intermediate, chondrocytes produce an initial cartilaginous bridge that is later replaced by bone in endochondral ossification once strain conditions have stabilized. Histologically, this sequence is synonymous with soft callous, which becomes hard callous over time. If strain conditions are high, strain conditions are not stabilized, or if tensile forces exist, then fibrous tissue is formed (leading to nonunion or pseudarthrosis). In both direct and indirect bone formation, the initial bridge is replaced and reorganized by remodeling according to Wolff's law until eventually mature lamellar bone is left. The initial goal of lumbar fusion surgery is to create a vascularized low strain environment that facilitates direct ossification and graft incorporation.[7,18–23]

Bone healing and regeneration models are applicable for small defects or relatively nondisplaced fractures where reparative cells are close to a vascular supply. They therefore have access to substrate molecules (e.g., glucose, oxygen, amino acids), and metabolic products (e.g., CO_2, lactate, urea) are cleared from the environment. At distances greater than 200 μm (the typical maximum distance between lacunae in haversian bone and the width of individual trabeculae in cancellous bone), mass transport becomes a limiting factor for cell survival.[24] The transport of oxygen and glucose to the center of most autograft sites must occur over distances on the order of 5 mm. Cells greater than 1 mm from the edge of the graft generally do not survive. Because cells are competing with each other for survival, reducing the number of cells can improve the maximum cellular depth of survival (inverse square relationship between cell concentration and the depth of cell survival).[24–26]

In normal bone marrow, MSCs and connective tissue progenitor cells exist at a concentration of 1:20,000. By concentrating MSCs and progenitor cells for transplantation into graft matrices, some of the metabolic competition is eliminated with resultant improved depth of survival of important osteoprogenitor cells. This is in part the basis behind selective retention device applications for augmentation of lumbar spine fusions. Such devices (e.g., CELLECT™ Graft Preparation Device, DePuy Spine, Warsaw, IN) concentrate osteoprogenitor cells from marrow aspirate three- to fourfold and deposit them on an allograft carrier. The concept is not only to increase the number of available osteoprogenitor cells at the site of fusion, but also to reduce the metabolic competition at the fusion site by relatively decreasing other marrow-derived cell populations from the graft material.[7,17]

Biology of Lumbar Fusion

Appropriate conditions must be present for bone healing and regeneration to take place. That is, appropriate mechanical conditions, a physiologic osteoconductive scaffold, adequate mass transport, correct cell signals, and abundant stem cell and progenitor cell populations must be present to predictably repair any given defect with bone. As in complex high-energy fracture situations with significant bone loss, the challenge of bone generation is expanded as the required osteogenic jumping distance exceeds normal physiologic conditions.

Bore hole studies in rabbits have shown that rapid bridging of defects via primary ossification does not occur in defects exceeding roughly 1 mm. Bore holes less than 200 μm are quickly filled by woven bone. Larger holes (200 μm to 1 mm) are bridged over the course of 2 weeks by a scaffold of woven bone. Parallel fibered lamellar bone is then layered upon this scaffold until the hole is completely filled by around 6 weeks. Larger holes (greater than 1 mm) were eventually filled with bone as well over a longer time course.[24] The structure is then altered via remodeling. However, in lumbar spine fusion, this longer time course of larger defects has important in vivo implications as osteogenesis must compete with fibrous ingrowth in a time sensitive fashion (particularly in posterolateral fusion). Clearly the interbody (8 to 12 mm) and intertransverse process distances (25 to 35 mm) in the lumbar spine exceed normal osteogenic jumping distances. Therefore, appropriate osteoinductive signals and the presence of an osteoconductive matrix are essential to bridge these supraphysiologic distances. This is accomplished either through the use of composite autograft (bone and bone marrow) via osteogenic transfer or through the use of allograft augmented with appropriate osteoinductive growth factors.[24,25]

The osteoconductive matrix required for lumbar spine fusion is similar to that required for bone healing and regeneration at other sites. The gold standard matrix is that of trabecular bone that has a bone volume density of about 20 to 30% (porosity of 70 to 80%). The average trabecular width is around 200 μm with an average intertrabecular pore size of around 500 μm with ample pore interconnections. As one would logically expect, these distances are within the body's osteogenic jumping distance. Besides these structural features, the surface properties of trabecular bone demonstrate bioactivity that attracts bone ongrowth and bone matrix apposition.[11,25]

Mechanically, a rigid construct must be achieved for the attainment of reliable lumbar fusion rates. Laboratory studies have demonstrated improved direct bone generation and superior graft incorporation in a 500- to 2000-microstrain environment with adequate mass transport parameters. This can be achieved reliably either by interbody fusion techniques or by modern posterior pedicle screw fixation constructs. Intermediate strain environments promote the formation of a cartilage intermediate with chondrocyte proliferation. High strain environments encourage fibrous tissue generation. All other conditions being equal, both of the latter two scenarios put patients at high risk for the development of a pseudarthrosis. Histologic studies of lumbar pseudarthroses demonstrate microtrabecular bone fracture, fibrous tissue with proliferation of fibroblasts, and fibrocartilaginous metaplasia.[27]

The precise rigidity of the lumbar spine postoperative construct affects the quality of the lumbar fusion mass and the time course of achieving fusion. Variations in the local strain environment, even within the range for direct ossification, have important implications for the fusion mass. This has been vividly demonstrated with cage interbody fusion techniques. Intervertebral cage devices have become a standard procedure for achieving interbody fusion **(Fig. 14.2)**. Currently materials range from radiopaque titanium and tantalum to radiolucent carbon fiber (or polyether-ether-ketone, PEEK), machined cortical allograft, and resorbable poly L-lactic acid (PLLA) cages. There are theoretical advantages to each material, and a full discussion is beyond the scope of this chapter. Briefly, the mechanical stability of the fused segment is mainly set by the geometry and size of the cage. The device material, and specifically its Young's modulus, plays a role in mechanical loading of the transplanted bone or graft within the cage and therefore is an important factor in stress shielding.[1,21,27,28]

Assuming all requisite conditions are met for successful fusion, graft material at fusion sites is replaced by a bridge of trabecular bone in a process called creeping substitution.[21] This new bone is typically immature woven bone that is remodeled into lamellar trabecular bone in accordance with environmental mechanical cues. The time course for this remodeling can take up to 2 years under ideal strain conditions. Stress shielding can delay or prevent this from happening.

In addition to an appropriate mechanical construct and osteoconductive matrix, reliable fusion requires an adequate vascular supply for convection and mass transport as well as access to a plentiful supply of MSCs and

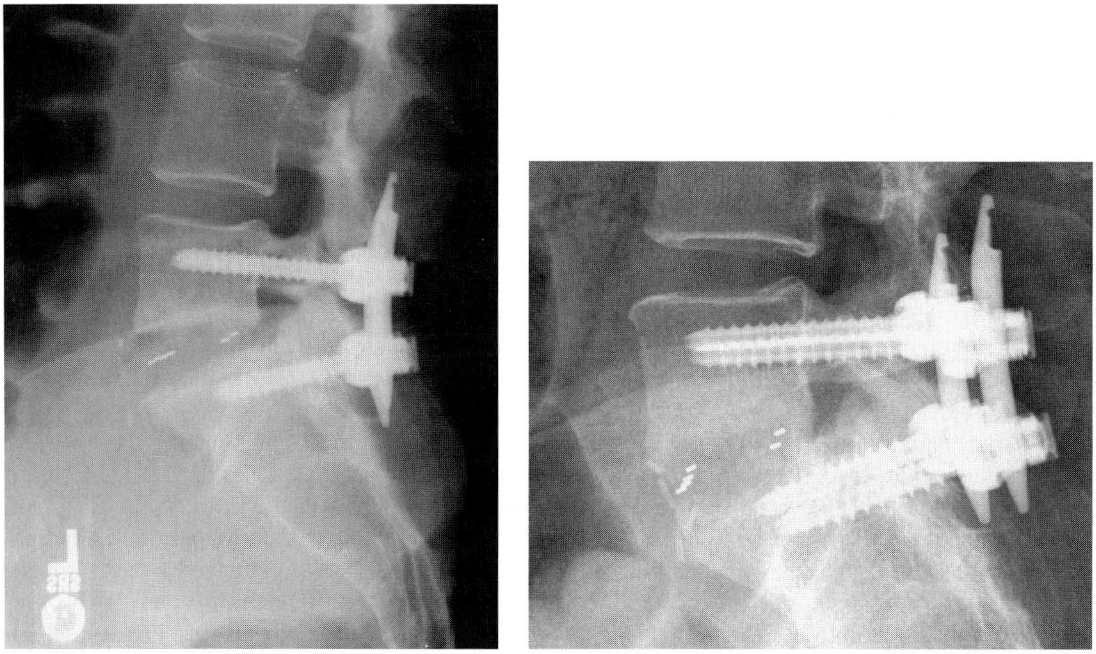

A B

Fig. 14.2 (A) Immediate postoperative lateral lumbar spine radiograph of a 50-year-old woman who underwent an anterior L5-S1 fusion using a polyether-ether-ketone (PEEK) cage filled with bone morphogenetic protein (BMP) and percutaneous pedicle screws. **(B)** Radiograph obtained 7 months postsurgery demonstrates bony bridging and a solid fusion.

osteoprogenitor cells. Intervertebral fusion mass access to the rich blood supply of the vertebral bodies and their trabecular bone contents is created by removing the cartilaginous end plates of the surrounding superior and inferior vertebra. This gives the fusion bed direct contact with the well-perfused intertrabecular vascular channels of the vertebral body and its abundant osteoprogenitor cell populations. Similarly, for posterior intertransverse process fusion, fusion mass access to this same rich blood supply and the trabecular bone contents of the vertebral bodies is achieved by decorticating the superior and inferior transverse processes at each level of desired fusion. It should be remembered that the transverse process and superior articular facet are appendages of the vertebral body and similarly consist largely of trabecular bone. This is in direct contrast to the dense, relatively poorly perfused, cortical-like posterior elements. Nearly all of the blood supply to an intertransverse process fusion mass is derived from the transverse processes/vertebral bodies themselves, with little contribution from the posterior elements **(Fig. 14.3).** Recent studies demonstrate a small but present vascular contribution to intertransverse process lumbar fusion mass from the paraspinal muscles themselves.[12,13]

The synthetic requirements of fusion outstrip the capacity of local osteoblasts that may be present as a result of decortication or even osteoblasts that are present via osteogenic transfer (use of composite autograft). Furthermore, as previously discussed, transplanted osteoblasts may not survive depending on graft depth and rate of neovascularization. Rather, the formation of a successful fusion mass relies largely on the recruitment of MSCs and osteoprogenitor cells via chemotactic cell signaling and neovascularization to the fusion site to generate new osteoblast cell populations. Once at the site, local growth factors (either embedded in allograft or autograft matrix or augmented recombinant BMP) then induce osteoprogenitors into osteoblasts and encourage the production of bone matrix.[7,17,26]

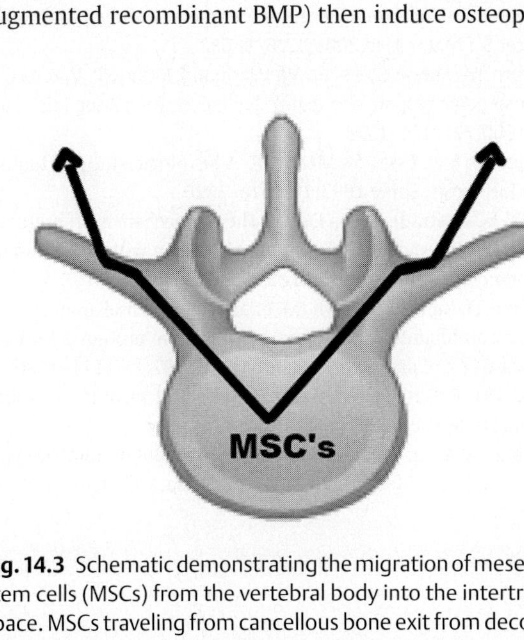

Fig. 14.3 Schematic demonstrating the migration of mesenchymal stem cells (MSCs) from the vertebral body into the intertransverse space. MSCs traveling from cancellous bone exit from decorticated transverse processes to intertransverse process fusion gutter.

With the advent of recombinant osteogenic protein 1 (OP-1 or BMP-2), an asterisk has been attached to this paradigm. Studies have suggested that osteoinduction can occur in a dose-dependent fashion via recruitment of undifferentiated progenitor cells from ectopic tissues or periosteum. This was demonstrated in an animal model in which successful intertransverse process fusion was achieved using high-dose OP-1 without decortication of the surrounding transverse processes.[29] Lower doses failed to achieve fusion. Of course, the standard remains to perform decortication of the surrounding transverse processes of a given fusion segment to maximize the fusion time course and fusion potential of a given segment.[13,15]

The time course for the achievement of a solid fusion mass is important for several reasons. First, if successful fusion does not occur within a given time frame, mechanical failure of construct will occur at some point. Second, fusion is a race between the rate of creeping substitution of graft material by woven bone and the ingrowth of fibrous tissue from surrounding tissue. Especially in intertransverse process fusion, the longer it takes for trabecular bridging to occur in a fusion segment, the more likely fibrous tissue ingrowth from surrounding paraspinal muscle sources will occur.

Factors that are known to delay fusion should be eliminated if possible in the preoperative period. Systemic medical conditions should be carefully managed with special consideration given to recombinant growth factors. Smoking, nicotine in any form, early postoperative daily nonsteroidal antiinflammatory drugs (NSAIDs), systemic steroids, obesity, alcohol abuse, diabetes, osteoporosis, renal failure, cancer, systemic chronic illness, and immune compromise are conditions that require special consideration. Nicotine demonstrates in animal models a direct inhibitory effect on osteoblast synthetic capacity and promotes the formation of structurally inferior bone.[30] Daily NSAID administration has been shown to have a deleterious effect on fusion rates especially if taken during the healing phase or initial phases of ossification in fusion models. However, it has recently been shown that the limited perioperative use of intravenous ketorolac has no deleterious effects on lumbar fusion rates.[31] Animal models have demonstrated inferior graft incorporation and increased pseudarthrosis rates in the setting of systemic steroids. Systemic disease can function to hinder fusion by metabolic disruption of the synthetic or reparative capacity of the body, by a calcium or phosphate imbalance, or by increasing the likelihood of postoperative infection.

■ Conclusion

A comprehensive understanding of bone biology and the biology of lumbar fusion is essential for maximizing the potential for fusion of each patient. By dissecting each factor that contributes to achieving reliable surgical outcomes and identifying risk factors for failures, new algorithms are constantly being written as our knowledge expands. Recent advances in molecular biology, new laboratory techniques for producing recombinant growth factors, and improved implant materials have ushered in an exciting new era of understanding and possibility for lumbar fusion.

References

1. Roy ME, Rho JY, Ting YY, et al. Mechanical and morphological variation of the human lumbar vertebral cortical trabecular bone. J Biomed Mater Res 1999;44:191–197
2. Nakamura M, Sekijima Y, Nakamura S, et al. Role of blood coagulation components as intermediators of high osteoconductivity of electrically polarized hydroxyapatite. J Biomed Mater Res A 2006;79:627–634
3. Brown A, Stock G, Patal A, et al. Osteogenic protein-1: a review of its utility in spinal applications. BioDrugs 2006;20:243–251
4. Carlisle E, Fischgrund JS. Bone morphogenetic proteins for spinal fusion. Spine J 2005;5:240S–249S
5. Foldes J, Napastek E, Statter M, Menczel J, Bab I. Osteogenic response to marrow aspiration: increased serum osteocalcin and alkaline phosphatase in human bone marrow donors. J Bone Miner Res 1989;4:643–646
6. Kanaan RA, Kanaan LA. Transforming growth factor beta-1, bone connection. Med Sci Monit 2006;12:RA164–RA169 [Epub ahead of print]
7. Kapur T, Kadiyala S, Urbahns D. Autologous growth factors and progenitor cells as effective components in bone grafting products for spine. In: Lewandrowski K-U, ed. Advances in Spinal Fusion: Molecular Science, Biomechanics, and Clinical Management. New York: Marcel Dekker, 2004
8. Okamoto M, Murai J, Yoshikawa H, Tsumaki N. Bone morphogenetic proteins in bone stimulate osteoclasts and osteoblasts during bone development. J Bone Miner Res 2006;21:1022–1033
9. Whyte MP. Paget's disease of bone and genetic distorders of RANKL/OPG/RANK/NF-KappaB signaling. Ann N Y Acad Sci 2006; 1068:143–164
10. Scapinelli R. Morphological and functional changes of the lumbar spinous processes in the elderly. Surg Radiol Anat 1989;11:129–133
11. Zerne R, Levy M. Endocrine regulation of calcium and phosphate metabolism. In: Physiology, 4th ed. St. Louis: Mosby, 848–870
12. Bawa M, Schimizzi AL, Leek B, et al. Paraspinal muscle vasculature contributes to posterolateral spinal fusion. Spine 2006;31:891–896
13. Toribatake Y, Hutton WC, Tomita K, Boden SD. Vascularization of the fusion mass in a posterolateral intertransverse process fusion. Spine 1998;23:1149–1154
14. Hempfing A, Dreimann M, Krebs S, et al. Reduction of vertebral blood flow by segmental vessel occlusion: an intraoperative study using laser Doppler flowmetry. Spine 2005;30:2701–2705
15. Slappey G, Toribatake Y, Ganey TM, Ogden JA, Hutton WC. Guidelines to decortication in posterolateral spine fusion. J Spinal Disord 1998;11:102–109
16. Vraney RT, Phillips FM, Wetzel FT, Brustein M. Peridiscal vascular anatomy of the lower lumbar spine. An endoscopic perspective. Spine 1999;24:2183–2187
17. Kraus KH, Kirker-Head C. Mesenchymal stem cells and bone regeneration. Vet Surg 2006;35:232–242
18. Bidner SM, Rubins IM, Desjardins JV, Zukor DJ, Goltzman D. Evidence for a humoral mechanism for enhanced osteogenesis after head injury. J Bone Joint Surg Am 1990;72:1144–1149
19. Nakase T. Gene expression profiling during osteochondrogenic events in the spinal region: use in the development of promising spinal fusion. In: Lewandrowski K-U, ed. Advances in Spinal Fusion: Molecular Science, Biomechanics, and Clinical Management. New York: Marcel Dekker, 2004
20. Patel TC, Erulkar JS, Grauer JN, et al. Osteogenic protein-1 overcomes the inhibitory effect of nicotine on posterolateral fusion. Spine 2001;26:1656–1661
21. Smit TH, Muller R, Martijn V, et al. Changes in bone architecture during spinal fusion: three years follow up and the role of cage stiffness. Spine 2003;28:1802–1808
22. Vaccaro AR, Anderson DG, Patel T, et al. Comparison of OP-1 putty (rhBMP-7) to iliac crest autograft for posterolateral lumbar arthrodesis: a minimum 2 year follow-up pilot study. Spine 2005;30:2709–2716
23. Varkey M, Kucharski C, Haque T, Sebald W, Uludag H. In vitro osteogenic response of rat bone marrow cells to bFGF and BMP-2 treatments. Clin Orthop Relat Res 2006;443:113–123
24. Habibovic P, Huipin Y, Mirella D, et al. Relevance of osteoinductive biomaterials in critical-sized orthotopic defect. J Orthop Res 2006;24:867–876
25. Flautre B, Descamps M, Delecourt C, Delecourt C, Blary MC, Hardouin P. Porous HA ceramic for bone replacement: Role of the pores and interconnections- experimental study in the rabbit. J Mater Sci Mater Med 2001;12:679–682
26. Einhorn TA, Simon G, Devlin VJ, Warman J, Sidhu SP, Vigorita VJ. The ostegenic response to distal skeletal injury. J Bone Joint Surg Am 1990;72:1374–1378
27. Heggeness MH, Esses SI, Mody DR. A histologic study of lumbar pseudarthrosis. Spine 1993;18:1016–1020
28. Benzel EC, Lastra JJ, Kalfas I, et al. The biomechanics of interbody fusion and the shortcomings of lumbar fusion with cages and interbody dowels. Clin Neurosurg 2000;47:557–588
29. Sandhu HS, Kamim LE, Toth JM, et al. Experimental spinal fusion with recombinant human bone morphogenic protein-2 without decortication of osseous elements. Spine 1997;22:1171–1180
30. Silcox DH, Daftari T, Boden SD. The effect of nicotine on spinal fusion. Spine 1995;20:1549–1553
31. Pradhan B, Wang J, Dawson E. Effect of Toradol on lumbar spine fusion when used for perioperative analgesia. Philadelphia: NASS, 2005

15 Bone Graft Extenders and Substitutes

Daniel J. Hoh and Michael Y. Wang

Spinal fusion surgery by orthopedic and neurologic surgeons has been steadily increasing over the last few decades. In the United States alone, it is estimated that 200,000 spinal fusion surgeries are performed annually.[1] The rising incidence of surgical management for degenerative low back pain has led to a concomitant increase in lumbar fusions, with lumbar interbody and posterolateral arthrodeses being the most common operations.[2] These fusion procedures are performed for a wide range of painful degenerative conditions including discogenic and facet mediated disease. In addition, stabilization of spinal segments is often a necessary adjunctive measure in treating several other spinal pathologies including infection, trauma, tumors, rheumatologic conditions, and spinal deformities.

Until recently, autogenous bone has definitively been the graft material of choice for spinal arthrodesis. Autograft combines osteogenic, osteoinductive, and osteoconductive properties to maximize bone healing without the risks of provoking an immunogenic response or viral disease transmission. Generally, autograft bone is harvested from the iliac crest or in certain indications from a resected rib or fibula. Although autograft is an optimal agent for promoting arthrodesis, several factors limit its use. The morbidity of harvesting iliac bone is reported to be as high as 30% and includes complications such as donor-site pain, infection, fractures, hematoma, necessity of a separate incision, increased operative time, and blood loss.[3–8] Another limitation of using autogenous bone is the availability of sufficient graft material. Multilevel fusions for deformity, particularly in children, may require more bone graft than can be reasonably harvested.

Local autograft from the primary surgical site is an alternative to iliac crest bone. Laminectomy bone, spinous processes, and facet joints are frequently removed as part of lumbar decompressive and fusion procedures, and provide an autogenous bone source without the risks associated with iliac crest harvest. Cortical bone shavings following use of a high-speed cutting burr is an additional method for obtaining autogenous bone.[9] Studies have demonstrated good results using local bone for lumbar interbody and posterolateral arthrodeses.[10–13] The quantity of local bone available from the surgical site, however, is limited, and evidence suggests that local bone alone may be ineffective for multilevel fusions.[14]

With the rising popularity of spinal fusion surgery, attention has focused on developing new synthetic and biologic agents that can substitute for autograft. The complexity of various current graft options is predicated on the notion that successful arthrodesis is influenced by many local and systemic factors that compose the biologic milieu in which the graft is placed. Therefore, these graft alternatives have different intrinsic biochemical and structural properties that affect their potential for enhancing fusion. In addition, graft substitutes are subject to a variety of mechanical stresses depending on where and how they are used, which in turn affect their ability to promote arthrodesis. Ultimately, choosing the ideal bone graft substitute is dependent on understanding the complex interaction of biologic and biomechanical forces that occur in spinal fusion.

The biology of bone fusion is a multifactorial process, in which three basic graft properties have been identified. *Osteogenicity* is the presence of viable precursor stem cells that will differentiate into osteoblasts, thereby directly forming new bone. Autogenous bone marrow is the primary example of an osteogenic graft. *Osteoinductivity* relies on growth factors, namely bone morphogenetic proteins (BMPs), that recruit precursor cells to the graft site and induce their differentiation into osteoblasts. Recombinant BMP and demineralized bone matrix are osteoinductive substitutes. *Osteoconductivity* is the structural scaffold in which neovascularization and infiltration of osteogenic stem cells occurs. Osteoconductive grafts assist with bone formation, but do not directly provide precursor cells or growth factors. Osteoconduction depends on the graft's specific porosity and interconnectivity to allow for ingrowth of blood vessels and new bone. Osteoconductive implants include allograft, ceramics, collagen, and polymers.

In addition to properties of the graft, the graft–host environment plays an important role in promoting new bone formation. Local and systemic factors, surgical preparation of the host bone, and mechanical stabilization are critical issues affecting new bone growth. Systemic conditions such as diabetes and osteoporosis, the use of nicotine or antiinflammatory medications, and prior radiation treatments significantly inhibit bone healing.[15,16] Excessive muscle stripping during surgery devascularizes tissue, thereby limiting angiogenesis and the supply of oxygen, nutrients, and precursor cells to the developing fusion mass.[17] Inadequate decortication of the host bone surface reduces exposure of the fusion site to essential bone marrow, vascularity, and osteoprogenitor cells.[18] Mechanical instability and excessive motion injures fragile new blood vessels and disrupts graft–host apposition, leading to fibroblastic nonunion. The improvement in fusion rates with spinal

Table 15.1 Properties of Bone Graft Materials

Bone Graft Substitute	Osteogenic Cells	Osteoinductive Factors	Osteoconductive Matrix	Initial Biomechanical Strength	Donor-Site Morbidity
Autogenous bone, cancellous	+++	++	+++	−	++
Autogenous bone, cortical	+	+	+	+++	++
Allograft, frozen	−	+	+	++	−
Allograft, lyophilization	−	+	+	+	−
Ceramics	−	−	+++	+	−
Demineralized bone matrix	−	++	+	−	−
Osteoinductive growth factors	−	+++	−	−	−
Unfractioned bone marrow	++	+	−	−	+
Mesenchymal stem cells	+++	−	−	−	+
Autologous platelet concentrate	−	++	−	−	−
Gene therapy, in vivo	−	+++	−	−	−
Gene therapy, ex vivo	++	+++	−	−	+

Source: From Whang PG, Wang JC. Bone graft substitutes for spinal fusion. Spine 2003;3:155–165. Copyright 2003, with permission from Elsevier.

fixation underscores the benefit of mechanical rigidity in promoting arthrodesis.[19]

In choosing the appropriate bone graft, several important factors need to be considered. The ideal bone graft is a material that possesses the properties of osteogenesis, osteoinduction, and osteoconduction without the risk of donor complications or disease transmission **(Table 15.1)**. The graft should be easy to use and cost-effective, it should provide structural stability, and it should be readily available in a reliable and reproducible form. For a given clinical indication, the graft alternative should either *extend* the amount of autograft available or entirely *substitute* for autograft with the same fusion rate. Ultimately, however, new bone forms via different mechanisms in various locations in the spine. Therefore, the ideal graft alternative may differ considerably on where and how it is used.

■ Allograft

Allograft bone obtained from cadaveric sources is the most widely used substitute for autogenous graft in spinal fusion surgery.[20] Allograft is primarily an osteoconductive scaffold with limited or minimal osteoinductive potential. Tissue preparation and processing eliminates all precursor stem cells and therefore osteogenicity. Advantages to allograft include the lack of donor-site morbidity, increased availability, and in some instances greater structural support (e.g., allograft femoral rings versus tricortical iliac crest). Allograft also can be customized via precision machine tooling and pressing into threaded bone dowels, wedges, and cancellous chips for a variety of indications. Disadvantages of allograft include a longer incorporation and remodeling time than autograft, resulting in delayed fusion and greater graft resorption. Extensive graft sterilization and preparation also compromises the graft's structural integrity. Lastly, allogeneic transplantation of tissue carries the potential risk of disease and infection transmission.

The risk of disease transmission from allograft bone in spinal surgery is estimated to be less than one in one million.[21] This low incidence of viral transmission is dependent on rigorous and thorough donor screening for human immunodeficiency virus (HIV), hepatitis B virus (HBV), and hepatitis C virus (HCV).[22] The only documented cases of viral transmission due to allograft implantation involved frozen unprocessed grafts.[23] The extensive sterilization process entails high-dose gamma irradiation or ethylene oxide gas, which consequently also destroys osteoinductive growth factors. After sterilization, allograft bone is then either frozen or lyophilized, which alters the antigenicity and structural integrity of the graft. In comparison, fresh frozen grafts have preserved structural integrity, but will also provoke an immunogenic response. Lyophilized grafts are substantially less immunogenic and can be stored for longer periods of time; however, their mechanical strength can be decreased by up to 50%.[24]

Allograft is available in cortical, cancellous, or as a composite corticocancellous form. Structural differences between cortical and cancellous grafts influence how they are incorporated into host bone, and thereby impact ultimately how they are used clinically. Cortical grafts provide strong mechanical support; however, they incorporate via a slow process of callus formation and periosteal bone growth around the graft. The lattice network of cancellous graft confers less mechanical strength, but provides a large surface area for ingrowth of new bone and vessels. Cancellous bone thereby incorporates more rapidly and eventually completely remodels over time. Consequently, cortical allografts such as femoral rings or fibular struts are used to occupy a disk space or corpectomy defect where they are placed under compressive loads. Cancellous allograft (e.g., cancellous chips) is generally used in posterolateral fusions where the forces are primarily tensile. New hybrid corticocancellous allografts have been developed to maximize the advantages of both cortical and cancellous bone forms.

Clinical studies comparing the use of autograft and allograft for spinal fusions have generated varied results. Cortical allograft in anterior lumbar surgery has demonstrated comparable fusion rates to iliac crest autograft.[25] Barnes et al[26] implanted either allograft cylindrical threaded cortical bone dowels (TCBDs) or impacted allograft wedges in patients undergoing posterior lumbar interbody fusion. Both groups of patients had excellent radiographic fusion rates (TCBD 95.4%, impacted wedges 88.9%), with patients receiving wedges having a higher rate of satisfactory outcomes. The use of allograft for posterolateral arthrodesis, however, has demonstrated less favorable outcomes. Autograft alone was found to be superior to mixed autograft and allograft, as well as fresh frozen allograft in achieving solid arthrodesis.[27] Freeze-dried allograft alone was inadequate in promoting posterolateral fusion. Use of allograft for posterolateral fusion has primarily been successful in children undergoing surgery for deformity correction.[28] Effective use of cancellous autograft for posterolateral fusion may only be as a graft extender of autogenous bone, and not as a sole bone graft substitute.

■ Demineralized Bone Matrix

Marshall Urist[29] first identified that demineralized bone matrix (DBM) that, when implanted in the subcutaneous muscle of mice, led to ectopic osteogenesis. Further studies revealed that DBM contains growth factors, later identified as BMPs, that are capable of inducing precursor cells down the osteoblastic pathway toward new bone formation. BMPs, however, represent only about 0.1% by weight of all bone proteins in DBM.[30] The majority of DBM is a composite of type 1 collagen (93%) and other soluble noncollagenous proteins (5%) that serve as osteoconductive carriers for growth factors.[31]

The extensive processing and demineralization of DBM reduces its immunogenicity and renders it nonosteogenic. After processing, DBM is primarily in powder form and lacks any structural integrity. Therefore, DBM is often combined with several carriers to modify its consistency and improve ease of handling. Crushed granules, putty, flexible wafers, or gel-packed syringes represent the variety of forms in which DBM is available **(Fig. 15.1)**. The types of carriers used with DBM include glycerol, poloxamer, gelatin, calcium sulfate, lecithin and hyaluronic acid.

Various DBM products differ significantly in their osteoinductivity. Different sterilization and demineralization techniques may alter the graft's intrinsic BMP potential. The handling characteristics of the various carriers may also impact the ability of the graft to maintain localization at the fusion site. Grafton (Osteotech, Eatontown, NJ), one of the first commercially available DBMs, is suspended in glycerol. Glycerol, however, is acidic, which may be harmful to host precursor cells necessary for osteoblastic differentiation, and in high doses in rats were found to be toxic.[32] Hyaluronic preparations have a more neutral pH that may be more conducive to host tissue.

Animal studies of spinal fusion using DBM have shown varied results. In a rabbit posterolateral fusion model, implantation of a flexible wafer form of DBM alone led to a 100% fusion rate.[33] In another rabbit posterolateral fusion study, Grafton, when combined with a less than standard amount of autograft, achieved fusion rates comparable to autograft alone.[34] In addition, DBM combined with autograft resulted in more rapid fusion both radiographically and biomechanically than with autograft alone.

Other studies, however, have revealed conflicting results. Cook et al[35] showed that DBM, either alone or combined with allograft, did not produce reliable fusion in dogs. In a dog model of posterolateral fusion, autograft was combined with a variety of graft extenders including DBM, type I collagen, and recombinant human bone morphogenetic protein-2 (rhBMP-2). The groups with DBM showed markedly lower rates of fusion and decreased biomechanical strength compared with groups without DBM.[36]

In humans, a multicenter prospective study was performed comparing allograft with DBM versus autograft for cervical spine fusion. Graft collapse and pseudarthrosis occurred more commonly with allograft and DBM, which may suggest that allograft and DBM may be unreliable as a graft substitute.[37] In another prospective randomized study, iliac crest autograft was compared with three parts DBM and one-third the standard amount of iliac crest autograft for posterolateral lumbar fusion.[38] At follow-up, the DBM autograft composite demonstrated similar fusion mineralization compared with autograft alone.

Because DBM lacks osteogenicity and is only weakly osteoinductive, it has limited capacity as a bone graft substitute. DBM may have a more effective role as a bone graft extender in the setting of insufficient autograft and has been demonstrated to be successful even in 3:1 ratios with autograft. DBM may also serve a valuable function as a carrier for more osteoinductive substances such as recombinant BMP or osteogenic sources like bone marrow aspirate.

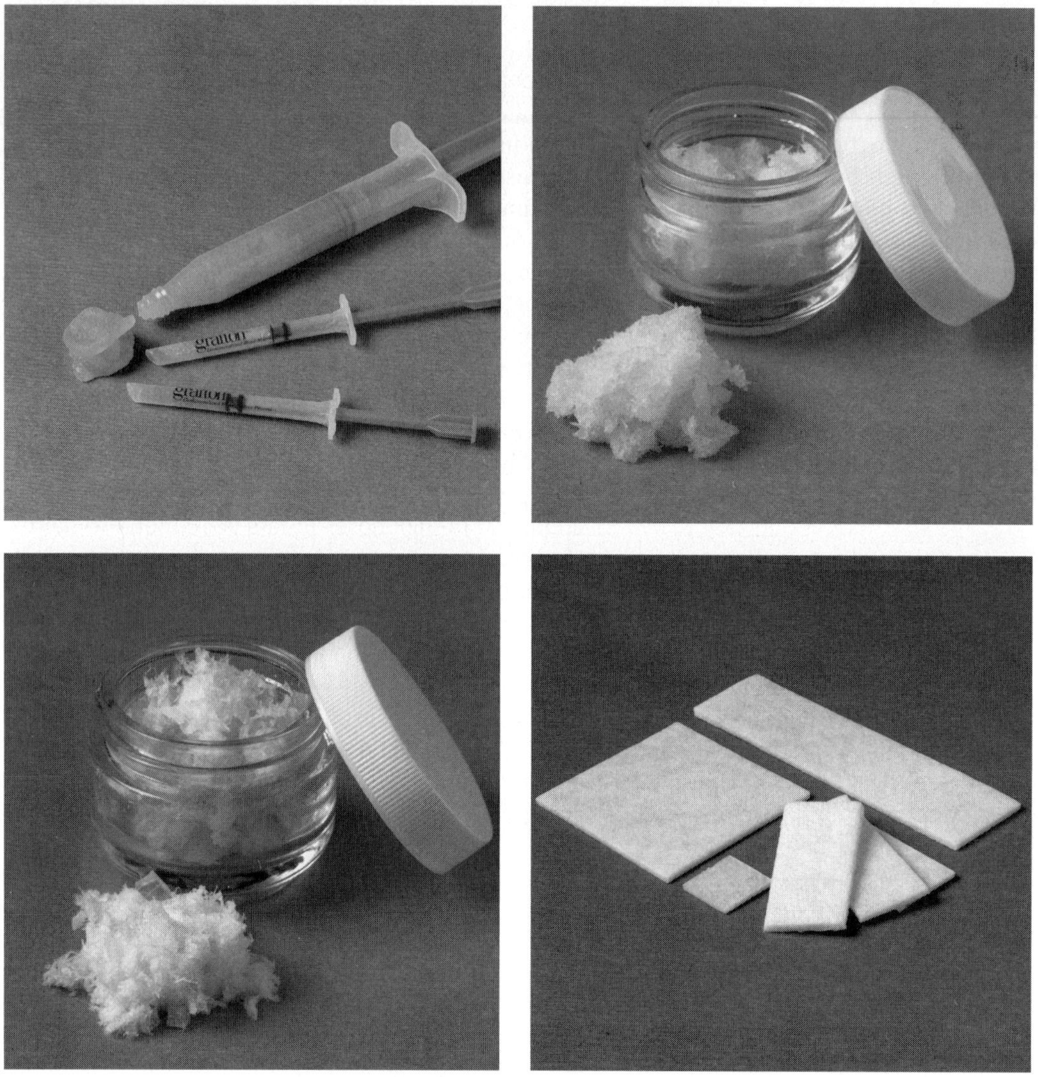

A B C D

Fig. 15.1 A variety of commercially available forms of demineralized bone matrix (DBM) (Grafton, Osteotech, Eatontown, NJ). **(A)** Gel. **(B)** Putty. **(C)** Combined DBM fibers and bone cubes. **(D)** Flexible wafer.

■ Ceramics

Ceramics include a broad array of natural or synthetic materials that were first identified as graft alternatives due to their close resemblance in chemical and structural architecture to human cancellous bone. Hydroxyapatite (HA), β-tricalcium phosphate (TCP), and biphasic calcium phosphate (composite of HA and TCP) are three forms of ceramics that are used for spinal fusion. HA of natural origin is processed via hydrothermal conversion from the coral exoskeleton of *Porites astreoides*. Synthetic TCP composites are developed by compacting TCP powder with naphthalene, which is later removed, leaving a porous structure. The unique mineral composition, porosity, and interconnectivity of ceramics allow for a high affinity for binding proteins, tissue ingrowth, cell attachment, and diffusion of nutrients into the fusion mass. In addition, the high porosity creates a large surface area for the migration of bony ingrowth. Ideally, the remodeling and biodegradation of ceramic grafts matches the rate of new bone formation.

The bioresorbability and mechanical strength of ceramics depend on their specific chemical and structural composition. In general, ceramics are brittle with a low fracture resistance. Increasing the material density of the ceramic results in greater structural integrity, but impedes graft resorption and subsequent remodeling. In contrast, greater porosity with a macropore interconnectivity resembling cancellous bone facilitates bone ingrowth and biodegradation of the graft material. HA has a higher material density, resulting in slow resorption and prolonged graft retention. Because of this, HA alone is rarely used as a bone graft extender. Conversely, TCP is rapidly resorbing and degrades as quickly as 6 weeks postimplantation. Biphasic composites of HA and TCP attempt to optimize material strength while closely matching the rate of graft degradation with the formation of new bone.

Ceramics offer many advantages. Because ceramics do not contain human tissue, they have no associated risk of disease transmission or of eliciting an immunogenic response. Synthetic ceramics can be produced in a reliable and consistent manner, are easy to sterilize, and are available in virtually limitless supply. They can also be machined into a variety of functional shapes for several different clinical applications (**Fig. 15.2**). Ceramics, however, are purely osteoconductive and generally need to be combined with autograft or used as a delivery vehicle for osteoinductive growth factors. Ceramics also are intrinsically brittle and confer little structural stability. Therefore, ceramics are only placed under neutral loading forces unless used in conjunction with a mechanical device such as a cage to provide primary structural support.

Animal studies using ceramics for spinal fusion have yielded varied results. Toth et al[39] tested biphasic calcium phosphates of increasing porosity versus autograft in a goat model of anterior cervical fusion. All calcium phosphate groups achieved fusion rates that were equal to or better than those for autograft. Animals treated with grafts with greater porosity demonstrated higher fusion rates; however, these grafts also resulted in more graft fractures. Baramki et al[40] studied HA in an instrumented posterolateral lumbar fusion model in sheep. Sheep were implanted with no graft, autograft, HA alone, or a mixture of HA and autograft. Autograft alone resulted in 100% fusion, followed by the autograft/HA composite, which achieved arthrodesis in 72% of animals. Only 50% of animals treated with HA alone demonstrated fusion.

The introduction of several new techniques for using and preparing ceramic grafts has demonstrated promising results. Boden et al[41,42] separately studied HA/TCP as a delivery vehicle for rhBMP-2 and HA as a carrier for osteoinductive bone protein extract in monkey and rabbit fusion models, respectively. Both HA/TCP/rhBMP-2 and HA/osteoinductive bone protein extract demonstrated superior fusion rates when compared with autograft. A novel silicated calcium phosphate (Actifuse, Apatech, London, UK) has also recently been developed in which a portion of the phosphate groups are replaced with silicate ions (**Fig. 15.3**). This concept is based on studies suggesting that dietary silicon plays a significant role in bone mineral density and new bone formation.[43] In an instrumented posterolateral fusion model in sheep, silicated calcium phosphate resulted in a robust fusion equivalent to autograft at 2 and 6 months.[44]

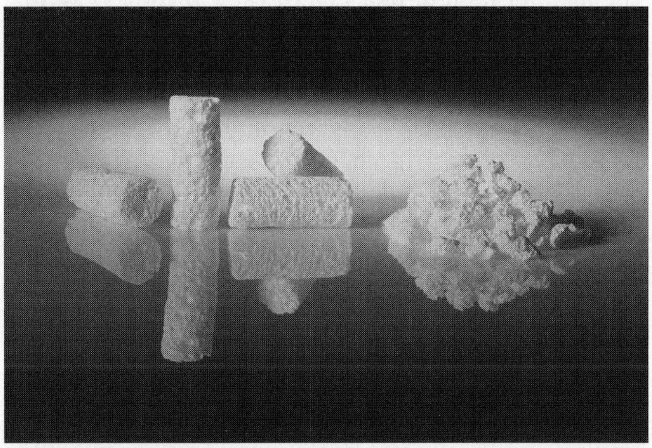

Fig. 15.2 Beta-tricalcium phosphate blocks and morsels (Vitoss, Orthovita, Malvern, PA).

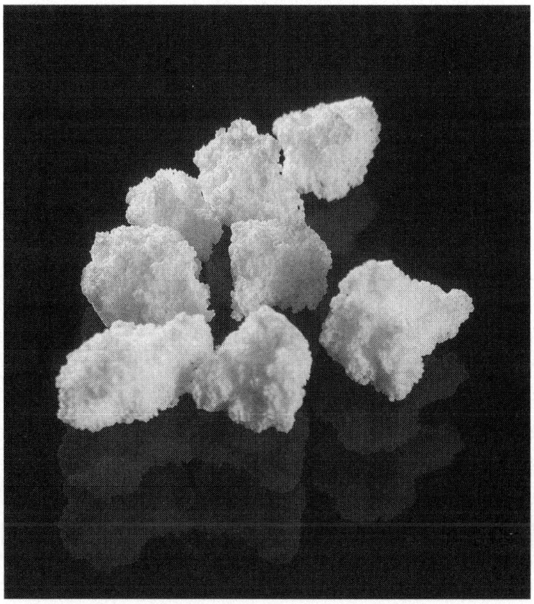

Fig. 15.3 Actifuse (Actifuse, Apatech, London, UK) silicated calcium phosphate granules.

Clinically, Thalgott et al[45] implanted coralline HA in patients undergoing anterior cervical diskectomy and fusion with rigid plate fixation and found a 100% fusion rate. The same coralline HA in patients undergoing anterior lumbar interbody fusion with posterior instrumentation and fusion demonstrated a 93.8% fusion rate.[46] Cho et al[47] randomly assigned patients undergoing anterior cervical diskectomy and fusion with a cage packed with either autograft or biphasic calcium phosphate. They found that prior to 6 months, the biphasic calcium phosphate group had significantly lower fusion rates. However, at 6 months, 100% of patients implanted with biphasic calcium phosphate demonstrated solid arthrodesis. Hsu et al[48] prospectively studied patients undergoing instrumented posterolateral lumbar fusion in which all patients received autogenous iliac bone graft (AIBG) on one side, and one of the following three on the contralateral side: AIBG mixed with laminectomy bone, HA mixed with AIBG, and HA mixed with laminectomy bone. HA mixed with AIBG demonstrated successful fusion rates comparable to AIBG and laminectomy bone. HA mixed with laminectomy bone, however, resulted in poor fusion rates.

■ Bone Marrow Aspirate

Autologous bone marrow is a source of osteoprogenitor cells and growth factors. Conventional methods of harvesting autogenous iliac crest bone marrow are associated with significant donor-site morbidity.[3–8] Bone marrow aspiration, however, is an alternative method for procurement of mesenchymal stem cells (MSCs) via a less invasive approach.[49] The bone marrow of healthy adults contains only one mesenchymal stem cell per 50,000 nucleated cells.[50] As bone marrow is aspirated, this concentration of stem cells is further diluted by peripheral blood. Muschler et al[50] found that 4 cc of bone marrow aspirate (BMA) has a 9% lower concentration of MSCs compared with 2 cc of BMA from the same patient. Therefore, no more than 2 cc of bone marrow should be harvested from any single site to avoid further dilution of precursor cells.

Recently, a commercially available device (Cellect, Depuy Acromed, Raynham, MA) has been developed to maximize the number of MSCs obtained during bone marrow aspiration **(Fig. 15.4)**. Selective cell retention technology uses the properties of an affinity column to result in a three to fourfold increase in MSCs by eliminating nucleated cells. During surgery, Cellect can be used to process bone marrow aspirate to optimize the concentration of osteoprogenitor cells. The same device then populates an allograft, ceramic, or collagen matrix with the increased MSCs prior to implantation in a fusion site.

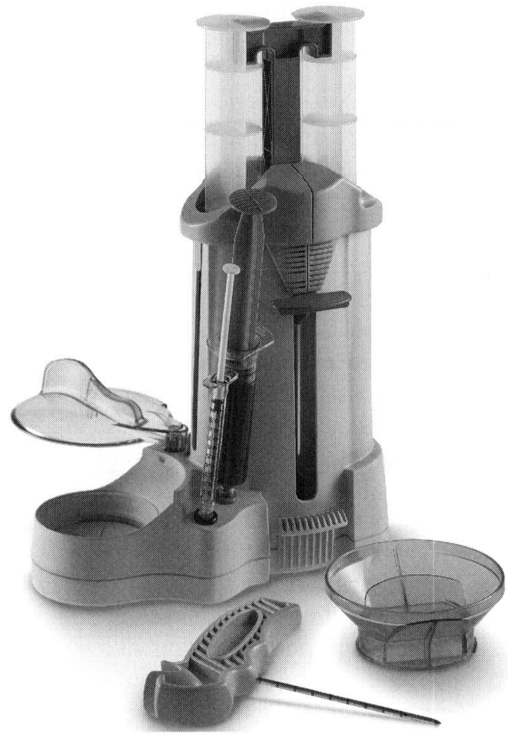

Fig. 15.4 Selective cell retention technology (Cellect, Depuy Acromed, Raynham, MA) designed to optimize the concentration of osteoprogenitor cells from bone marrow aspirate.

Preclinical studies have demonstrated optimistic results for the use of BMA as a bone graft substitute. Tay et al[51] implanted BMA and a collagen matrix mineralized with hydroxyapatite (Healos, Depuy Acromed, Raynham, MA) **(Fig. 15.5)** in a rabbit posterolateral fusion model. At 8 weeks postsurgery, 100% of rabbits receiving BMA and Healos demonstrated fusion, compared with only 18% of rabbits implanted with Healos alone. Griffith et al[52] studied baboons undergoing anterior lumbar interbody fusion with either BMA and Healos or autologous bone. Both groups had similar fusion rates at both 3 and 6 months, with identical biomechanical strength and amount of trabecular bone seen.

Clinically, Kitchel[53] investigated BMA in 25 patients undergoing posterior lumbar interbody fusion and instrumented posterolateral fusion. All patients received mineralized collagen matrix and BMA on one side of the posterolateral fusion and autograft on the contralateral side. Patients were followed at 12 and 24 months. Computed tomography reconstructions and flexion/extension radiography demonstrated an 84% fusion rate on the autograft side and an 80% fusion rate with BMA.

Bone marrow aspiration is a method in which autologous mesenchymal stem cells can be harvested, and, when combined with an appropriate carrier, provides both an osteogenic and osteoconductive graft. The benefit of bone marrow aspiration is that it eliminates many of the typical donor-site morbidities associated with conventional autologous graft harvesting techniques. The capability of BMA to function as a bone graft substitute and its appropriate indications remain to be fully elucidated in clinical trials.

■ Bone Morphogenetic Proteins

The identification of BMPs dates back to early work first pioneered by Urist.[29] He found that the organic matrix of bone contained proteins that serve to induce precursor cells to differentiate into osteoblasts and form new bone. These proteins are capable of initiating the multitude of cellular events leading to osteogenesis, such as recruiting stem cells, neovascularization, new bone formation, remodeling, and marrow formation. These proteins were later identified as bone morphogenetic proteins (BMPs).

The BMPs are multifunctional signaling proteins that are in the family of the transforming growth factor-β (TGF-β) cytokines. BMPs bind to the two types of serine/threonine kinase receptors, which then phosphorylate intracellular substrates known as Smads. These Smads subsequently affect transcription of BMP-specific genes within the nucleus. In this manner, they serve a role in a variety of different processes including embryogenesis, skeletal

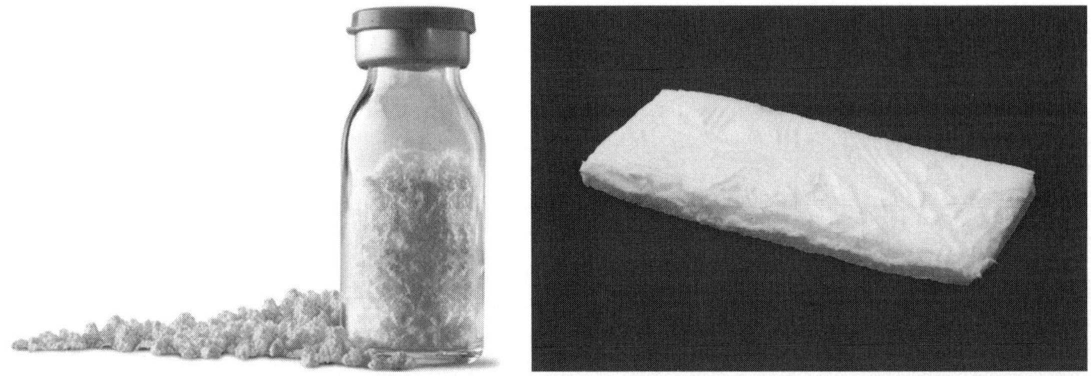

A B

Fig. 15.5 Healos (Depuy Acromed, Raynham, MA) collagen matrix mineralized with hydroxyapatite. **(A)** Granules. **(B)** Sponge.

morphogenesis, angiogenesis, and tissue homeostasis. In addition, BMPs are the only known cytokines that can induce de novo bone formation.

Methods of extracting and purifying bone matrix to obtain BMP result in a low yield of osteoinductive material. Only 20 μg of purified osteoinductive graft can be extracted from a 10-kg source of bone. Molecular cloning techniques, however, resulted in the identification and subsequent recombinant expression of a few BMPs specifically capable of osteoinduction. BMP-2 (InFuse, Medtronic Sofamor Danek, Memphis, TN), BMP-4, and BMP-7 (OP-1, Stryker Biotech, Hopkinton, MA) are recognized as molecules responsible for forming new cartilage and bone. Recombinant formulations allow the possibility of a virtually unlimited quantity of BMP. In addition, these recombinant growth factors can be produced reliably without impurities or irrelevant factors as are seen in bone-derived BMP extracts.

The practical use of BMP, however, requires a carrier or delivery vehicle to maintain a concentration of these growth factors at the intended fusion site. The best studied carrier for BMP is type 1 collagen that is derived from bovine or porcine connective tissue. Collagen delivery vehicles bind BMP well, but do not provide biomechanical support. Biodegradable polymers such as polylactic acid (PLA) and polyglycolic acid (PLG) are synthetic carriers that can be created into a variety of shapes, but they are less osteoconductive than collagen, they result in acidic by-products, and in some animal studies have demonstrated low-grade inflammatory reactions.[54] Inorganic matrices include hydroxyapatite, tricalcium phosphate, and biphasic calcium phosphates. HA alone is slowly resorbed and may interfere with osteogenesis. TCPs and biphasic calcium phosphates are more rapidly resorbed and may be more ideally suited to serve as a carrier for BMP. Cortical allograft (i.e., femoral ring) remodels quickly with rhBMP-2 and has been used successfully as a carrier for rhBMP-2 in anterior interbody fusions.[55]

Preclinical studies comparing the benefit of BMP versus autograft have shown promising results in a variety of animal spinal fusion models. In a rabbit posterolateral fusion model, Schimandle et al[56] demonstrated a 100% fusion rate with rhBMP-2 combined with a type 1 collagen sponge compared with a 42% fusion rate with iliac crest autograft. These results were confirmed by both radiographic and histologic studies that showed increased and more rapid bone formation, consolidation, and remodeling with rhBMP-2. Zdeblick et al[57] placed Bagby and Kuslich (BAK) cages (Spine-Tech, Minneapolis, MN) with rhBMP-2 and collagen sponge in a goat anterior cervical fusion model and demonstrated a 95% fusion rate. Only 48% of goats implanted with a BAK cage and autograft also achieved spinal fusion.

Bone morphogenetic protein has also been successful in achieving fusion in settings in which autograft is known to be poorly effective. Sandhu et al[58] demonstrated that posterolateral fusion in dogs with rhBMP-2 and a collagen sponge occurred even without decortication of the transverse processes. rhBMP-7 was studied in a posterolateral fusion model in New Zealand rabbits and found a 100% fusion rate, even when exposed to systemic nicotine.[59,60] In the same model, arthrodesis with autograft dropped from 63% to 25% when similarly exposed to nicotine.

Initial nonhuman primate studies with BMP and a collagen sponge for posterolateral fusion were less successful, suggesting that either the rhBMP dose was too low or the collagen sponge may be too compressible a carrier in the paraspinal muscles. Boden et al[41] combined rhBMP-2 and a bulkier HA/TCP (60/40) carrier in adult rhesus monkeys undergoing laminectomy and posterolateral fusion. All rhBMP-2 groups had 100% fusion, with a greater amount and quality of bone with increasing doses of rhBMP-2 (6, 9, and 12 mg). Akamaru et al[61] used rhBMP-2 and a collagen sponge layered with allograft bone chips or ceramic granules as bulking agents. This method resulted in 100% fusion in a nonhuman primate posterior fusion model, whereas only one of three animals treated with autograft achieved arthrodesis.

Bolstered by preclinical success, a prospective multicenter randomized trial was conducted comparing a lumbar tapered (LT) cage (Medtronic Sofamor Danek, Memphis, TN)

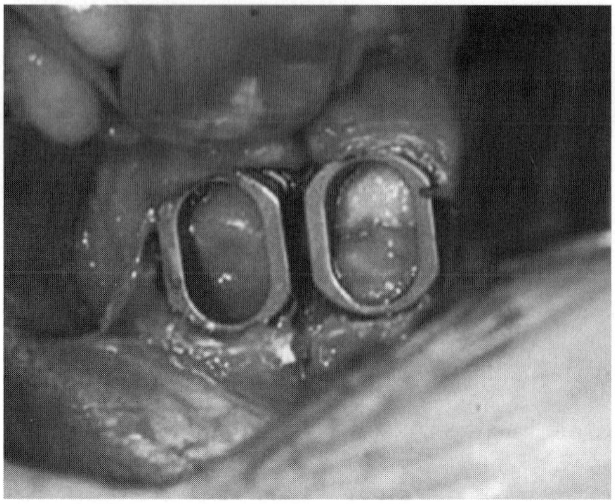

Fig. 15.6 Anterior lumbar interbody fusion with lumbar tapered (LT) cage (Medtronic Sofamor Danek, Memphis, TN) and InFuse bone morphogenetic protein- 2 (Medtronic Sofamor Danek).

with rhBMP-2 on a type 1 collagen sponge (InFuse bone graft, Medtronic Sofamor Danek) versus autograft for anterior lumbar interbody fusion (ALIF) **(Fig. 15.6)**.[62] At 2-year follow-up, the rhBMP-2 group demonstrated 100% radiographic fusion compared with 95.6% fusion in the autograft group. Standard clinical outcome measures (Oswestry Disability Index, Short Form [SF]-36, and back pain scores) were not statistically different between the two groups. These data have subsequently been replicated with similar success using an allograft bone dowel packed with rhBMP-2.[63]

Boden et al[64] further studied rhBMP-2 in a posterolateral lumbar fusion setting. Patients were randomized to receive autograft with Texas Scottish Rite Hospital (TSRH) pedicle screw instrumentation, rhBMP-2 with biphasic calcium phosphate carrier and TSRH, or rhBMP-2 without instrumentation. All patients treated with rhBMP-2 demonstrated radiographic fusion, compared with only 40% of patients with autograft and instrumentation. The rhBMP-2 (without TSRH) group showed earliest evidence of significant improvement in the Oswestry score (at 6 weeks). The rhBMP-2/TSRH group followed with improvement in the Oswestry score at 3 months. The autograft/TSRH group did not demonstrate improvement in Oswestry score until 6 months. The most improvement in Oswestry score at final follow up was achieved in the rhBMP-2 only group.

Similar clinical studies have been performed investigating the efficacy of BMP-7 for spinal fusion. Vaccaro et al[65] compared rhBMP-7 (OP-1) putty to iliac crest autograft in patients undergoing noninstrumented posterolateral lumbar fusion. Patients receiving rhBMP-7 demonstrated successful fusion in 55% of patients versus only 40% of patients implanted with autograft. The rhBMP-7 group also resulted in higher rates of improvement in Oswestry score compared with the autograft group. Kanayama et al[66] studied rhBMP-7 versus local autograft and ceramic bone substitute in patients undergoing posterolateral lumbar fusion with pedicle screw fixation. The patients with rhBMP-7 demonstrated comparable rates of radiographic fusion compared with the autograft/ceramic group. Interestingly, however, upon open surgical exploration, the rhBMP-7 group demonstrated solid fusion in only four of seven patients despite evidence of new bone formation in all patients.

Other BMP studies have demonstrated less than favorable results. A prospective randomized controlled study investigated patients receiving either rhBMP-2 or autograft in a cylindrical titanium cage for stand-alone posterior lumbar interbody fusion.[67] Oswestry disability, back pain, and leg pain scores were similar in both treatment groups. However, the fusion rate was lower in the rhBMP-2 group at 12 months compared with the autograft group. In addition, extravertebral bone was seen adjacent to the cage in the anterior portion of the spinal canal. Pradhan et al[68] prospectively studied a cohort of patients undergoing anterior lumbar interbody fusion with a femoral ring allograft (FRA) combined with rhBMP-2. After only nine patients, the authors terminated the study secondary to suboptimal results compared with their cohort of patients receiving FRA and autograft. Pradhan et al found that the patients implanted with FRA and rhBMP-2 had a noticeably higher nonunion rate (56%) as opposed to the FRA and autograft group (36%). In addition, they noted that patients in the rhBMP-2 group had evidence of early and aggressive resorption of the FRA with some instances of graft fracture and disintegration. The authors attributed this untoward effect to osteoclastic activity induced by the rhBMP-2. The study was terminated early due to these findings, and therefore statistical significance was not attained in comparing the two treatment groups.

The identification and subsequent recombinant expression and cloning of BMPs has led to a surge of interest in the development of BMPs as a bone graft substitute for spinal surgery. Initial overwhelming successes with BMP in both preclinical and clinical models have been met with great enthusiasm. However, the appropriate clinical settings, dosages, and delivery vehicles still need to be further studied before this powerful biologic agent is approved for the variety of needs of the spinal surgeon.

■ Platelet Growth Factors

The pursuit of growth factors involved in new bone formation has led to recent study of platelets and their release of specific signaling molecules in response to tissue repair. These growth factors, distinct from BMPs, are thought to be responsible for chemotaxis of various undifferentiated progenitor stem cells to an injury site. Platelet-derived growth factor (PDGF) and TGF-β are two such factors that are implicated in tissue repair. Further examination reveals that increasing the concentration of PDGF and TGF-β at an injury site enhances healing and thereby may potentially serve as an autologous osteoinductive graft source. This enthusiasm has been validated by in vitro and animal studies demonstrating that platelet concentrate stimulates bone growth.[69–72]

Recently, commercially available techniques have been developed to filtrate and sequester platelets from autologous whole blood (Symphony Platelet Concentrate System, Depuy Acromed, Raynham, MA) **(Fig. 15.7)**. By this process, platelets and their associated growth factors are reportedly concentrated in plasma several times that of whole blood. This platelet-rich plasma is then combined with a fibrin clot or an osteoconductive carrier matrix for implantation in a spinal fusion bed.

Clinical studies using autologous platelet growth factors have demonstrated mixed results. Lowery et al[73] reported a 100% arthrodesis rate when retrospectively reviewing their series of anterior and posterior lumbar fusions combining platelet growth factors with allograft or autograft. Jenis et al[74] prospectively studied patients undergoing lumbar interbody fusion with either iliac crest bone graft or allograft combined with autogenous growth factors. At 1- and 2-year follow-up, the allograft/growth factor group had an 89% fusion rate, and no statistical difference radiographically or clinically with autograft.

Other studies, however, have found an inhibitory effect of platelet growth factors on lumbar fusion. Weiner and Walker[75] augmented iliac crest autograft with autologous growth factors in patients undergoing single-level noninstrumented lumbar fusion. The control group, consisting of patients receiving only autograft, had a fusion rate of 91% compared with a 62% fusion rate in patients augmented with growth factors. Carreon et al[76] performed a similar study in patients undergoing instrumented posterolateral fusion. They found a higher nonunion rate in the iliac crest/growth factor group (25%) versus the autograft only group (17%). These paradoxical results are possibly explained by

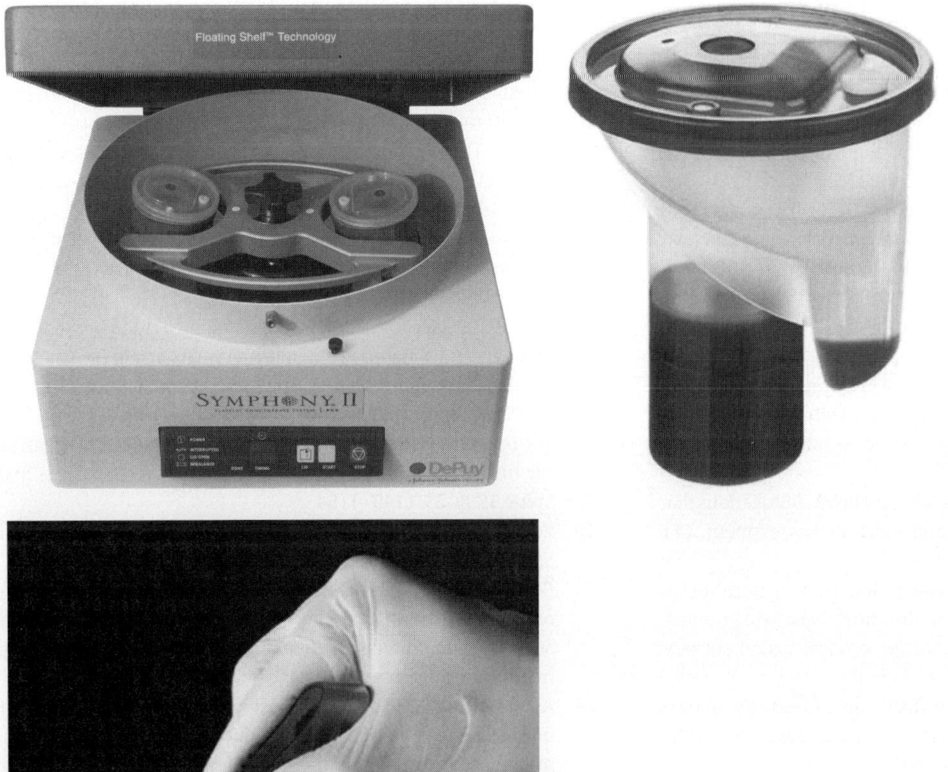

A

B

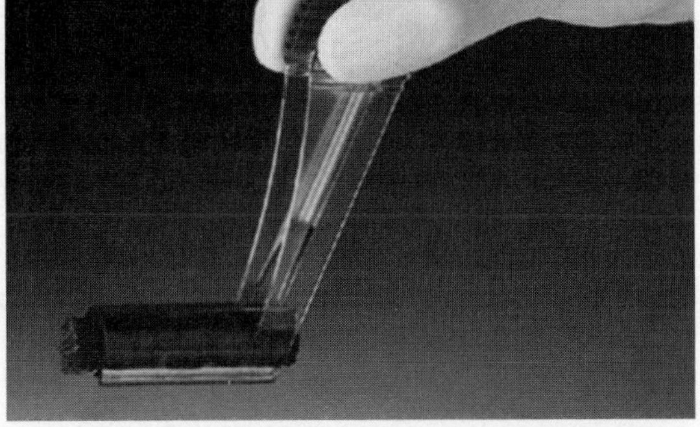

C

Fig. 15.7 Platelet concentration system for the preparation of autologous growth factors. **(A)** Symphony II (Depuy Acromed, Raynham, MA) platelet-rich plasma filtration device. **(B)** Disposable chamber with platelet-rich plasma. **(C)** Graft log with platelet concentrate in forceps.

an inhibitory effect on bony repair found when unnatural amounts of PDGF are combined with BMP.[75,77]

Several issues remain to be answered before platelet growth factors can play a major role in spinal surgery. The threshold concentration of platelets necessary to provide an enhanced effect on bone healing is yet to be determined. Also, the ideal carrier material for stable gradual release of platelet growth factors has not been identified in laboratory or clinical testing. Ultimately, though, the safe and autologous nature of harvesting platelet concentrate makes for a promising bone graft enhancer for spinal fusion.

■ Conclusion

An exciting new era of discovery is occurring in spinal surgery. The advent of new technology, such as improved spinal fixation, minimally invasive techniques, neuromonitoring, and 3D navigation systems, allows for the surgical management of an expanding number of patients and diseases. The current rise in spinal operations has been met with an increasing need for improved bone grafting alternatives for fusion procedures. Consequently, a surging interest has developed in spine biologics to provide spinal surgeons with a variety of graft options in their armamentarium. Each graft alternative possesses distinct cellular and biomechanical properties that dictate its clinical indication. The appropriate application of each bone graft material to optimize patient outcomes will be borne out only through rigorous, prospective, randomized clinical testing. The future holds the possibility of performing consistently successful spinal arthrodesis with minimized risk or morbidity to the patient.

References

1. Katz JN. Lumbar spinal fusion: surgical rates, costs, complications. Spine 1995;20:78S–83S
2. Boden SD. Overview of the biology of lumbar spine fusion and principles for selecting a bone graft substitute. Spine 2002;27(suppl): S26–S31
3. Kuhn DA, Moreland MS. Complications following iliac crest bone grafting. Clin Orthop Relat Res 1986;209:224–226
4. Kurz LT, Garfin SR, Booth RE. Harvesting autogenous iliac bone grafts: a review of complications and techniques. Spine 1989;14: 1324–1331
5. Summers BN, Eisenstein SM. Donor site pain from the ilium: a complication of lumbar spine fusion. J Bone Joint Surg Br 1989;71:677–680
6. Fernyhough JC, Schimandle JJ, Weigel MC, Edwards CC, Levine AM. Chronic donor site pain complicating bone graft harvesting from the posterior iliac crest for spinal fusion. Spine 1992;17:1474–1480
7. Goulet JA, Senunas LE, DeSilva GL, Greengield ML. Autogenous iliac crest bone graft. Complications and functional assessment. Clin Orthop Relat Res 1997;339:76–81
8. Wang MY, Levi AD, Shah S, Green BA. Polylactic acid mesh reconstruction of the anterior iliac crest after bone harvesting reduces early postoperative pain after anterior cervical fusion surgery. Neurosurgery 2002;51:413–416
9. Wang MY, Liu CY. Resorbable polylactic acid interbody spacers with vertebral autograft for anterior cervical discectomy and fusion. Neurosurgery 2005;57:135–140
10. Couture DE, Branch CL. Posterior lumbar interbody fusion with bioabsorbable spacers and local autograft in a series of 27 patients. Neurosurg Focus 2004;16:E8
11. Violas P, Chapuis M, Bracq H. Local autograft bone in the surgical management of adolescent idiopathic scoliosis. Spine 2004;29:189–192
12. Kai Y, Oyama M, Morooka M. Posterior lumbar interbody fusion using local facet joint autograft and pedicle screw fixation. Spine 2004;29:41–46
13. Chen WJ, Tsung-Ting T, Lih-Huei C, et al. The fusion rate of calcium sulfate with local autograft bone compared with autologous iliac bone graft for instrumented short-segment spinal fusion. Spine 2005;30:2293–2297
14. Sengupta DK, Truumees E, Patel CK, et al. Outcome of local bone versus autogenous iliac crest bone graft in the instrumented posterolateral fusion of the lumbar spine. Spine 2006;31:985–991
15. Daftari TK, Whitesides TE, Heller JG, Goodrich AC, McCarey BE, Hutton WC. Nicotine on the revascularization of bone graft. Spine 1994;19:904–911
16. Silcox DH, Daftari T, Boden SD, Schimandle JH, Hutton WC, Whitesides TE. The effect of nicotine on spinal fusion. Spine 1995;20:1549–1553
17. Boden SD, Schimandle JH. Fusion. Biology of lumbar spine fusion and bone graft materials. In: International Society for Study of the Lumbar Spine Editorial Committee, eds. The Lumbar Spine, 2nd ed. Philadelphia: WB Saunders, 1996:1284–1306
18. Toribatake Y, Hutton WC, Boden SD, et al. Revascularization of the fusion mass in a posterolateral intertransverse process fusion. Spine 1998;23:1149–1154
19. Zdeblick TA. A prospective, randomized study of lumbar fusion. Spine 1993;18:983–991
20. Berven S, Tay B, Kelinstueck FS, Bradford DS. Clinical applications of bone graft substitutes in spine surgery: consideration of mineralized and demineralized preparations and growth factor supplementation. Eur Spine J 2001;10:S169–S177
21. Asselmeier MA, Casperi RB, Bottenfeld S. A review of allograft processing and sterilization techniques and their role in transmission of the human immunodeficiency virus. Am J Sports Med 1993;21:170–175
22. Marthy S, Ricther M. Human immunodeficiency virus activity in rib allografts. J Oral Maxillofac Surg 1998;56:474–476
23. Tomford WW. Transmission of disease through transplantation of musculoskeletal allografts. J Bone Joint Surg Am 1995;77:1742–1754
24. Hamer AJ, Strachan JR, Black MM, Ibbotson CJ, Stockley I, Elson RA. Biomechanical properties of cortical allograft bone using a new method of bone strength measurement: a comparison of fresh, fresh-frozen, and irradiated bone. J Bone Joint Surg Br 1996;78: 363–368

25. Kozak JA, Heilman AE, O'Brian JP. Anterior lumbar fusion options: techniques and graft materials. Clin Orthop Relat Res 1994;300:45–51
26. Barnes B, Rodts GE, Haid RW, Subach BR, McLaughlin MR. Allograft implants for posterior lumbar interbody fusion: results comparing cylindrical dowels and impacted wedges. Neurosurgery 2002;51:1191–1198
27. An HS, Lynch K, Toth J. Prospective comparison of autograft vs. allograft for adult posterolateral lumbar spine fusion: differences among freeze-dried, frozen, and mixed grafts. J Spinal Disord 1995;8:131–135
28. Dodd CA, Ferguson CM, Freedman K. Allograft versus autograft in scoliosis surgery. J Bone Joint Surg Br 1988;70:431–434
29. Urist MR. Bone formation by autoinduction. Science 1965; 150:893–899
30. Sandhu HS, Grewal HS, Parvataneni H. Bone grafting for spinal fusion. Orthop Clin North Am 1999;30:685–698
31. Lee KJH, Roper JG, Wang JC. Demineralized bone matrix and spinal arthrodesis. Spine J 2005;5:217S–223S
32. Wang JC, Davies M, Kanim LEA, Ukatu CJ, Dawson EG, Lieberman JR. Prospective comparison of commercially available demineralized bone matrix for spinal fusion. Paper presented at the annual meeting of the North American Spine Society, October 2000, New Orleans
33. Martin GJ, Boden SD, Morone MA, Titus L, Scarborough NL. New formulations of demineralized bone matrix as a more effective graft alternative in experimental posterolateral lumbar spine arthrodesis. Spine 1999;24:637–645
34. Morone MA, Boden SD. Experimental posterolateral lumbar spinal fusion with a demineralized bone matrix gel. Spine 1998;23:159–167
35. Cook SD, Dalton JE, Prewett AB, Whitecould TS. In vivo evaluation of demineralized bone matrix as a bone graft substitute for posterior spine fusion. Spine 1995;20:877–886
36. Helm GA, Sheehan JM, Sheehan JP, et al. Utilization of type I collagen gel, demineralized bone matrix, and bone morphogenetic protein-2 to enhance autologous bone lumbar spinal fusion. J Neurosurg 1997;86:93–100
37. An HS, Simpson JM, Glover JM, Stephany J. Comparison between allograft plus demineralized bone matrix versus autograft in anterior cervical fusion: a prospective multi-center study. Spine 1995;20:2211–2216
38. Cammisa FP, Lowery G, Garfin SR, et al. Two-year fusion rate equivalency between Grafton DBM gel and autograft in posterolateral spine fusion: a prospective controlled trial employing a side-by-side comparison in the same patient. Spine 2004;29:660–666
39. Toth JM, An HS, Lim TH, et al. Evaluation of porous biphasic calcium phosphate ceramics for anterior cervical interbody fusion in a caprine model. Spine 1995;20:2203–2210
40. Baramki HG, Steffen T, Lander P, Chang M, Marchesi D. The efficacy of interconnected porous HA in achieving posterolateral lumbar fusion in sheep. Spine 2000;25:1053–1060
41. Boden SD, Martin GJ, Morone MA, Ugbo JL, Moskovitz PA. Posterolateral lumbar intertransverse process spine arthrodesis with recombinant human bone morphogenetic protein 2/HA-TCP after laminectomy in the nonhuman primate. Spine 1999;24:1179–1185
42. Boden SD, Martin GJ, Morone M, Ugbo JL, Titus L, Hutton WC. The use of coralline HA with bone marrow, autogenous bone graft, or osteoinductive bone protein extract for posterolateral lumbar spine fusion. Spine 1999;24:320–327
43. Eisinger J, Clariet D. Effects of silicon, fluoride, etidronate and magnesium on bone mineral density: a retrospective study. Magnes Res 1993;6:247–249
44. Wheeler DL, Jenis LG, Kovach ME, et al. Efficacy of silicated calcium phosphate graft in posterolateral lumbar fusion in sheep. Spine J 2007;7:308–317
45. Thalgott JS, Fritts K, Giuffre JM, Timlin M. Anterior interbody fusion of the cervical spine with coralline hydroxyapatite. Spine 1999;24:1295–1299
46. Thalgott JS, Klezl Z, Timlin M, Giuffre JM. Anterior lumbar interbody fusion with processed seal coral (coralline hydroxyapatite) as part of a circumferential fusion. Spine 2002;27:E518–E525
47. Cho DY, Lee WY, Sheu PC, Chen CC. Cage containing a biphasic calcium phosphate ceramic (Triosite) for the treatment of cervical spondylosis. Surg Neurol 2005;63:497–503
48. Hsu CJ, Chou WY, Teng HP, Chang WN, Chou YJ. Coralline hydroxyapatite and laminectomy-derived bone as adjuvant graft material for lumbar posterolateral fusion. J Neurosurg Spine 2005;3:271–275
49. Kitchel SH, Wang MY, Lauryssen CL. Techniques for aspirating bone marrow for use in spinal surgery. Neurosurgery 2005;57(ONS suppl 3):ONS286–ONS289
50. Muschler GF, Boehm C, Easley KA. Aspiration to obtain osteoblast progenitor cells from human bone marrow: the influence of aspiration volume. J Bone Joint Surg Am 1997;79:1699–1709
51. Tay BK, Le AX, Heilman M, et al. Use of a collagen-hydroxyapatite matrix in spinal fusion: a rabbit model. Spine 1998;23:2276–2281
52. Griffith S, Criscitello A, Cunningham B, et al. Non-human primate evaluation of an osteoconductive bone substitute in an interbody fusion cage. Paper presented at EuroSpine, 1999, Munich, Germany
53. Kitchel SH. A preliminary comparative study of radiographic results using mineralized collagen and bone marrow aspirate versus autologous bone in the same patients undergoing posterior lumbar interbody fusion with instrumented posterolateral lumbar fusion. Spine J 2006;6:405–411
54. Sandhu HS, Kanim LE, Kabo JM, et al. Evaluation of rhBMP-2 with an OPLA carrier in a canine posterolateral (transverse process) spinal fusion model. Spine 1995;20:2669–2682
55. Hecht BP, Fischgrund JS, Herkowitz HN, Penman L, Toth JM, Shirkhoda A. The use of recombinant human bone morphogenetic protein 2 (rhBMP-2) to promote spinal fusion in a nonhuman primate anterior interbody fusion model. Spine 1999;24:629–636
56. Schimandle JH, Boden SD, Hutton WC. Experimental spinal fusion with recombinant human bone morphogenetic protein-2. Spine 1995;20:1326–1337
57. Zdeblick TA, Ghanayem AJ, Rapoff AJ, et al. Cervical interbody fusion cage: An animal model with and without bone morphogenetic protein. Spine 1998;23:758–766
58. Sandhu HS, Kanim LEA, Toth JM, et al. Experimental spinal fusion with recombinant bone morphogenetic protein-2 without decortication of osseous elements. Spine 1997;22:1171–1180
59. Grauer JN, Patel TC, Erulkar JS, Troiano NW, Panjabi MM, Friedlaender GE. Evaluation of OP-1 as a graft substitute for intertransverse process lumbar fusion. Spine 2001;26:127–133
60. Patel TC, Erulkar JS, Grauer JN, Troiano NW, Panjabi MM, Friedlaender GE. OP-1 overcomes the inhibitory effect of nicotine on posterolateral lumbar fusion. Presented at the 15th annual meeting of the North American Spine Society, October 25–28, 2000, New Orleans
61. Akamaru T, Suh D, Boden SD, et al. Simple carrier matrix modifications can enhance delivery of recombinant human bone

morphogenetic protein-2 for posterolateral spine fusion. Spine 2003;28:429–434

62. Burkus JK, Gornet MF, Dickman CA, Zdeblick TA. Anterior lumbar interbody fusion using rhBMP-2 with tapered interbody cages. J Spinal Disord Tech 2002;15:337–349
63. Burkus JK, Transfeldt EE, Kitchel SH, Watkins RG, Balderston RA. Clinical and radiographic outcomes of anterior lumbar interbody fusion using recombinant human bone morphogenetic protein-2. Spine 2002;27:2396–2408
64. Boden SD, Kang J, Sandhu H, Heller JG. Use of recombinant human bone morphogenetic protein-2 to achieve posterolateral lumbar spine fusion in humans: A prospective, randomized clinical pilot trial: 2002 Volvo Award in clinical studies. Spine 2002;27:2662–2673
65. Vaccaro AR, Anderson DG, Patel T, et al. Comparison of OP-1 putty (rhBMP-7) to iliac crest autograft for posterolateral lumbar arthrodesis: a minimum of 2-year follow-up pilot study. Spine 2005;30:2709–2716
66. Kanayama M, Hashimoto T, Shigenobu K, et al. A prospective randomized study of posterolateral lumbar fusion using osteogenic protein-1 (OP-1) versus local autograft with ceramic bone substitute: emphasis of surgical exploration and histologic assessment. Spine 2006;31:1067–1074
67. Alexander JT, Branch CL Jr, Haid RW Jr, et al. An analysis of the use of rhBMP-2 in PLIF constructs: clinical and radiographic outcomes. Presented at the 18th annual meeting of the American Association of Neurological Surgeons and Congress of Neurological Surgeons Section on Disorders of the Spine and Peripheral Nerves, Orlando, FL, February 27 to March 2, 2002
68. Pradhan BB, Bae HW, Dawson EG, Patel VV, Delamarter RB. Graft resorption with the use of bone morphogenetic protein: lessons from anterior lumbar interbody fusion using femoral ring allografts and recombinant human bone morphogenetic protein-2. Spine 2006;31:E277–E284
69. Marx RE, Carlson ER, Eichstaedt RM, et al. Platelet-rich plasma: growth factor enhancement for bone graft. Oral Surg Oral Med Oral Pathol Oral Radiol Endod 1998;85:638–646
70. Gruber R, Varga F, Fischer MB, et al. Platelets stimulate proliferation of bone cells: involvement of platelet-derived growth factor, microparticles and membranes. Clin Oral Implants Res 2002;13:529–535
71. Kim ES, Park EJ, Choung PH. Platelet concentration and its effect on bone formation in calvarial defects: an experimental study in rabbits. J Prosthet Dent 2001;86:428–433
72. Siebrecht MA, De Rooij PP, Arm DM, et al. Platelet concentrate increases bone ingrowth into porous hydroxyapatite. Orthopedics 2002;25:169–172
73. Lowery GL, Kulkarni S, Pennisi AE. Use of autologous growth factors in lumbar spinal fusion. Bone 1999;25:47S–50S
74. Jenis LG, Banco RJ, Kwon B. A prospective study of autologous growth factors (AGF) in lumbar interbody fusion. Spine J 2006;6:14–20
75. Weiner BK, Walker M. Efficacy of autologous growth factors in lumbar intertransverse fusions. Spine 2003;28:1968–1971
76. Carreon LY, Glassman SD, Anekstein Y, Puno RM. Platelet gel (AGF) fails to increase fusion rates in instrumented posterolateral fusions. Spine 2005;30:E243–E246
77. Marden LJ, Fan RSP, Pierce GF, et al. Platelet derived growth factors inhibit bone regeneration induced by osteogenin, a BMP, in rat craniotomy defects. J Clin Invest 1993;92:2897–2905

16 Growth Factors for Spinal Fusion

Thomas E. Mroz

Over 185,000 spinal fusions are performed annually in the United States, and the reported failure rates range from 5 to 45% and continue to be problematic.[1] Arthrodesis is a technique used to treat various spinal pathologies, including deformity, instability, trauma, infection, and tumor. Traditionally, fusions are performed with either allogenic or autogenous bone graft, the latter of which is superior in promoting arthrodesis. The ideal bone graft has three primary properties: osteogenic, osteoinductive, and osteoconductive. Autogenous bone (e.g., iliac crest) contains osteoblasts, supplies regulatory factors that promote bone formation, and is a natural lattice that supports new osseous growth. Hence it has all three components of an ideal graft, and as such, it is considered the gold standard source of bone for fusion procedures. However, bone graft harvest from the iliac crest has been fraught with considerable morbidity, and complication rates that are as high as 30% have been reported. Reports of excessive blood loss,[2,3] neuropathy,[4,5] hernia,[6–8] ureteral injury,[9] arteriovenous fistula formation,[2,9] pseudoaneurysm of the pelvic vasculature,[2] pelvic instability,[10] and infection[11] all have been reported. This associated morbidity, with a procedure that occurs 200,000 times annually in this country,[11] underscores the avid interest in developing reliable bone graft substitutes to use in spinal fusions.

■ Bone Morphogenetic Protein

Bone is composed of approximately 65 to 70% inorganic components (i.e., calcium phosphates, calcium carbonate, sodium, magnesium, fluoride) and 30 to 35% organic components. The latter is, in turn, composed of 90% collagen (mainly type I), and 10% mixture of noncollagenous matrix proteins (glycoproteins, phospholipids, phosphoproteins), growth factors, and cytokines.

Marshall R. Urist is credited with the discovery of bone morphogenetic proteins (BMPs). In 1965, he reported on the ability of demineralized bone matrix (DBM) to induce differentiation of cartilage and bone and bone formation in ectopic sites in multiple species, including mice, rats, rabbits, and guinea pigs.[12–14] Urist later became the first to extract an osteoinductive glycoprotein (i.e., the first BMP) from DBM.[15] Since this report, a multitude of BMPs have been identified, and many have been shown to have osteoinductive potential.[16]

Bone morphogenetic proteins are secreted polypeptides that have regulatory effects on various cell lineages, and belong to the transforming growth factor-β (TGF-β) superfamily. It is well known that DBM and purified or recombinant BMPs affect many cell lines, including pluripotent mesenchymal stem cells, bone marrow cells, osteoblast precursors, neural cells, fibroblasts, and myoblasts. In addition to their osteoinductive effects, this influential group of proteins has been demonstrated to play roles in nervous system development,[17,18] atherosclerosis,[19] primary pulmonary hypertension,[20] and prostate cancer.[21] BMPs are further subdivided according to their primary amino acid sequence. Intact bone contains small amounts of BMP, and successful extraction is difficult.[16] Wozney and colleagues[24] overcame this hurdle in 1988, when they successfully cloned BMP-1 through -4; since then, a myriad of other BMP genes have been cloned. These advances have paved the way for the production of larger quantities of recombinant BMP for preclinical and clinical use.

Molecular Biology of Bone Morphogenetic Protein

Bone morphogenetic proteins are synthesized as propeptides in the range of 400 to 500 amino acids, and post-translational alterations result in a typical secreted protein of 100 to 140 amino acids in length. Although the amino acid sequence differs among the various BMPs, seven cysteine residues are usually conserved for each subtype. The protein dimerizes extracellularly through a single disulfide bond to its biologically active form, and will usually form homodimers; however, biologically active heterodimers and multidimers are known to occur.

There are two main types of transmembrane serine/threonine BMP receptors, types I and II, which exist independently in the cell membrane. In their native state, these receptors have a low affinity for BMP (type I has better affinity than type II when considered separately), but when complexed together, the affinity is much higher. BMP binding to type II receptors result in transphosphorylation, and activation, of type I receptors. The latter then phosphorylate and activate various Smads, which are a group of intracellular signaling mediators, or second messengers, that can be classified into three subtypes by structure and function: (1) receptor-regulated, (2) common-mediator, and (3) inhibitory. The type of Smad activation depends on which of type I receptor is activated. For example, Smads 1 and 5 are activated by BMP-Ia and –Ib receptors, and Smads 1, 5, and 8 are activated by ALK-2 receptors. The various BMP receptor subtypes and intracellular messengers translate into considerable signaling range within a particular cell or across different cell lines.

Osteoinduction is thought to be signaled by Smads 1, 5, and 8, primarily. These activated factors become associated with Smad 4, a co-Smad, a complex that then translocates into the nucleus. Nuclear transcription that follows is selective, and again is predicated upon the type of signaling cascade that induced it. BMP-2 has been shown to stimulate the transcription of osteopontin, osteocalcin, and type I collagen genes in mesenchymal marrow cells. Although regulation of the signaling cascade is incompletely defined, inhibition of Smad-mediated transcription is thought to occur, in part, via the competition of Smads 6 and 7 with co-Smad 4.

Bone morphogenetic protein–induced osteogenesis follows three sequential and critical phases: (1) migration and mitosis of mesenchymal cells, (2) differentiation of mesenchymal cells into chondroblasts that begin to synthesize cartilage, and (3) mineralization of cartilage to produce bone. This process of endochondral ossification is initiated by the binding of fibronectin to demineralized bone matrix. Chondrogenesis can be observed at 5 days, and peaks at about 8 days. Cartilage hypertrophy and mineralization begins at 9 days. Angiogenesis is critical for osteoblast differentiation, and the former peaks after 10 to 11 days.[23] The endochondral bone then is remodeled, and becomes a site for hematopoiesis.

As mentioned, BMPs have effects on many cell lines. Mesenchymal and embryonic cells are induced by BMP to differentiate into osteoblasts. However, this effect on mesenchymal cells is dose dependent. That is, in vitro work has demonstrated that lower dose exposure of BMP results in differentiation into adipocytes, whereas larger dose exposure induces osteoblastic differentiation. The osteogenic potential of BMP has been well studied with osteoblasts. An increase in DNA synthesis, reflecting a stimulatory effect on transcription, and a subsequent increase in alkaline phosphatase, osteopontin, bone sialoprotein, and osteocalcin have all been reported following the stimulation of osteoblasts with BMP.[24]

It is typical for BMPs to promote target cell differentiation into osteoblast-like cells. However, other studies have demonstrated an increase in bone resorption via a stimulatory effect of BMP on osteoclasts.[25] The clinical relevance of this has not yet been defined, and further delineation of the effect of BMP on fusion biology is necessary.

Osteogenic protein-1, also known as BMP-7 and OP-1, is also within the TGF-β family. Its amino acid sequence is 60% similar to BMP-2, and like BMP-2, it is a homodimeric glycoprotein stabilized by disulfide bonds. OP-1 induces chondrogenic and osteoblastic differentiation, and increases chondrocyte proliferation and collagen synthesis.

Preclinical Studies

Extensive research with multiple animal models using the various BMPs has preceded clinical use. The preclinical research will be subdivided in accordance with the type of fusion and the animal model.

Interbody Fusion Models

Cervical

Relative to thoracic and lumbar models, there is a paucity of literature that evaluates the utility of BMP in the cervical spine. Zdeblick and colleagues[26] compared fusion rates in 21 goats that underwent three-level diskectomy and fusion using the Bagby and Kuslich (BAK) cage (Spine-Tech, Minneapolis, MN) with autograft, a BAK cage with hydroxyapatite and autograft, or a BAK cage with rhBMP-2 in a collagen sponge. The fusions in the BMP-treated animals were both qualitatively and quantitatively superior to the other groups. BMP-treated animals had a 95% fusion rate, compared to autograft alone (48%) and hydroxyapatite/autograft (62%) groups. In the same animal and surgical model, Takahashi et al[27] demonstrated a 100% fusion rate using a hydroxyapatite carrier and 50 μg rhBMP-2, compared with a 50% fusion rate in animals that received hydroxyapatite/5 μg rhBMP-2 or hydroxyapatite alone.

Thoracic and Lumbar

Multiple authors have reported on the osteoinductive properties of BMPs in various animal models for thoracic and lumbar fusions. Sandhu et al[28] performed interbody lumbar fusions in sheep via a retroperitoneal approach using cylindrical, threaded cages filled with either rhBMP-2 with a collagen sponge carrier or with iliac crest autograft. The animals were evaluated both radiographically and histologically. Although all animals demonstrated successful fusions at 6 months radiographically, the BMP-treated animals demonstrated a 100% histologic fusion rate compared with 37% fusion rate in the control group. Notably, analysis of the fusion masses demonstrated less fibrous tissue ingrowth in the BMP group as well. Cunningham et al[29] performed anterior thoracic interbody fusions in 12 sheep and compared BAK/rhBMP-7 to diskectomy alone, BAK device alone, autograft alone, and BAK with autograft. No group obtained 100% fusion; however, the BMP group results were equivalent to the results of the BAK/autograft and autograft alone groups. Magin and Delling[30] reported on their experience using rhBMP-7 for instrumented posterior lumbar interbody fusion in 33 sheep. Animals were either treated with rhBMP-7 and hydroxyapatite or autogenous bone alone, and evaluated by manual testing and histology at 6 months.

Human Trials of Bone Morphogenetic Protein

Most of the reports in the literature to date have investigated the role of BMP-2 in spinal fusion. There are a plethora of citations (over 3000) on BMPs; however, as of this writing there are only 16 randomized clinical trials pertaining to the use of BMP in spinal arthrodesis in humans. The majority of these studies have demonstrated BMP to be beneficial in promoting fusion. However, research in this arena has elicited distinct differences in the applications of BMP to various fusion procedures. For example, the type of protein, the dosage, and the carrier used for anterior lumbar interbody fusion (ALIF) may not have the same benefit when applied to posterolateral lumbar fusions.

Anterior Lumbar Interbody Fusion The results of the pilot clinical study comparing fusion and clinical outcomes using the lumbar tapered (LT) cage (Medtronic Sofamor Danek, Memphis, TN) filled with rhBMP-2 combined with Helistat absorbable collagen sponge (Integra Life Sciences, Plainsboro, NJ) to outcomes using the LT cage filled with autograft were published in 2000.[31] The safety and efficacy data derived from the pilot clinical trial was used to launch the larger, multicenter, prospective, randomized trial;[32] 279 patients were enrolled, with 143 randomized to the experimental group that received the rhBMP-2. No significant differences were realized in Oswestry Disability Index scores between the experimental and control groups at any time point. Arthrodesis rates were higher in the rhBMP-2 group at 6, 12, and 24 months postoperatively. The fusion rates at terminal follow-up were 94.5% and 88.7% for the BMP and autograft groups, respectively. Based on these results, rhBMP-2 (InFUSE Bone Graft, Medtronic Sofamor Danek) was approved by the Food and Drug Administration (FDA) in 2002 for use with the LT cage for single-level ALIF.

A similar study was done using rhBMP-2 or autograft placed in threaded bone dowels for single-level ALIF.[33] This multicenter, prospective, randomized controlled trial enrolled 131 patients, 79 of whom received rhBMP-2 with an absorbable collagen sponge carrier, and the remaining patients received iliac crest autograft. At 6, 12, and 24 months the experimental group has significantly more improvement than the control group patients with regard to the Oswestry Disability Index scores, the physical component summary scores of the Short Form (SF)-36, and to the back and leg pain scores. At 2-year follow-up, the fusion rates were 99% and 76% for the rhBMP-2 and autograft groups, respectively.

Not all applications of rhBMP-2 for ALIF procedures have been associated with favorable results. Pradhan et al[34] reported their results of a prospective study that involved nine patients who underwent stand-alone ALIF with femoral ring allograft (FRA) filled with rhBMP-2/absorbable collagen sponge (ACS), and compared them to 26 patients who underwent the same procedure using FRA with autograft. The pseudarthrosis rate for the autograft group was 36% compared with 56% in the BMP group. The authors also reported an early resorption of the FRA when used with BMP, a finding not characteristic in the autograft group.

Posterior Lumbar Interbody Fusion There are no published randomized controlled clinical trials on the safety or utility of BMP with transforaminal lumbar interbody fusion (TLIF). Villavicencio et al[35] reported clinical and radiographic outcomes from a prospective study of 74 patients who underwent TLIF procedures with BMP-7/ACS. They reported a 100% fusion rate at both 12 and 24 months, and an improvement in clinical outcomes.

Haid et al[36] performed a randomized controlled nonblinded study involving 67 patient who underwent posterior lumbar interbody fusion (PLIF) with two titanium cages filled with either rhBMP-2/ACS or autogenous bone. All clinical outcomes scores for both groups were improved from the preoperative scores; however, there was no statistically significant difference between the two groups. The fusion rates at 24 months were 92.3% and 77.8% for the BMP and autograft groups, respectively (the difference was not statistically significant).

There is a paucity of randomized controlled data that adequately assesses the efficacy and safety of BMP for use PLIF and TLIF surgery.

Posterolateral Lumbar Fusion Vaccaro and colleagues[37] studied the clinical and radiographic outcomes in patients with symptomatic stenosis associated with degenerative lumbar spondylolisthesis treated with decompression and uninstrumented posterolateral fusion with either autogenous bone or BMP-7. This prospective randomized controlled multicenter clinical trial involved 20 investigational and 11 control patients. Clinical success was defined as a 20% improvement in the preoperative Oswestry score, and it was obtained in 85% and 64% of BMP-7 and autograft patients, respectively. Fusion analysis was performed by blinded, independent radiologists and was achieved in 55% and 40% of the investigational and control patients, respectively.

Posterolateral instrumented lumbar fusion rates using rhBMP-2 with a compression-resistant matrix have been compared with autogenous iliac crest bone graft.[38] This prospective randomized unblinded analysis involved 74 patients, and fusion analysis was performed with computed tomography at 6 and 12 months. The authors reported 81% solid, bilateral fusion rate in BMP-treated individuals at 1 year, compared with a 43% fusion rate in patients who received autograft.

Although these results are encouraging, more research is necessary to further define the role of BMP in posterolateral fusion. The dosage, carrier, and the application method are all critically important in the use of these growth factors.

Cervical Fusion There are fewer published reports that assess the utility of BMP in cervical fusion compared with lumbar fusion. One prospective randomized controlled clinical trial involving 33 patients compared anterior cervical fusion using fibular allograft packed with either autogenous bone or rhBMP-2/ACS.[39] All patients in this study were deemed fused at 6 months. There was no difference in blood loss between the two groups, and graft harvest site pain was negligible at 3 months in the control group. There were no reported device-related adverse events. At 24 months, the control group had higher mean improvement in both neck and arm disability scores ($p < .03$). In a retrospective study, Boakye et al[40] reported 100% fusion rate using polyetheretherketone (PEEK) spacers filled with rhBMP-2 in 23 patients who underwent single or multilevel anterior cervical fusion. Clinical outcome, as assessed by Odom's criteria, was good/excellent in 22 patients (95%) and fair in one (5%).

Potential Complications of Bone Morphogenetic Protein Use

Anterior Cervical Spine The anatomy of the neck is unique due to the proximity of the vital organs to the spinal column. The use of BMP for anterior cervical fusions has been associated with exaggerated soft tissue edema, dysphagia, and airway compromise. Shields et al[41] published a retrospective analysis on 151 patients who underwent either anterior cervical diskectomy or corpectomy and fusion using rhBMP-2 (up to 2.1 mg/level). They reported a 23.2% (35 of 151) complication rate; 15 patients developed a hematoma, 13 required prolonged (>48-hour) hospitalization, or hospital readmission because of breathing/swallowing problems that were not associated with hematoma. The adverse side-effect profile of BMP use in the cervical spine has not been characterized completely, nor has an algorithm of complication treatment been developed to date.

Excessive Bone Growth Normally, the local cellular levels of BMP are in the nanogram range; however, the typical dose used in clinical studies is in the milligram range. This is a six orders of magnitude difference, or a millionfold increase, in the concentration of BMP. It is thought that the osteogenic inductivity of BMP is controlled by a negative feedback under physiologic circumstances, which is overridden by this supraphysiologic concentration of rhBMP. Evidence indicates that production of inhibitory proteins (e.g., SMADs) is increased with cellular exposure to BMP-2, which in theory, can serve as a check to developing unwanted, excess bone formation. However, the potential outcomes of excessive bone growth include nerve root compression, spinal cord compression, thecal sac compression, and various soft tissue complications. Preclinical evidence supports that notion that rhBMP has the potential to result in heterotopic bone formation. Studies have demonstrated the capacity of rhBMP-2[42] and -7[43] to form undesired bone directly over laminectomy defects. Other authors have induced spinal stenosis by placing BMP over the ligamentum flavum.[44,45]

Recombinant human BMP-2 was found in one study to cause intracanal bone formation when used in minimal access interbody fusion (TLIF and PLIF) surgery;[46] however, it was reported that no patients developed related symptoms in that trial. Heterotopic bone formation with the use of rhBMP-2 has not been reported to be problematic in ALIF, or posterolateral lumbar fusion surgery. Although its use in the anterior cervical spine has been associated with bone formation anterior to the spinal column, this has not been reported to be problematic to date. Of the data available on BMP-7, there does not appear to be an association between its use and heterotopic bone formation.

Antibody Formation Antibody formation to exogenously supplied BMP is a potential systemic complication, and currently the complete profile of this phenomenon is incompletely defined. Antibody formation to rhBMP-2 has been shown through various human trials to be negligible. In part, this is thought to be due to rapid clearance of the antibody from circulation. There have been no reports of adverse long-term sequelae from exposure to rhBMP-2. Antibody titers to rhBMP-7, on the other hand, have been shown to be present in 38% of patients treated with rhBMP-7 (European Public Assessment Report on Osteogenic Protein 1, from the Committee for Proprietary Medicinal Products, 2001). The reason for the heightened antibody response to rhBMP-7 is unclear, but delayed circulatory clearance may be responsible at least in part.

As mentioned, BMPs have a role in many cellular processes beside their role in osteoinduction. The impact of immune responses on them is less clear, and more research is required to ensure that the use of various BMPs in spinal surgery does not lead to perturbation(s) of other normal physiologic mechanisms.

■ Conclusion

There have been considerable advancements of our understanding of fusion biology, and the growth factors that are involved with this process. At the time of this writing, there is a plethora of reports that describe growth factor molecular biology, and potential preclinical and clinical applications. The need to develop a bone graft substitute is underscored by the potential morbidity that is known to be associated with the harvest of autogenous bone graft and radiographic failure of spinal fusion procedures. In order for growth factors to be accepted as bone graft substitutes or extenders, they need to pass the scrutiny of well-designed and executed randomized controlled trials that demonstrate them to be at least equal to autogenous bone in promoting union. Currently, there is ample evidence that BMP-2 used in conjunction with an LT cage for ALIF results in acceptable fusion rates and is safe, and can be used as a stand-alone technique. Research to date has not proven growth factors to be valid bone graft substitutes for other applications in spinal fusion procedures. However, there is a great deal of evidence that suggests that this technology may have a promising role in spinal surgery either as bone graft extenders or substitutes.

The osteogenic capability of BMP is highly dependent on the biologic environment in which it is placed, its carrier, and the dosage used. As our knowledge of this technology evolves, the optimal applications of it will be further defined. Similarly, more experience with BMP will also elucidate the local and systemic effects, and the short- and long-term side effects, if any, that are associated with its use in spinal surgery. In the interim, clinicians must be judicious and thoughtful with its use and properly educate the patient during informed consent about possible complications.

References

1. Boden SD. Bone repair and enhancement clinical trial design. Spine applications. Clin Orthop Relat Res 1998;(355, suppl):S336–S346
2. Catinella FP, De Laria GA, De Wald RL. False aneurysm of the superior gluteal artery. A complication of iliac crest bone grafting. Spine 1990;15:1360–1362
3. Kurz LT, Garfin SR, Booth RE. Harvesting autogenous iliac bone graft: a review of complication and techniques. Spine 1989;14:1324–1331
4. Guha SC, Poole MD. Stress fracture of the iliac bone with subfascial femoral neuropathy: unusual complications at a bone graft donor site: case report. Br J Plast Surg 1983;36:305–306
5. Ubhi CS, Morris DL. Fracture and herniation of bowel at bone graft donor site in the iliac crest. Injury 1984;16:202–203
6. Challis JH, Lyttle JA, Stuart AE. Strangulated lumbar hernia and volvulus following removal of iliac crest bone graft. Acta Orthop Scand 1975;46:230–233
7. Hamad MM, Majeed SA. Incisional hernia through iliac crest defects. Arch Orthop Trauma Surg 1989;108:383–385
8. Summers BN, Eisenstein SM. Donor site pain from the ilium: a complication of lumbar spine fusion. J Bone Joint Surg Br 1989;71:677–680
9. Escalas F, DeWald RL. Combined traumatic arteriovenous fistula and ureteral injury: a complication of bone grafting. J Bone Joint Surg Am 1977;59:270–271
10. Coventry MB, Tapper EM. Pelvic instability—a consequence of removing iliac bone for grafting. J Bone Joint Surg Am 1972;54:83–101
11. Goulet JA, Senunas LE, DeSilva GL, et al. Autogenous iliac crest bone graft: complications and functional assessment. Clin Orthop Relat Res 1997;339:76–81
12. Urist MR. Bone: Formation by autoinduction. Science 1965;150:893–899
13. Van de Putte KA, Urist MR. Osteogenesis in the interior of intramuscular implants of decalcified bone matrix. Clin Orthop Relat Res 1965;43:257–270
14. Urist MR, Dowell TA. The newly deposited mineral in cartilage and bone matrix. Clin Orthop Relat Res 1967;50:291–308
15. Urist MR, Huo YK, Brownell AG. Purification of bovine growth morphogenetic protein by hydroxyapatite chromatography. Proc Natl Acad Sci U S A 1984;81:371–375
16. Riley EH, Lane JM, Urist MR, et al. Bone morphogenetic protein-2: biology and applications. Clin Orthop Relat Res 1996;324:39–46
17. Mehler MF, Mabie PC, Zhang D, et al. Bone morphogenetic proteins in the nervous system. Trends Neurosci 1997;20:309–317
18. Monsoro-Burq AH, Duprez D, Watanabe Y, et al. The role of morphogenetic proteins in vertebral development. Development 1996;122:3607–3616
19. Bostrom K, Watson KE, Horn S, et al. Bone morphogenetic protein expression in human atherosclerotic lesions. J Clin Invest 1993;91:1800–1809
20. Morse JH. Bone morphogenetic protein receptor 2 mutations in pulmonary hypertension. Chest 2002;121:50S–53S
21. Kim IY, Lee DH, Ahn HJ, et al. Expression of bone morphogenetic protein receptors type IA, -IB, and –II correlates with tumor grade in human prostate cancer tissues. Cancer Res 2000;60:2840–2844
22. Wozney JM, Rosen V, Celeste AH, et al. Novel regulators of bone formation: molecular clones and activities. Science 1988;242:1528–1534
23. Pacicca DM, Patel N, Lee C, et al. Expression of angiogenic factors during distraction osteogenesis. Bone 2003;33:889–898
24. Wang EA, Israel DI, Kelly S, et al. Bone morphogenetic protein-2 causes commitment and differentiation in C3H0T1/2 and 3T3 cells. Growth Factors 1993;9:57–71
25. Kaneko H, Arakawa T, Mano H, et al. Direct stimulation of osteoclastic bone resorption by bone morphogenetic protein (BMP)-2 and expression of BMP receptors in mature osteoclasts. Bone 2000;27:479–486
26. Zdeblick TA, Ghanayem AJ, Rapoff AJ, et al. Cervical interbody fusion cages. An animal model with and without bone morphogenetic protein. Spine 1998;23:758–766
27. Takahashi T, Tominaga T, Watabe N, et al. Use of porous hydroxyapatite graft containing recombinant human bone morphogenetic protein-2 for cervical fusion in a caprine model. J Neurosurg 1999;90:224–230
28. Sandhu HS, Toth JM, Diwan AD. Histological evaluation of the efficacy of rhBMP-2 compared with autograft bone in sheep spinal anterior interbody fusion. Spine 2002;27:567–575
29. Cunningham BW, Kanayama M, Parker LM, et al. Osteogenic protein versus autologous interbody arthrodesis in a sheep thoracic spine. A comparative endoscopic study using the Bagby and Kuslich interbody fusion device. Spine 1999;24:509–518
30. Magin MN, Delling G. Improved lumbar vertebral interbody fusion using OP-1. Spine 2001;26:469–478
31. Boden SD, Zdeblick TA, Sandhu HS, Heim SC. The use of rhBMP-2 in interbody fusion cages. Definitive evidence of osteoinduction in humans: a preliminary report. Spine 2000;25:376–381
32. Burkus JK, Gornet MF, Dickman CA, Zdeblick TA. Anterior lumbar interbody fusion using rhBMP-2 with tapered interbody cages. J Spinal Disord Tech 2002;15:337–349
33. Burkus JK, Sandhu HS, Gornet MF, Longley MC. Use of rhBMP-2 in combination with structural cortical allografts: Clinical and radiographic outcomes in anterior lumbar spinal surgery. J Bone Joint Surg Am 2005;87:1205–1212
34. Pradhan BB, Bae HW, Dawson EG, Patel VV, Delamarter RB. Graft resorption with the use of bone morphogenetic protein: lessons from anterior lumbar interbody fusion using femoral ring allografts and recombinant human bone morphogenetic protein-2. Spine 2006;31:E277–E284

35. Villavicencio AT, Burneikiene S, Nelson EL, Bulsara KR, Favors M, Thramann J. Safety of transforaminal lumbar interbody fusion and intervertebral recombinant human bone morphogenetic protein-2. J Neurosurg Spine 2005;3:436–443
36. Haid RW, Branch CL, Alexander JT, Burkus JK. Posterior lumbar interbody fusion using recombinant human bone morphogenetic protein type 2 with cylindrical interbody cages. Spine J 2004;4:527–538
37. Vaccaro AR, Anderson DG, Patel T, et al. Comparison of OP-1 Putty (rhBMP-7) to iliac crest autograft for posterolateral lumbar arthrodesis: a minimum 2-year follow-up pilot study. Spine 2005;30:2709–2716
38. Glassman SD, Dimar JR, Carreon LY, Campbell MJ, Puno RM, Johnson JR. Initial fusion rates with recombinant human bone morphogenetic protein-2/compression resistant matrix and a hydroxyapatite and tricalcium phosphate/collagen carrier in posterolateral spinal fusion. Spine 2005;30:1694–1698
39. Baskin DS, Ryan P, Sonntag V, Westmark R, Widmayer MA. A prospective, randomized, controlled cervical fusion study using recombinant human bone morphogenetic protein-2 with the CORNERSTONE-SR allograft ring and the ATLANTIS anterior cervical plate. Spine 2003;28:1219–1225
40. Boakye M, Mummaneni PV, Garrett M, Rodts G, Haid R. Anterior cervical discectomy and fusion involving a polyetheretherketone spacer and bone morphogenetic protein. J Neurosurg Spine 2005;2:521–525
41. Shields LB, Raque GH, Glassman SD, et al. Adverse effects associated with high-dose recombinant human bone morphogenetic protein-2 use in anterior cervical spine fusion. Spine 2006;31:542–547
42. Meyer RA, Gruber HE, Howard BA, et al. Safety of recombinant human bone morphogenetic protein-2 after spinal laminectomy in the dog. Spine 1999;24:747–754
43. Paramore CG, Lauryssen C, Rauzzino MJ, et al. The safety of OP-1 for lumbar fusion with decompression—a canine study. Neurosurgery 1999;44:1151–1155
44. Mimatsu K, Kishi S, Hashizume Y. Experimental chronic compression on the spinal cord of the rabbit by ectopic bone formation in the ligamentum flavum with bone morphogenetic protein. Spinal Cord 1997;35:740–746
45. Miyamoto S, Takaoka K, Yonenobu K, Ono K. Ossification of the ligamentum flavum induced by bone morphogenetic protein. An experimental study in mice. J Bone Joint Surg Br 1992;74:279–283
46. Joseph V, Rampersand YR. Heterotropic bone formation with the use of rhBMP2 in posterior minimal access interbody fusion: a CT analysis, Spine 2007;32(25):2885–2890

17 Gene Therapy and Tissue Engineering for Spinal Fusion

Wellington K. Hsu and Jeffrey C. Wang

Despite advances in the use of internal fixation, pseudarthrosis still occurs in 10% to 15% of all spine fusion surgeries.[1–4] Furthermore, 500,000 autogenous bone grafting procedures are performed annually, of which nearly 50% are used for spinal fusion.[5] Because the procurement of autologous bone graft is fraught with significant morbidity and postoperative pain,[6–13] the study of bone graft substitutes in spine surgery has expanded to include recombinant growth factors, cell-based therapies, and the use of gene transfer strategies to enhance bone formation and improve fusion rates.

The optimal treatment regimen for spinal fusion requires the restoration of the biologic processes associated with bone healing. Four critical elements influence successful bony fusion: First, an osteoinductive signal that can stimulate the recruitment or differentiation of osteoprogenitor cells into osteoblasts is required. Second, responding cells that can react to an osteoinductive signal must either be present at the bone defect site or supplied by the surgeon. Third, an osteoconductive matrix providing a three-dimensional scaffold for new bone formation is necessary to accommodate the ingrowth of mineralized bone. Finally, an adequate vascular supply is critical for the early migration of progenitor cells, osteoclasts, and other critical inflammatory agents into the fusion bed.

The use of recombinant osteoinductive growth factors, such as bone morphogenetic protein (BMP) to induce spine fusion, has been studied thoroughly in several animal models and recently has been used successfully in clinical trials. Recombinant human BMP-2 (rhBMP-2) has been shown to reproducibly heal the lumbar spine in rodents and nonhuman primates,[14–24] whereas rhOP-1 (BMP-7) has also demonstrated bone healing in rodent and sheep models.[24–28] In fact, Food and Drug Administration (FDA) approval has been granted for the use of rhBMP-2 to enhance anterior spinal fusion[29] and rhOP-1 to supplement posterior spine fusions.[30] However, in humans, large doses of BMP are required to produce an adequate biologic response. The doses of BMP used in clinical trials are more than one million times greater than the level found in human bone.[31] For this reason, rhBMP is quite expensive, and further study is required to determine if it will be cost-effective in a variety of clinical scenarios.

Tissue engineering options are attractive as an adjunct to spine surgery because of their ability to closely approximate the biology of autologous bone graft. Furthermore, many of these treatment strategies offer a continuous delivery of recombinant protein, which may enhance spinal fusion rates in a compromised biologic environment. Protocols utilizing the combination of bone graft substitutes, recombinant proteins, and gene transfer systems could offer additional options for spine arthrodesis.

Gene therapy involves the in vitro transfer of genetic material to cells to stimulate in vivo expression of a targeted protein. Gene therapy systems are composed of the DNA sequence; a vector, such as a virus, to mobilize the genetic material in question; and target cells to express the protein. Transduction of target cells can occur in several different ways. In vivo techniques involve the direct injection of the vector into the site of bony repair, whereas ex vivo systems require the harvest of responding cells and transduction with a virus in an in vitro setting. In general, ex vivo systems have been studied more extensively because of higher transduction efficiencies when compared with in vivo methods.

There are several theoretical advantages with the use of genetic transfer systems over the use of recombinant protein. First, gene therapy offers greater availability of a growth factor such as BMP at the intended site of fusion. Gene delivery vehicles are available to deliver a protein to a local area continuously, thereby compensating for the rapid biodegradation of recombinant growth factors. Second, target cells have osteoinductive capabilities that increase the potential for bone formation. Third, target cells have the propensity of responding to the osteoinductive stimulus, thereby acting via both paracrine and autocrine mechanisms of action. These differences may prove to be critical in a stringent biologic environment where sustained BMP production is required for osseous repair.

The study of gene therapy strategies for spinal fusion has been aimed at developing a suitable regimen for use in clinical trials. Investigators have compared the utilization of different vectors, genes of interest, target cells, and carriers to develop an effective treatment strategy. The recent findings in the study of gene transfer systems and tissue engineering for spinal fusion are summarized in this chapter.

■ Adenoviral Vectors

Early results using BMP gene transfer via an in vivo technique revealed successful fusion only in immunocompromised animals.[32–34] Since then, several immunocompetent animal studies have demonstrated the efficacy of gene therapy in the healing of long bone defects[35–37] and spinal fusion.[38,39] Wang et al[18] reported the initial results with the use of ex vivo adenoviral gene transfer in a posterolateral spine fusion model in immunocompetent rats. BMP-2–producing target cells were created from syngeneic rat bone marrow cells and implanted with demineralized bone matrix and collagen sponge between the transverse processes of L4 and L5. All spines treated with BMP-2–producing bone marrow cells and recombinant BMP fused at 4 weeks postoperatively regardless of the carrier used, whereas none of the control groups fused. Histomorphometric analysis revealed that coarse trabecular bone had formed from cells generated by adenoviral gene transfer, whereas thin, lacelike bone formed from that of recombinant BMP.[18] This finding has also been confirmed in a rat femoral critical-sized defect model.[35]

A separate group of investigators reported the use of adenoviral gene transfer with a construct containing the complementary DNA (cDNA) for BMP-7 in a rat spine fusion model.[40] Syngeneic bone marrow cells modified with BMP-7 were combined with freeze-dried allograft bone and then implanted into immunocompetent rats. Successful fusion, deemed by manual palpation, was seen in eight of 10 rats in the treated groups as compared with zero of 10 in the control groups.[40] Using an adenoviral construct coding for the reporter gene β-galactosidase, the authors found maximal protein expression on postoperative day 3, and observed a progressive decline to background levels by postoperative day 14. This end point suggests that due to the episomal nature of the adenovirus genome, genetically modified cells are not permanently altered.[40] Further studies have proposed that gene expression is lost when genetically modified cells divide.[40]

The success of gene therapy has also been reported in higher animal models.[34,41,42] In one study, harvested mesenchymal stem cells from pigs were used as targets for adenoviral-mediated transfer of the BMP-2 gene.[41] The transduced cells were then used to successfully heal the thoracic disk spaces of three pigs through an anterior thoracoscopic injection. Radiographic and histologic examination confirmed bridging bone in all six disk spaces treated with adenovirus, whereas little bone formation was seen in the control injections.[41]

■ Alternative Delivery Vectors

Studies reporting the use of gene therapy systems in animal models of spine fusion have most often involved the use of the adenoviral vector.[18,39–41,43] Despite the widespread use of adenoviral vectors for the transfer of BMP genes, several limitations exist regarding its use in clinical trials. First, adenovirus has been found to offer short-term production of protein. In vivo data suggest that the delivery of growth factor falls to background levels 14 days after implantation.[40] There are concerns about the immunogenic response to adenoviral proteins, which can limit the duration of transgene expression.[44] Adenoviral vectors have also been found to induce a significant host immune response. Studies suggest that this immunogenicity may interfere with spine arthrodesis rates, especially if the host has been previously exposed to the vector.[45] Furthermore, some authors have shown that adenoviral gene transfer can induce spinal fusion in immunocompromised but not immunocompetent animals.[33] For this reason, the development of alternative vectors in the induction of bone formation has been explored.

Lentivirus, which is based on the human immunodeficiency virus, exhibits minimal immunogenicity when compared with gene therapy systems involving adenovirus.[46] Lentiviral vectors have also demonstrated high levels of stable gene transfer and target gene expression.[47] Furthermore, the use of lentiviral vectors in bone formation has led to the long-term production of BMP-2 in vitro for over 12 weeks after transduction.[48] Preliminary studies with the use of lentivirally based BMP-2 gene transfer in a critical-sized rat femoral defect model have shown the advantages of long-term BMP-2 production in vivo.[49] Reports of the use adeno-associated virus, which is derived from a parvovirus and believed to be innocuous to humans, have also been reported.[50]

■ Genes of Interest

The utilization of other BMPs with ex vivo gene therapy in bone formation has also been described. In addition to BMP-2 and BMP-7, recent reports have shown the successful use of other genes, such as BMP-4,[50] BMP-6,[51] and BMP-9.[52] Furthermore, Viggeswarapu et al[39] demonstrated solid posterolateral arthrodesis of the spine in a rabbit model from the adenoviral delivery of LIM mineralization protein 1 (LMP-1) into the fusion bed.[39] LMP-1 is an intracellular protein that has been shown to function as an upstream regulator for several BMPs.

Although recombinant BMP homodimers such as BMP-2 and BMP-7 have been used successfully in animal models of spinal fusion, studies have suggested that the coexpression of multiple BMPs can lead to the formation of heterodimeric BMPs.[53–55] These studies also suggest that heterodimeric BMPs may have more potent osteoblastic potential than their homodimeric counterparts. Using a rat posterolateral spine fusion model, Zhu and colleagues[40] tested the in vivo and in vitro capacity of combination gene transfer using BMP-2 and BMP-7 in comparison to single BMP gene transfer. A549 cells were cotransfected with adenoviral vectors encoding for BMP-2 and BMP-7, and with each vector alone. The authors found that the animals treated with cotransfection of both BMP genes experienced a significantly greater number of mechanically stable spinal fusions with higher

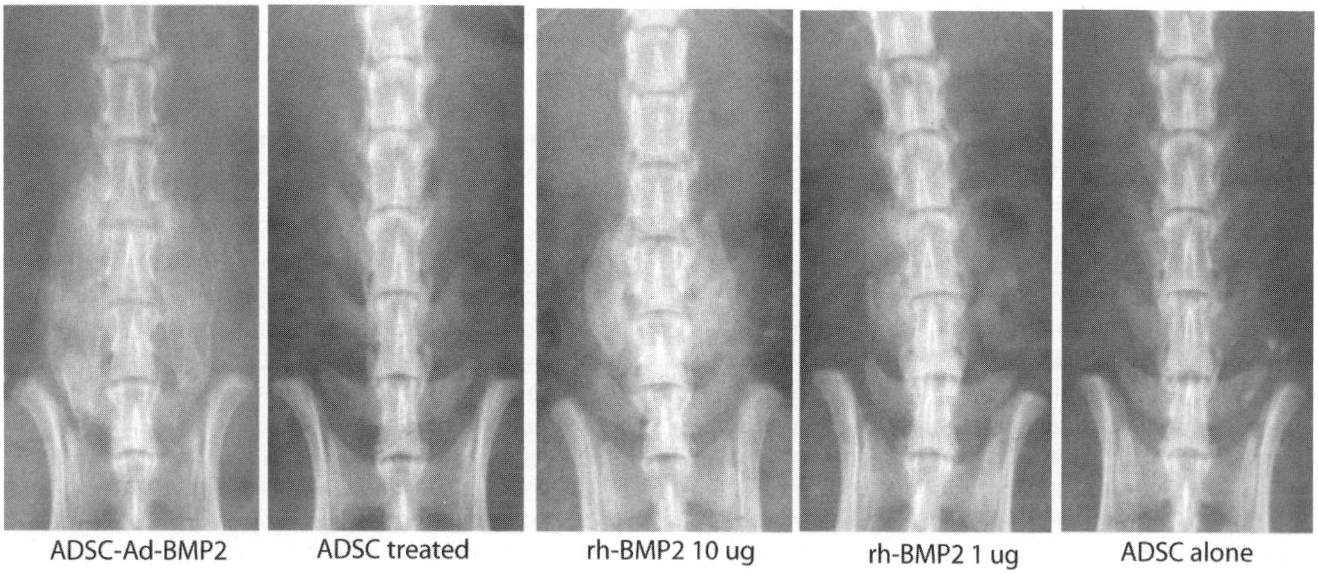

Fig. 17.1 Plain anteroposterior (AP) radiograph of representative rat spines 4 weeks after surgery. The adipose-derived stem cells (ADSC)–adenovirus (Ad)–bone morphogenetic protein-2 (BMP-2) and recombinant human BMP-2 (rhBMP-2) 10 μg groups show successful spine fusion, whereas ADSC alone and the cell-based therapy group (ADSC treated) show little new bone formation. Fusion masses formed from ADSC transduced with Ad-BMP-2 were far larger than that from rhBMP-2 10 μg.

bone fusion mass assessed via computed tomography (CT) scanning when compared with single gene transfer.[40] These findings suggest that the use of heterodimeric BMPs may possibly lead to lower required doses of recombinant protein and fewer responding cells in tissue engineering.

■ Cellular Delivery Vehicles

Further improvements to gene therapy systems have been directed at the use of different cellular delivery vehicles. Although multiple types of target cells have been used to deliver growth factors for bone formation, bone marrow stromal cells have been the most widely used. In fact, the successful use of human-derived bone marrow cells transduced with adenovirus in producing spinal arthrodesis in immunocompromised rats has also been described.[56] However, studies demonstrate that bone marrow contains a relatively low percentage of mesenchymal stem cells (MSCs) that have the capability of differentiating into osteoblasts.[57] Moreover, this ratio is further diminished in elderly patients, in those with metabolic diseases, and in those with osteoporosis.[58]

Because of the inherent limitations of bone marrow stromal cells, several other gene delivery vehicles have been utilized. Buffy coat cells, which are a concentrate of white blood cells and platelets derived from either bone marrow or blood, have been used successfully to produce spine fusions in both rat and rabbit models after transduction with LMP-1.[39] Other target cells used successfully in gene transfer strategies include periosteal cells,[42] C2C12 myoblasts,[59] and muscle-derived stem cells.[60,61]

Recent interest has been directed toward human liposuction aspirates, obtained from human fat, which contain an abundance of pluripotent progenitor cells termed processed lipoaspirate cells (PLAs). These cells can undergo purification steps to produce adipose-derived stem cells (ADSC) that have demonstrated the ability to differentiate into cells of chondrogenic, osteogenic, myogenic, and adipogenic lineage. The prospect of using PLAs is attractive because they offer a significantly higher yield of mesenchymal stem cells than bone marrow,[62] can be obtained through a minimally invasive procedure under local anesthesia, and are widely available among the patient population.[63]

Studies using adipose cells as gene delivery vehicles have reported initial success in the induction of bone formation in several different animal models.[43,64,65] One preliminary study from our laboratory has successfully described the use of ADSCs as cellular delivery vehicles in the induction of spine fusion in a rat posterolateral spine fusion model using an adenoviral vector.[43] Micro-CT and plain radiographic analysis of fusion masses revealed over twice as much bone formation in animals treated with ADSC transduced with the adenoviral vector carrying the BMP-2 gene when compared with those from high-dose recombinant BMP-2 (**Fig. 17.1**).[43]

■ Discussion

Spine arthrodesis often presents several quandaries including poor biologic environment, compromised bone stock, and structural instability. Bone graft and bone graft substitutes are vital to a spine surgeon's armamentarium in dealing with issues of bone loss, solid fusion, and clinical outcome. These substances vary widely in regard to available data, and careful evaluation is necessary to identify the appropriate use of various bone graft agents.

Despite excellent clinical results, many concerns still exist for cost-effectiveness from the routine use of recombinant growth factors. Recent study into the use of tissue engineering to deliver the sustained production of BMP may soon present an additional bone graft option for the spine surgeon. Delivery of protein through gene expression may be better suited in a biologically stringent environment than recombinant BMP, which may be degraded quickly. Offering a larger number of mesenchymal stem cells to the local area may also lead to a greater osteoinductive response.[66] Ultimately, this technique may prove to be more cost-effective in the local augmentation of spine arthrodesis. Further studies into the use of gene therapy may allow the delivery of upstream activators in the BMP production pathway, such as the expression of LMP-1.[38] This option may prove to be more efficacious in a rigorous setting.

■ Conclusion

Despite promising preclinical results from gene therapy, safety concerns have hindered the progress of tissue engineering in the clinical setting. Recent interest has been dedicated to characterizing the life span of transduced cells, duration of gene expression, and systemic effects on the host genome after the use of gene therapy. Additional studies in higher animal models are needed to assess the long-term effects of gene therapy before its clinical use in humans is widely accepted. With additional investigation into its safety profile in humans, the use of gene therapy may one day become a reality in the field of orthopedic surgery.

References

1. Bridwell KH, Sedgewick TA, O'Brien MF, Lenke LG, Baldus C. The role of fusion and instrumentation in the treatment of degenerative spondylolisthesis with spinal stenosis. J Spinal Disord 1993;6:461–472
2. McGuire RA, Amundson GM. The use of primary internal fixation in spondylolisthesis. Spine 1993;18:1662–1672
3. West JL, Bradford DS, Ogilvie JW. Results of spinal arthrodesis with pedicle screw-plate fixation. J Bone Joint Surg Am 1991;73:1179–1184
4. Zdeblick TA. A prospective, randomized study of lumbar fusion. Preliminary results. Spine 1993;18:983–991
5. Ludwig SC, Kowalski JM, Boden SD. Osteoinductive bone graft substitutes. Eur Spine J 2000;9(suppl 1):S119–S125
6. Banwart JC, Asher MA, Hassanein RS. Iliac crest bone graft harvest donor site morbidity. A statistical evaluation. Spine 1995;20: 1055–1060
7. Goulet JA, Senunas LE, DeSilva GL, Greenfield ML. Autogenous iliac crest bone graft. Complications and functional assessment. Clin Orthop Relat Res 1997;339:76–81
8. Reid RL. Hernia through an iliac bone-graft donor site. A case report. J Bone Joint Surg Am 1968;50:757–760
9. Coventry MB, Tapper EM. Pelvic instability: a consequence of removing iliac bone for grafting. J Bone Joint Surg Am 1972;54:83–101
10. Challis JH, Lyttle JA, Stuart AE. Strangulated lumbar hernia and volvulus following removal of iliac crest bone graft. Acta Orthop Scand 1975;46:230–233
11. Cowley SP, Anderson LD. Hernias through donor sites for iliac-bone grafts. J Bone Joint Surg Am 1983;65:1023–1025
12. Kuhn DA, Moreland MS. Complications following iliac crest bone grafting. Clin Orthop Relat Res 1986;(209):224–226
13. Kurz LT, Garfin SR, Booth RE. Harvesting autogenous iliac bone grafts. A review of complications and techniques. Spine 1989;14:1324–1331
14. Boden SD, Moskovitz PA, Morone MA, Toribitake Y. Video-assisted lateral intertransverse process arthrodesis. Validation of a new minimally invasive lumbar spinal fusion technique in the rabbit and nonhuman primate (rhesus) models. Spine 1996;21:2689–2697
15. Holliger EH, Trawick RH, Boden SD, Hutton WC. Morphology of the lumbar intertransverse process fusion mass in the rabbit model: a comparison between two bone graft materials–rhBMP-2 and autograft. J Spinal Disord 1996;9:125–128
16. Martin GJ, Boden SD, Titus L. Recombinant human bone morphogenetic protein-2 overcomes the inhibitory effect of ketorolac, a nonsteroidal anti-inflammatory drug (NSAID), on posterolateral lumbar intertransverse process spine fusion. Spine 1999;24:2188–2193 discussion 2193–2194
17. Schimandle JH, Boden SD, Hutton WC. Experimental spinal fusion with recombinant human bone morphogenetic protein-2. Spine 1995;20:1326–1337
18. Wang JC, Kanim LE, Yoo S, Campbell PA, Berk AJ, Lieberman JR. Effect of regional gene therapy with bone morphogenetic protein-2-producing bone marrow cells on spinal fusion in rats. J Bone Joint Surg Am 2003;85-A:905–911
19. Silcox DH, Boden SD, Schimandle JH, Johnson P, Whitesides TE, Hutton WC. Reversing the inhibitory effect of nicotine on spinal fusion using an osteoinductive protein extract. Spine 1998;23:291–296 discussion 297
20. Cook SD, Dalton JE, Tan EH, Whitecloud TS, Rueger DC. In vivo evaluation of recombinant human osteogenic protein (rhOP-1) implants as a bone graft substitute for spinal fusions. Spine 1994;19:1655–1663
21. Boden SD, Martin GJ, Morone M, Ugbo JL, Titus L, Hutton WC. The use of coralline hydroxyapatite with bone marrow, autogenous bone graft, or osteoinductive bone protein extract for posterolateral lumbar spine fusion. Spine 1999;24:320–327
22. Muschler GF, Hyodo A, Manning T, Kambic H, Easley K. Evaluation of human bone morphogenetic protein 2 in a canine spinal fusion model. Clin Orthop Relat Res 1994;(308):229–240
23. Hau WK, Wang JC, Liu NQ, Krenick L, Zuk PA, Hedrick MH, Benhaim P, Lieberman JR. Stem cells from human fat as cellular delivery vehicles in an ethymic rat posterolateral spine fusion model. J Bone Joint Surg Am 2008;90(5):1043–1052

24. Grauer JN, Patel TC, Erulkar JS, Troiano NW, Panjabi MM, Friedlaender GE. 2000 Young Investigator Research Award winner. Evaluation of OP-1 as a graft substitute for intertransverse process lumbar fusion. Spine 2001;26:127–133
25. Kalodiki EP, Hoppensteadt DA, Nicolaides AN, et al. Deep venous thrombosis prophylaxis with low molecular weight heparin and elastic compression in patients having total hip replacement. A randomised controlled trial. Int Angiol 1996;15:162–168
26. Magin MN, Delling G. Improved lumbar vertebral interbody fusion using rhOP-1: a comparison of autogenous bone graft, bovine hydroxylapatite (Biol-Oss), and BMP-7 (rhOP-1) in sheep. Spine 2001;26:469–478
27. Blattert TR, Delling G, Dalal PS, Toth CA, Balling H, Weckbach A. Successful transpedicular lumbar interbody fusion by means of a composite of osteogenic protein-1 (rhBMP-7) and hydroxyapatite carrier: a comparison with autograft and hydroxyapatite in the sheep spine. Spine 2002;27:2697–2705
28. Masuda K, Takegami K, An H, et al. Recombinant osteogenic protein-1 upregulates extracellular matrix metabolism by rabbit annulus fibrosus and nucleus pulposus cells cultured in alginate beads. J Orthop Res 2003;21:922–930
29. Boden SD, Zdeblick TA, Sandhu HS, Heim SE. The use of rhBMP-2 in interbody fusion cages. Definitive evidence of osteoinduction in humans: a preliminary report. Spine 2000;25:376–381
30. http://www.fda.gov/cdrh/pdf2/H020008a.pdf
31. Baltzer AW, Lieberman JR. Regional gene therapy to enhance bone repair. Gene Ther 2004;11:344–350
32. Alden TD, Pittman DD, Beres EJ, et al. Percutaneous spinal fusion using bone morphogenetic protein-2 gene therapy. J Neurosurg 1999;90(suppl):109–114
33. Helm GA, Alden TD, Beres EJ, et al. Use of bone morphogenetic protein-9 gene therapy to induce spinal arthrodesis in the rodent. J Neurosurg 2000;92(suppl):191–196
34. Riew KD, Wright NM, Cheng S, Avioli LV, Lou J. Induction of bone formation using a recombinant adenoviral vector carrying the human BMP-2 gene in a rabbit spinal fusion model. Calcif Tissue Int 1998;63:357–360
35. Lieberman JR, Daluiski A, Stevenson S, et al. The effect of regional gene therapy with bone morphogenetic protein-2-producing bone-marrow cells on the repair of segmental femoral defects in rats. J Bone Joint Surg Am 1999;81:905–917
36. Lieberman JR, Le LQ, Wu L, et al. Regional gene therapy with a BMP-2-producing murine stromal cell line induces heterotopic and orthotopic bone formation in rodents. J Orthop Res 1998;16:330–339
37. Lee JY, Musgrave D, Pelinkovic D, et al. Effect of bone morphogenetic protein-2-expressing muscle-derived cells on healing of critical-sized bone defects in mice. J Bone Joint Surg Am 2001;83:1032–1039
38. Boden SD, Titus L, Hair G, et al. Lumbar spine fusion by local gene therapy with a cDNA encoding a novel osteoinductive protein (LMP-1). Spine 1998;23:2486–2492
39. Viggeswarapu M, Boden SD, Liu Y, et al. Adenoviral delivery of LIM mineralization protein-1 induces new-bone formation in vitro and in vivo. J Bone Joint Surg Am 2001;83:364–376
40. Zhu W, Rawlins BA, Boachie-Adjei O, et al. Combined bone morphogenetic protein-2 and -7 gene transfer enhances osteoblastic differentiation and spine fusion in a rodent model. J Bone Miner Res 2004;19:2021–2032
41. Riew KD, Lou J, Wright NM, Cheng SL, Bae KT, Avioli LV. Thoracoscopic intradiscal spine fusion using a minimally invasive gene-therapy technique. J Bone Joint Surg Am 2003;85:866–871
42. Breitbart AS, Grande DA, Mason JM, Barcia M, James T, Grant RT. Gene-enhanced tissue engineering: applications for bone healing using cultured periosteal cells transduced retrovirally with the BMP-7 gene. Ann Plast Surg 1999;42:488–495
43. Hsu W, Wang J, Feeley B, et al. Gene therapy utilizing stem cells from human fat in a rat posterolateral spine fusion model. Spine J 2004;4(suppl):51S
44. Planes A, Vochelle N, Mazas F, et al. Prevention of postoperative venous thrombosis a randomized trial comparing unfractionated heparin with low molecular weight heparin in patients undergoing total hip replacement. Thromb Haemost 1988;60: 407–410
45. Kim HS, Viggeswarapu M, Boden SD, et al. Overcoming the immune response to permit ex vivo gene therapy for spine fusion with human type 5 adenoviral delivery of the LIM mineralization protein-1 cDNA. Spine 2003;28:219–226
46. Naldini L, Blomer U, Gallay P, et al. In vivo gene delivery and stable transduction of nondividing cells by a lentiviral vector. Science 1996;272:263–267
47. Naldini L, Blomer U, Gage FH, Trono D, Verma IM. Efficient transfer, integration, and sustained long-term expression of the transgene in adult rat brains injected with a lentiviral vector. Proc Natl Acad Sci U S A 1996;93):11382–11388
48. Sugiyama O, An DS, Kung SP, et al. Lentivirus-mediated gene transfer induces long-term transgene expression of BMP-2 in vitro and new bone formation in vivo. Mol Ther 2005;11:390–398
49. Hsu W, Sugiyama O, Feeley B, et al. Lentiviral-mediated BMP-2 gene transfer enhances healing of segmental femoral defects in rats. Bone 2007;40:931–938
50. Luk KD, Chen Y, Cheung KM, Kung HF, Lu WW, Leong JC. Adeno-associated virus-mediated bone morphogenetic protein-4 gene therapy for in vivo bone formation. Biochem Biophys Res Commun 2003;308:636–645
51. Laurent JJ, Webb KM, Beres EJ, et al. The use of bone morphogenetic protein-6 gene therapy for percutaneous spinal fusion in rabbits. J Neurosurg Spine 2004;1:90–94
52. Dumont RJ, Dayoub H, Li JZ, et al. Ex vivo bone morphogenetic protein-9 gene therapy using human mesenchymal stem cells induces spinal fusion in rodents. Neurosurgery 2002;51:1239–1244 discussion 1244–1245
53. Aono A, Hazama M, Notoya K, et al. Potent ectopic bone-inducing activity of bone morphogenetic protein-4/7 heterodimer. Biochem Biophys Res Commun 1995;210:670–677
54. Hazama M, Aono A, Ueno N, Fujisawa Y. Efficient expression of a heterodimer of bone morphogenetic protein subunits using a baculovirus expression system. Biochem Biophys Res Commun 1995;209:859–866
55. Israel DI, Nove J, Kerns KM, et al. Heterodimeric bone morphogenetic proteins show enhanced activity in vitro and in vivo. Growth Factors 1996;13:291–300
56. Peterson B, Iglesias R, Zhang J, Wang JC, Lieberman JR. Genetically modified human derived bone marrow cells for posterolateral lumbar spine fusion in athymic rats: beyond conventional autologous bone grafting. Spine 2005;30:283–289 discussion 289–290
57. Muschler GF, Boehm C, Easley K. Aspiration to obtain osteoblast progenitor cells from human bone marrow: the influence of aspiration volume. J Bone Joint Surg Am 1997;79:1699–1709

58. Muschler GF, Nitto H, Boehm CA, Easley KA. Age- and gender-related changes in the cellularity of human bone marrow and the prevalence of osteoblastic progenitors. J Orthop Res 2001;19:117–125
59. Okubo Y, Bessho K, Fujimura K, Iizuka T, Miyatake SI. In vitro and in vivo studies of a bone morphogenetic protein-2 expressing adenoviral vector. J Bone Joint Surg Am 2001;83-A(suppl 1, pt 2):S99–S104
60. Musgrave DS, Pruchnic R, Bosch P, Ziran BH, Whalen J, Huard J. Human skeletal muscle cells in ex vivo gene therapy to deliver bone morphogenetic protein-2. J Bone Joint Surg Br 2002;84:120–127
61. Shen HC, Peng H, Usas A, Gearhart B, Fu FH, Huard J. Structural and functional healing of critical-size segmental bone defects by transduced muscle-derived cells expressing BMP4. J Gene Med 2004;6:984–991
62. Fraser JK, Wulur I, Alfonso Z, Hedrick MH. Fat tissue: an underappreciated source of stem cells for biotechnology. Trends Biotechnol 2006;24:150–154
63. Zuk PA, Zhu M, Mizuno H, et al. Multilineage cells from human adipose tissue: implications for cell-based therapies. Tissue Eng 2001;7:211–228
64. Dragoo JL, Choi JY, Lieberman JR, et al. Bone induction by BMP-2 transduced stem cells derived from human fat. J Orthop Res 2003;21:622–629
65. Peterson B, Zhang J, Iglesias R, et al. Healing of critically sized femoral defects, using genetically modified mesenchymal stem cells from human adipose tissue. Tissue Eng 2005;11:120–129
66. Einhorn TA. Clinical applications of recombinant human BMPs: early experience and future development. J Bone Joint Surg Am 2003;85(suppl 3):82–88

18 Tissue Engineering and Strategies for Disk Regeneration

Corey A. Pacek, Gwendolyn A. Sowa, and James D. Kang

Low back pain is one of the most common complaints of patients presenting to physicians today. Approximately $91 billion was spent in 1998 on health care expenditures for patients with low back pain in the United States, which represented 1% of the gross domestic product that year.[1] Intervertebral disk degeneration (IVDD) is one of the most common and most important causes of low back pain. Multiple modalities, both operative and nonoperative, exist for the treatment of IVDD. Nonoperative therapies include medications, physical therapy, nerve root injections, and chronic pain management. Operative therapies consist of diskectomy, laminectomy, fusion, disk replacement, and others. Although all of these techniques have varying success with regard to the treatment of low back pain and IVDD, they all focus on the terminal stages of an as of yet unclear pathologic process. The goal of regenerative disk research is to discover therapies for IVDD in earlier stages of the degenerative cascade in an effort to preserve and restore normal intervertebral biology and biomechanics.

The focus of this chapter thus lies not in removing a degenerated disk and replacing it with a stable construct of metal and bone, but in regenerating the disk by repopulating or replacing it with healthy disk cells and tissue through techniques of tissue engineering. Tissue engineering as defined by Hunter et al[2] entails using "living cells, manipulated through their extracellular environment or even genetically, to develop biological substitutes for implantation into the body or to foster the remodeling of tissue in some other active manner. The purpose is to either repair, replace, maintain, or enhance the function of a particular tissue or organ." This chapter reviews intervertebral disk (IVD) biology to illuminate the anatomy and physiology, and discusses different strategies for tissue engineering, from the injection of isolated growth factor, to the complex creation of three-dimensional tissue scaffold implants.

Disk Biology

Structure

The IVD is made up of two main structures, the centrally located nucleus pulposus (NP) and the peripherally located anulus fibrosus (AF). The AF is composed of laminar layers of primarily type I collagen arranged in alternating oblique angles with respect to the axis of the spine. The collagen fibers in adjacent layers of AF are arranged perpendicular to one another, allowing for maximal tensile strength. The NP consists of a gelatinous matrix of primarily type II collagen, proteoglycans, and up to 90% water by weight in the healthy IVD. This construct allows for the axial compressive force seen by the NP to be transformed to a tensile force in the AF. Additionally, the gelatinous nature of the NP acts as a natural shock absorber, resulting in a more even distribution of force and strain.

Nutrition

In the mature adult, the IVD is the largest avascular organ in the body. It is flanked rostrally and caudally by cartilaginous end plates, and it is these end plates, along with the periphery of the AF, from which the IVD garners its nutrition and rids itself of metabolic by-products.[3] This avascularity has two great implications: (1) lack of blood flow results in the IVD being relatively immunogenically isolated; and (2) the nutrition of the disk depends entirely on diffusion, and anything that disrupts the diffusion leads to disruption of disk nutrition. This has important consequences when considering tissue engineering of the disk.

The main metabolic pathway for energy production of the disk is that of glycolysis, with the main by-product being lactic acid. This leads to a lower pH in the central NP as compared with the periphery of the IVD and other tissues. Additionally, the dependence on diffusion for oxygen leads to a relatively hypoxic environment for the IVD. This results in unique challenges when considering tissue regeneration and repair.

Applied Biochemistry of the Disk

The majority of the IVD consists of extracellular matrix produced by AF and NP cells. As mentioned, the matrix of the NP consists largely of type II collagen and proteoglycans, particularly aggrecan. Aggrecan molecules have a large number of negatively charged side chains, which give the disk its ability to imbibe water. It is this water that gives the disk its biomechanical advantage. However, as the disk degenerates, the proteoglycan content declines, leading to a subsequent decrease in hydration as well.

The overall content of matrix in the NP is believed to be a well-controlled equilibrium between degradative and

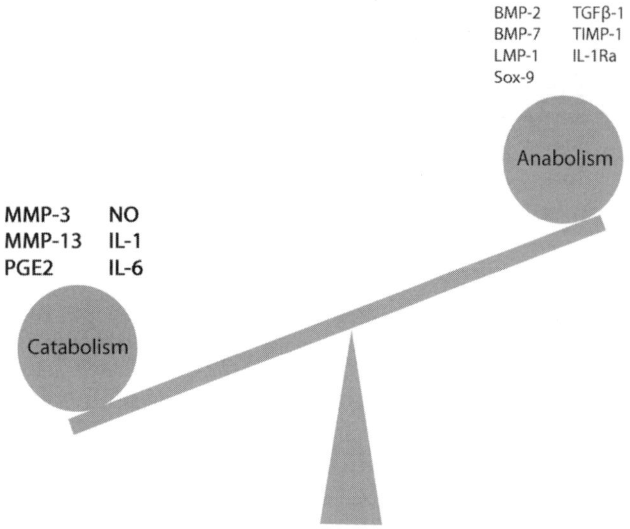

Fig. 18.1 A major theory of intervertebral disk degeneration (IVDD) is that increased levels of catabolism lead to an imbalance of degradation and synthesis, tipping the scale toward degradation. MMP, matrix metalloproteinase; PGE_2, prostaglandin E_2; NO, nitric oxide; IL, interleukin; TIMP, tissue inhibitor of metalloproteinases; BMP, bone morphogenetic protein; LMP, Lim mineralization protein; IL-1Ra, interleukin-1 receptor antagonist; TGF-β1, transforming growth factor-β1; Sox9, sex determining region Y, box 9.

synthetic pathways. Many proteins are involved in this equilibrium **(Fig. 18.1)**. Within the healthy disk there is a constant turnover of matrix, and maintenance of disk tissue relies on a balance of the system. Degradative enzymes such as matrix metalloproteinases (MMPs), particularly MMP-3 and MMP-13 (also known as stromelysin-1 and collagenase 3, respectively), have been found to be at increased levels in degenerated human disks. Likewise, mediators of inflammation such as nitric oxide (NO) and prostaglandin E_2(PGE_2), as well as the cytokines interleukin-1 (IL-1) and IL-6, have also been found to be increased in degenerated disks.[4] It is believed that the synthetic capabilities of the cells of the NP are unable to sustain appropriate levels of aggrecan and collagen in the face of this increased catabolism, which leads to the degeneration of the disk **(Fig. 18.1)**.

■ Protein Therapies

The most basic strategy for stimulating regeneration of IVD tissue lies in treating these cells with a specific protein aimed at increasing or decreasing a specific biochemical action. As applied to actual therapy, the proposed treatment would consist of intradiskal injections of the specific protein. Several candidates have been described in the literature with regard to what specific proteins are suitable for treatment, as well as the method of delivery, both in vitro and in vivo.

Transforming Growth Factor-β1

Thompson et al[5] were one of the earliest groups to demonstrate that transforming growth factor-β1 (TGF-β1) was capable of increasing proteoglycan synthesis in canine NP cells cultured in vitro. The authors concluded that the degeneration of the disk could in theory be countered with this increased expression of proteoglycan.

Bone Morphogenetic Protein 2

The potential utility of another growth factor, bone morphogenetic protein 2 (BMP-2), has also been demonstrated. Kim et al[6] were able to show in vitro that treatment of human IVD cells with BMP-2 leads to the upregulation of messenger RNA (mRNA) expression of aggrecan and type II collagen, as well as increased production of newly synthesized proteoglycan. Additionally, they showed that osteocalcin, an osteogenic marker, was not increased. This suggested that BMP-2 appeared capable of stimulating a more chondrogenic response by the NP cells as opposed to an osteogenic response.

Bone Morphogenic Protein 7 (Osteogenic Protein 1)

Another bone morphogenic protein, BMP-7 (also known as osteogenic protein 1 [OP-1]) has also been found to have significant stimulatory effects on proteoglycan synthesis in the IVD. Masuda et al[7] showed that introduction of BMP-7 to an in vitro culture of both NP and AF cells upregulated the production of proteoglycans. Following this work, An et al[8] showed that intradiskal injections of BMP-7 were able to increase disk height in healthy, skeletally mature rabbits. Subsequent biochemical analysis showed increased production of proteoglycan by the IVD. Taking this one step further, researchers then injected BMP-7 into rabbit IVD that had degeneration induced via an annular stab. It was shown in this study that the disk space narrowing that was seen at 4 weeks was restored following injection of BMP-7 and was maintained through the duration of the experiment, 24 weeks.[9] **(Fig. 18.2)** It is hypothesized that the increase in proteoglycan leads to increased attraction for water in the IVD, thus leading to the increased disk height. These were the first studies to show that not only could growth factor injection have an effect on IVDD, but it could produce a more lasting effect than a one-time injection of the growth factor would suggest.

Discussion

Intradiskal injection of growth factors into the IVD is one strategy for induction of regeneration in the IVD. Multiple growth factors show promise as far as the biochemical possibilities. The positive aspects of this strategy include

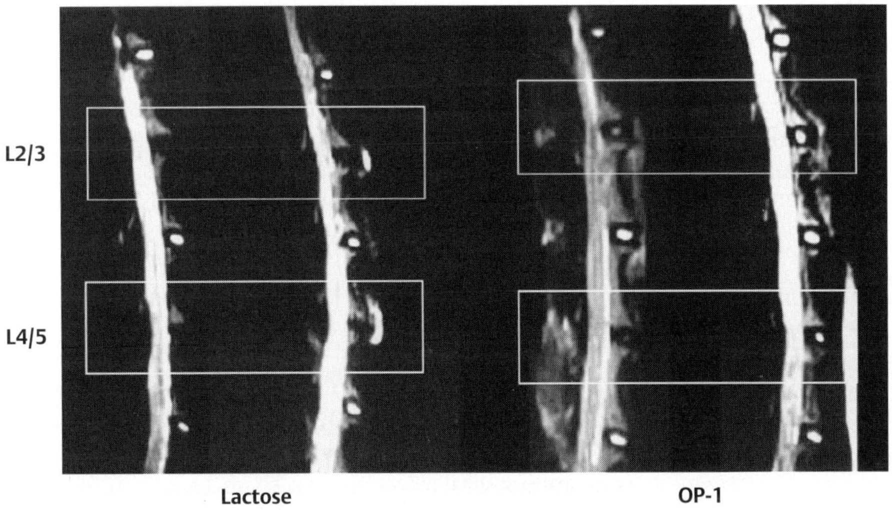

Fig. 18.2 Magnetic resonance imaging of degenerated rabbit spines is shown for the lactose-injected controls and the BMP-7 (OP-1) injected spines. Signal intensity of the stabbed disks (L2–L3 and L4–L5) is increased in the BMP-7 (OP-1) cohort versus the control. The best and worst spines are shown for each group for comparison. (From Masuda K, Imai Y, Okuma M, et al. Osteogenic protein-1 injection into a degenerated disc induces the restoration of disc height and structural changes in the rabbit anular puncture model. Spine 2006;31:742–754, with permission.)

ease of delivery of agent, as well as ease of production of injectable protein. Then main negative aspect involves the length of the therapeutic effect. The half-life of growth factors injected subcutaneously is approximately 20 minutes.[10] Although this half-life is likely to be extended in an avascular structure such as the IVD for reasons already discussed, in a chronic process such as IVDD it is unknown if such a short period would allow for a significant regeneration over the long term. It is this concern that leads to the next strategy for regeneration of the IVD: vector-mediated gene therapy.

■ In Vivo Gene Therapies

The second strategy of tissue engineering to be discussed is in vivo gene therapy. The goal of this strategy is to transfer a target gene to the IVD cells, which will subsequently lead to overproduction of the target gene product, resulting in a stable, continuous supply of that gene product **(Fig. 18.3)**. Vector loaded with the target gene is injected into the IVD as the method of delivery in this proposed technique.

■ Vectors

The initial step to this therapy involves choosing a method of introducing the target gene into the cells. Vectors may first be divided into nonviral and viral categories. Nonviral constructs include liposomes, biolistics (also know as the gene gun), and DNA-ligand complexes, where the most common viral vectors are retroviruses, adenovirus, and adeno-associated virus (AAV). These methods shall be discussed in turn.

Nonviral Vectors

Liposomes

Liposomes as vectors consist of phospholipid bilayers arranged in spheres and they contain target genes in plasmid form. Liposomes are simple, safe, and inexpensive to produce, but their main drawbacks are limited efficiency of transfection, limited target gene expression, and toxicity at high levels, which is why they have not been used in gene therapy for the IVD.[11]

Biolistics

Biolistics employ particles coated in plasmids of the target gene, which are then literally fired into the target cells.

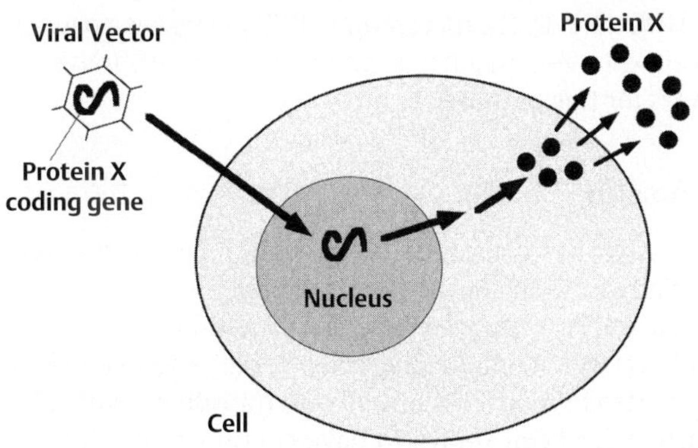

Fig. 18.3 Gene therapy using a viral vector to deliver protein X to the cell. The cell, as a result, produces large quantities of protein X. (From Nishida K, Kang JD, Gilbertson LG, et al. Modulation of the biologic activity of the rabbit intervertebral disc by gene therapy: an in vivo study of adenovirus-mediated transfer of the human transforming growth factor beta 1 encoding gene. Spine 1999;24:2419–2425, with permission.)

Transfection efficiencies for in vivo dermal injections range from 10 to 20%.[12] Although this method has merit in other gene therapy applications, the structure of the IVD make this technique problematic, in that transfecting cells within the center of the disk is difficult, has low efficiency of transfection, and could lead to more cell death and damage.

DNA-Ligand Complexes

DNA-ligand complexes employ protein or polymer constructs bound to plasmids containing the target gene. Again, although this technique does show merit in gene therapy as a whole,[13] the limited target gene expression and limited efficiency of transfer make this nonviral vector, along with the others, less desirable for gene therapy of the IVD.

Viral Vectors

Viral vectors are commonplace in gene therapy. The natural history of a viral infection performs the exact task called for in gene therapy. The key lies in removing viral proteins necessary for replication, keeping only those necessary for proper delivery of the target gene into the cell, and not allowing for continued viral replication or production of viral proteins. Viruses allow for typically the highest efficiencies of target gene transfer (90 to 95%, and even as high as 100%[14]) and allow for the longest periods of transcription of target gene product; hence their extensive use.

Retroviruses

Retroviruses have great utility in gene therapy, especially with regard to cancer therapy. This is due to their selective ability to infect only actively dividing cells. Although this is quite advantageous with regard to cancer, which involves such actively dividing cells, it is quite disadvantageous with regard to the IVD. The mature adult IVD undergoes a paucity of cell division, making retroviruses less attractive as vectors for this purpose.

Adenovirus

Adenovirus has been used extensively for gene therapy, especially in terms of the IVD. It is easily used with both in vivo and in vitro experimental conditions and infects a wide variety of nondividing cells. It is also quite efficient with regard to gene transfer, and cells transduced with adenovirus have been shown to have continuing production of transgene product for as long as 1 year.[15] One limiting factor of the use of adenovirus is that of immunogenicity. Expression of any viral proteins leads to an inflammatory reaction by the host and potentially to apoptosis, which can result in a decline in expression of the target gene over time.[16] This problem can be alleviated somewhat through the production of adenoviral vectors with more and more of the preexisting viral genome deleted. The newest adenoviral vectors consist only of beginning and end terminal repeats surrounding the target gene, thus inducing the least theoretical immune response by the host. As previously mentioned the avascularity of the IVD leads, in part, to a decreased immune response, which in and of itself would lead to a less vigorous response to the viral vector. However, this concern has led to the investigation of other viral vectors.

Adeno-Associated Virus

Adeno-associated virus is a virus that is rapidly becoming a more popular vector. It lacks the viral machinery to self-replicate, and can reproduce only in association with concomitant viral infection. This characteristic makes AAV a less immunogenic particle, which would, in theory, lead to longer and more continuous viral expression. The drawback of AAV lies in a slight decrease in efficiency of transfection, requiring an increased number of particles to achieve the efficiency of adenovirus.

Discussion

The characteristics of the ideal vector regarding gene therapy of the IVD are highly efficient target gene transfer, no immunogenicity, and a lack of viral protein production. Although that ideal vector does not exist, the closest to that ideal currently are adenovirus and AAV. A large amount of the research on gene therapy of the IVD has focused on adenovirus, whereas there is currently a growing interest in AAV as well.

■ Gene Therapy

TGF-β1

Nishida et al[17] successfully transferred TGF-β1 to the IVD of the rabbit through the injection of adenovirus loaded with the gene. The lumbar disk levels L2-L3, L3-L4, and L4-L5 were injected with the virus, whereas disk levels L1-L2 and L5-L6 were left untouched as controls. The cells of the injected disk levels proceeded to produce large levels of TGF-β1 (**Fig. 18.4**), whereas the control disk levels showed no significant increase in production, nor were controls transduced with a marker gene, indicating that it was indeed the transfected gene that caused the increased production. Additionally, the injected disk levels showed a 200% increase in newly synthesized proteoglycan production, showing that the transfected cells were in fact manufacturing new matrix.

Bone Morphogenetic Protein 2

Some preliminary evidence is available showing that gene therapy using bone morphogenetic protein 2 (BMP-2) may

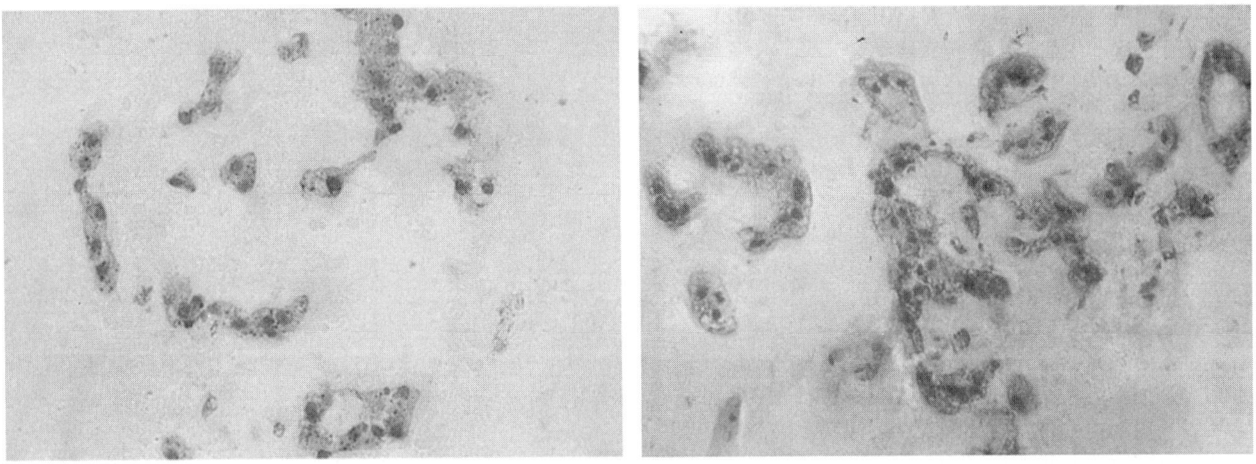

Fig. 18.4 Immunohistochemical staining for TGF-β1 in a control disk **(A)** and a disk 1 week following injection of adenovirus loaded with the TGF-β1 gene **(B)**. The increase in positive stain is evident in the injected disk. (From Nishida K, Kang JD, Gilbertson LG, et al. Modulation of the biologic activity of the rabbit intervertebral disc by gene therapy: an in vivo study of adenovirus-mediated transfer of the human transforming growth factor beta 1 encoding gene. Spine 1999;24:2419–2425, with permission.)

slow the degenerative process. In an abstract at the Orthopaedic Research Society meeting in 2005, Shimer et al[18] showed slowing of degeneration in BMP-2 transduced rabbit IVDs as compared with controls. This was the first time that gene therapy was shown to affect the natural history of a degenerative model.

Lim Mineralization Protein-1

Lim mineralization protein-1 (LMP-1) is another growth factor of interest with respect to gene therapy. LMP-1 has the unique action of stimulating the production of both BMP-2 and BMP-7, which have both already been shown to lead to increased synthesis of proteoglycan.[6,8] This makes LMP-1 particularly attractive in that through the transfection of one gene, two growth factors could be stimulated. This was evaluated by Yoon et al.[20] They showed that intradiskal injection of adenovirus loaded with LMP-1 was able to lead to the increased production of BMP-2, BMP-7, and subsequently aggrecan.

Tissue Inhibitor of Metalloproteinase-1

Tissue inhibitor of metalloproteinase-1 (TIMP-1) is a unique factor in the research on IVD regeneration in that its main action is not the synthesis of matrix, but rather the inhibition of its degradation. To date it has been shown in vitro to have action with respect to the human IVD tissue. Wallach et al[21] showed that degenerated human IVD tissue culture could be successfully transfected with adeno/TIMP-1, and this culture could subsequently increase its net production of proteoglycan. This study showed that the anti-catabolic effect of TIMP-1 could be taken advantage of and serves as an additional target for gene therapy.

Discussion

This strategy for the regeneration of the IVD involves the injection of a vector loaded with a target gene directly into the IVD. This has the advantage of direct delivery of the target gene to the cells, and then by using an efficient vector, inserting that gene into the target cells. By using appropriate vectors and genes, it has been shown that increased proteoglycan synthesis can be stimulated, as well as the degenerative process slowed. However, this modality still has the concern of side effects due to the use of viral vectors. Despite the relatively immunologically isolated nature of the IVD, the possibility of leakage of virus, and an ensuing adverse event in a patient, other modalities are currently being researched as well.

■ Cellular Therapies

The previous strategies have relied essentially on direct delivery, in the case of protein injections, or indirect delivery, in the case of in vivo gene therapy, of growth factors to the IVD for the purposes of tissue regeneration. The strategy of cellular therapy involves the introduction of entire cells, rather than protein or viral particles, into the IVD. These implanted cells are then intended to lead to the regeneration of the entire disk. Within this broad strategy there are many individual techniques that may be employed with the objective of disk regeneration.

Ex Vivo Gene Therapy

Ex vivo gene therapy shares the same goal as the in vivo treatment, except that the transfection of the cells takes place in vitro and transduced cells are subsequently injected rather than vector being injected. Cells are first harvested from the host, transfected in vitro, and then injected back into the host. The obvious disadvantage is that this technique would involve two separate procedures for the potential patient. However, this method's great significance is that the transfection takes place outside the body. This decreases the concern for the in vivo adverse effects of virus, in that no virus itself is directly introduced into the host.

This approach was used by Le Maitre et al[22] to evaluate the effectiveness of an IL-1 receptor antagonist (IL-1Ra). The hypothesis behind the use of this anticatabolic agent lies in the ability of IL-1Ra to block the activity of IL-1, a known inflammatory cytokine that leads to the upregulation of degradative pathways. Le Maitre et al first showed that IL-1Ra transfected cells were able to decrease the expression of MMP-3 and MMP-13 in cell culture, molecules known to degrade the extracellular matrix of the IVD. These cells were then labeled with green fluorescent protein and injected into in disk explants.[23] These cells were then identified and shown to still be producing statistically significant amounts of IL-1Ra up to 2 weeks postinjection.

The importance of ex vivo gene therapy lies in its ability to keep viral constructs out of the host and only in the laboratory. Given the concerns for side effects with the introduction of viral particles into hosts, the ability to achieve the same effect without the direct exposure of host to virus is of particular benefit. However, this strategy is limited by the necessity for a source of cells to be harvested. The healthy, adult IVD has a paucity of cells, and the degenerated IVD has even less, creating a problem with the cell source for ex vivo gene therapy.

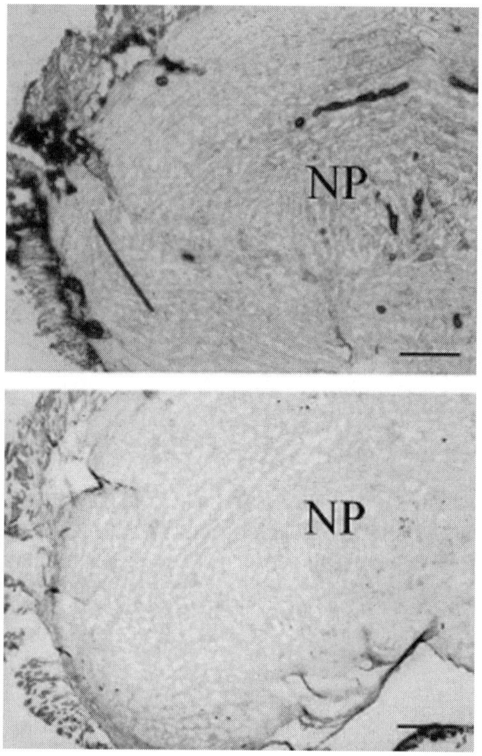

Fig. 18.5 Histologic section of an intervertebral disk (IVD) following injection of mesenchymal stem cells (MSCs) shows **(A)** no adipose differentiation evident with oil red O staining and **(B)** no osteogenesis with Von Kossa staining. (From Sakai D, Mochida J, Iwashina T, et al. Differentiation of mesenchymal stem cells transplanted to a rabbit degenerative disc model: potential and limitations for stem cell therapy in disc regeneration. Spine 2005;30:2379–2387, with permission.)

Mesenchymal Stem Cells

Mesenchymal stem cells (MSCs) are found in bone marrow aspirates and represent a cell type capable of division and differentiation to several cells types including bone, cartilage, muscle, and adipose tissue.[24,25] There has been much interest as to their ability for regenerating the IVD given their ability to differentiate into these multiple cell types. Steck et al[25] cultured MSC in the presence of TGF-β1 and showed that their phenotypic change was very chondrocytic in nature, but more similar to that of the IVD as opposed to hyaline cartilage.

Risbud et al[26] showed that MSCs could differentiate to cells with a phenotype indicative of chondrocytic cells by mimicking an environment even more similar to the IVD. They cultured bone-marrow–derived MSCs in the presence of decreased oxygen tensions and stimulated them with TGF-β1 and showed that these cells then upregulated their expression of chondrocytic-like proteins such as aggrecan and type II collagen.

As proof of the concept for therapeutic use, Sakai et al[24] labeled MSCs with green fluorescent protein and then injected them into the aging IVD of the rabbit. When the rabbits were sacrificed at the last time point of 48 weeks, the presence of and an increase in cells containing the stain were noted when compared with earlier time points. When these cells were analyzed, the cells again showed phenotypic behavior characteristic of the NP, and did not show histologic signs of differentiation toward adipose tissue or bone **(Fig. 18.5)**. This represents an exciting option for disk regeneration in the future, in that a patient's own MSCs could be harvested, cultured and expanded, and then injected into degenerated or damaged disks, allowing for the native environment to drive their phenotype toward that of the IVD, thus leading to the creation of new, healthy tissue.

Cocultures

Yet another cellular strategy involves coculture of cells. In this strategy, degenerated disk cells can be cocultured alongside healthy NP cells with the intent of stimulating the cells to proliferate or to increase their production of proteoglycan, or both. This was done by Okuma et al[27] using an

NP aspiration model of disk degeneration. The aspirated NP cells were cocultured with AF cells and then reinjected into the IVD. The experimental group showed a mild slowing of degeneration as compared with untreated, aspiration-only controls. In another study by the same group, injection of aspirated NP into degenerated disks (again the NP aspiration degeneration model) was shown to be superior to injection of NP cells that had been cocultured with AF cells. The group concluded that the extracellular matrix was an important component in slowing degeneration.[28] Although this technique has potential, the problems with a limited source of healthy NP cells as well as with cell viability after injection serve as major obstacles.

A promising use for this therapeutic strategy is combining it with MSC technology. This combined strategy involved coculturing MSC with IVD cells with the hope that the IVD cells will drive the differentiation of the MSC. The results of this strategy have shown the ability of the AF cells to stimulate an increase in proteoglycan production by the MSCs; however, this was not seen in coculture with the NP cells.[29] Richardson et al[30] were able to show an increase in NP marker gene expression following coculture of NP cells with MSCs, and that this effect was not dependent on cell-cell contact. Although much work still needs to be done in this area, the preliminary results in the literature thus far show yet another exciting area of hope for IVD regeneration.

Extracellular Scaffolds

Extracellular scaffolds represent one of the most challenging methods of IVD regeneration. As the name implies, scaffolds are created from various materials such as collagen/hyaluronate and chitosan,[31] calcium polyphosphate,[32] polyglycolic acid polymer,[33] and andalginate/calcium sulfate,[33] to name a few, in an effort to re-create the natural cellular microenvironment and thus foster the development of a new IVD grown in vitro, which would in turn be implanted to replace a damaged or degenerated disk.[34]

The feasibility of this design was shown by Alini et al[31] when they were able to successfully culture cells in a three-dimensional scaffold of collagen and hyaluronate. They concluded that although it was possible to three-dimensionally culture disk cells, the newly synthesized proteoglycan did not completely remain within the synthetic scaffold. Seguin et al[32] cultured bovine NP cells in a calcium polyphosphate scaffold and although the proteoglycan levels did not climb as high as native tissue, they did find that the construct had similar compressive mechanical properties to a native bovine disk. Mizuño et al[33] were likewise able to culture both AF and NP cells in a scaffold consisting of an outer region of polyglycolic acid polymer and an inner region of alginate/calcium sulfate. These scaffolds were implanted subcutaneously in athymic mice for the purposes of culturing

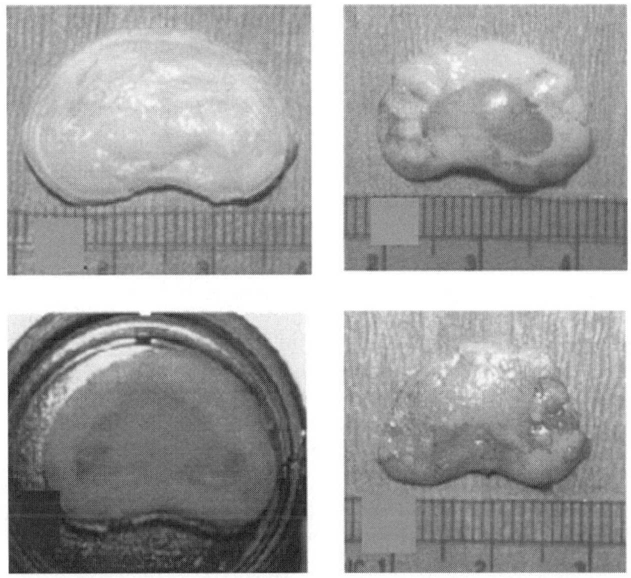

Fig. 18.6 Gross morphology **(A)** of native bovine lumber IVD and a tissue engineered disk **(B)** before implantation into athymic mice, postharvest after 4 weeks in vivo in athymic mice **(C)**, and postharvest after 12 weeks in vivo in athymic mice **(D)**, showing IVD cell growth throughout the scaffold. (From Mizuno H, Roy AK, Vacanti CA, et al. Tissue-engineered composites of anulus fibrosus and nucleus pulposus for intervertebral disc replacement. Spine 2004;29:1290–1297; discussion 1297–1298, with permission.)

the cells and harvested for analysis at differing time points **(Fig. 18.6)**. Again, although the cells did produce matrix components very similar to that of native disk tissue as well as showing the ability of cells to infiltrate into and reproduce within the scaffold at later time points, their level of proteoglycan synthesis still fell short of that in a native disk.

Cellular scaffolds, although yet another exciting strategy for disk regeneration, still remain an area of active research, with one of the main problems being maintenance of appropriate levels of extracellular proteoglycan. Nevertheless, the studies mentioned, as well as many others, show the potential of this technique.

Discussion

Cellular therapies for regeneration of the IVD consist of a collection of many individual strategies, with each carrying its own inherent obstacles and benefits. The key to success in this overall scheme of disk regeneration lies in the survivability of the cells once implanted. Care must be taken with techniques of injection such that the cells are not damaged or lysed in the process. However, this strategy provides the researchers the opportunity to perform a large amount of the regenerative work in vitro in a more controllable environment. It is this advantage that makes many of the cellular approaches enticing options for the treatment of IVDD.

Conclusion

The large amount of research that is currently being done on tissue engineering for the regeneration of IVD indicates the overwhelming problem of back pain and IVDD in today's world. Likewise, the variety of therapies currently being investigated signifies the fact that no one method has been shown to be far superior to the others. Each particular technique possesses its own pros and cons, its own risks and benefits. Although the majority of the strategies mentioned in this chapter are still years away from clinical trials, they have the potential to offer a great deal of hope to those suffering from low back pain.

References

1. Luo X, Pietrobon R, Sun SX, Liu GG, Hey L. Estimates and patterns of direct health care expenditures among individuals with back pain in the United States. Spine 2004;29:79–86
2. Hunter CJ, Matyas JR, Duncan NA. The notochordal cell in the nucleus pulposus: a review in the context of tissue engineering. Tissue Eng 2003;9:667–677
3. Urban JP, Smith S, Fairbank JC. Nutrition of the intervertebral disc. Spine 2004;29:2700–2709
4. Kang JD, Georgescu HI, McIntyre-Larkin L, et al. Herniated lumbar intervertebral discs spontaneously produce matrix metalloproteinases, nitric oxide, interleukin-6, and prostaglandin E2. Spine 1996;21:271–277
5. Thompson JP, Oegema TR, Bradford DS. Stimulation of mature canine intervertebral disc by growth factors. Spine 1991;16:253–260
6. Kim DJ, Moon SH, Kim H, et al. Bone morphogenetic protein-2 facilitates expression of chondrogenic, not osteogenic, phenotype of human intervertebral disc cells. Spine 2003;28:2679–2684
7. Masuda K, Takegami K, An H, et al. Recombinant osteogenic protein-1 upregulates extracellular matrix metabolism by rabbit annulus fibrosus and nucleus pulposus cells cultured in alginate beads. J Orthop Res 2003;21:922–930
8. An HS, Takegami K, Kamada H, et al. Intradiscal administration of osteogenic protein-1 increases intervertebral disc height and proteoglycan content in the nucleus pulposus in normal adolescent rabbits. Spine 2005;30:25–31
9. Masuda K, Imai Y, Okuma M, et al. Osteogenic protein-1 injection into a degenerated disc induces the restoration of disc height and structural changes in the rabbit anular puncture model. Spine 2006;31:742–754
10. Sprugel KH, McPherson JM, Clowes AW, Ross R. Effects of growth factors in vivo. I. Cell ingrowth into porous subcutaneous chambers. Am J Pathol 1987;129:601–613
11. Sobajima S, Kim JS, Gilbertson LG, Kang JD. Gene therapy for degenerative disc disease. Gene Ther 2004;11:390–401
12. Biewenga JE, Destree OH, Schrama LH. Plasmid-mediated gene transfer in neurons using the biolistics technique. J Neurosci Methods 1997;71:67–75
13. Ziady AG, Kim J, Colla J, Davis PB. Defining strategies to extend duration of gene expression from targeted compacted DNA vectors. Gene Ther 2004;11:1378–1390
14. Moon SH, Gilbertson LG, Nishida K, et al. Human intervertebral disc cells are genetically modifiable by adenovirus-mediated gene transfer: implications for the clinical management of intervertebral disc disorders. Spine 2000;25:2573–2579
15. Nishida K, Moon SH, Gilbertson LG, et al. Immune-privilege of the intervertebral disc: long-term transgene expression following direct adenovirus-mediated gene transfer. Presented at the International Society for the Study of Lumbar Spine, 2000, Adelaide, Australia
16. Yang Y, Nunes FA, Berencsi K, et al. Cellular immunity to viral antigens limits E1-deleted adenoviruses for gene therapy. Proc Natl Acad Sci U S A 1994;91:4407–4411
17. Nishida K, Kang JD, Gilbertson LG, et al. Modulation of the biologic activity of the rabbit intervertebral disc by gene therapy: an in vivo study of adenovirus-mediated transfer of the human transforming growth factor beta 1 encoding gene. Spine 1999;24:2419–2425
18. Shimer AL, Sobajima S, Chadderdon RC, et al. BMP-2 gene transfer favorably alters course of disc degeneration in rabbit model. Presented at the 51st annual meeting of the Orthopaedic Research Society, 2005, Washington, DC
19. Sobajima S, Kompel JF, Kim JS, et al. A slowly progressive and reproducible animal model of intervertebral disc degeneration characterized by MRI, X-ray, and histology. Spine 2005;30:15–24
20. Yoon ST, Park JS, Kim KS, et al. ISSLS prize winner: LMP-1 upregulates intervertebral disc cell production of proteoglycans and BMPs in vitro and in vivo. Spine 2004;29:2603–2611
21. Wallach CJ, Sobajima S, Watanabe Y, et al. Gene transfer of the catabolic inhibitor TIMP-1 increases measured proteoglycans in cells from degenerated human intervertebral discs. Spine 2003;28:2331–2337
22. Le Maitre CL, Freemont AJ, Hoyland JA. A preliminary in vitro study into the use of IL-1Ra gene therapy for the inhibition of intervertebral disc degeneration. Int J Exp Pathol 2006;87:17–28
23. Le Maitre CL, Hoyland JA, Freemont AJ. Studies of human intervertebral disc cell function in a constrained in vitro tissue culture system. Spine 2004;29:1187–1195
24. Sakai D, Mochida J, Iwashina T, et al. Differentiation of mesenchymal stem cells transplanted to a rabbit degenerative disc model: potential and limitations for stem cell therapy in disc regeneration. Spine 2005;30:2379–2387
25. Steck E, Bertram H, Abel R, et al. Induction of intervertebral disc-like cells from adult mesenchymal stem cells. Stem Cells 2005;23:403–411
26. Risbud MV, Albert TJ, Guttapalli A, et al. Differentiation of mesenchymal stem cells towards a nucleus pulposus-like phenotype in vitro: implications for cell-based transplantation therapy. Spine 2004;29:2627–2632
27. Okuma M, Mochida J, Nishimura K, et al. Reinsertion of stimulated nucleus pulposus cells retards intervertebral disc degeneration: an in vitro and in vivo experimental study. J Orthop Res 2000;18:988–997
28. Nomura T, Mochida J, Okuma M, et al. Nucleus pulposus allograft retards intervertebral disc degeneration. Clin Orthop Relat Res 2001;(389):94–101
29. Le Visage C, Kim SW, Tateno K, et al. Interaction of human mesenchymal stem cells with disc cells: changes in extracellular matrix biosynthesis. Spine 2006;31:2036–2042

30. Richardson SM, Walker RV, Parker S, et al. Intervertebral disc cell-mediated mesenchymal stem cell differentiation. Stem Cells 2006;24:707–716
31. Alini M, Li W, Markovic P, et al. The potential and limitations of a cell-seeded collagen/hyaluronan scaffold to engineer an intervertebral disc-like matrix. Spine 2003;28:446–454
32. Seguin CA, Grynpas MD, Pilliar RM, et al. Tissue engineered nucleus pulposus tissue formed on a porous calcium polyphosphate substrate. Spine 2004;29:1299–1306
33. Mizuno H, Roy AK, Vacanti CA, et al. Tissue-engineered composites of anulus fibrosus and nucleus pulposus for intervertebral disc replacement. Spine 2004;29:1290–1297
34. Anderson DG, Li X, Tannoury T, et al. Cellular therapy for disc degeneration. Spine 2005;30(suppl):S14–S19

19 Cost-Effectiveness of Lumbar Fusion

Paul G. Matz

Over the last two decades, the rate of spinal fusion per capita has been increasing.[1,2] Between 1993 and 2003, rates for lumbar fusion rose 80% in those 20 to 39 years, 137% in those 40 to 59 years, and 156% in those older than 60 years.[1] The leading diagnoses associated with spinal fusion increases were degenerative disk disease (183%) and spondylolisthesis (148%).[1] Between 1990 and 2001, the rate of fusion surgery increased from 19.1 surgeries per 100,000 adults to 61.1 surgeries per 100,000 (220%).[2]

The rate of increase has been accelerating as well. The rate of increase between 1996 and 2005 was far greater than the rate of increase observed between 1988 and 1996.[2] The rate of fusion accelerated for all types of lumbar disease but was far greater for herniated disk than for spondylolisthesis.[2] Rate increases were especially prevalent in those older than 60 years.[1,2]

The driving force behind these increases may be manifold. Advancements in radiographic imaging may enhance diagnostic sensitivity and accuracy. Innovations in surgical technique may reduce morbidity and augment success. In essence, lumbar instability may be more readily diagnosed and easily treated, especially in an aging population. However, lumbar fusion is an expensive procedure and health care resources are limited. For these reasons, it is important to examine the efficacy of lumbar fusion from both clinical as well as economic viewpoints. This chapter discusses the cost-effectiveness of lumbar fusion.

■ Overall Costs and Immediate Financial Impact

Quantifying cost and risk is paramount for any procedure. If the cost of a procedure is minimal and the complication rate low, then the expected efficacy need not be as high. Malter et al[3] reviewed data on 6376 patients who underwent lumbar surgery. Within this group were 1041 patients who were coded as having had lumbar fusion using data from the Washington State Department of Health. These authors analyzed costs (in 1988 dollars) as well as rates of complications and reoperation. The overall hospital costs averaged $7101 per patient treated with fusion compared with $4161 for patients who underwent surgery without fusion. The length of stay (LOS) in the hospital was 7 days for fusion patients compared with 5.1 days for nonfusion patients ($p < .001$). Complications rates were also higher in the fusion group (18% versus 7%, $p < .001$).

Deyo and colleagues[4] examined 18,122 hospitalizations for lumbar surgery in Washington State between 1986 and 1988. Most of these surgeries (84%) were undertaken for degenerative spinal stenosis or disk displacement. The authors compared the 15% of these patients who underwent surgical fusion to the remainder. The rates of complication (17.4% vs. 7.6%, $p < .0005$, chi-squared test), and LOS (7.6 days vs. 5.4 days, $p < .0005$) were higher in the fusion group. Cost was also higher with fusion ($6491 vs. $3793, $p = .0005$).

Deyo and colleagues[5] analyzed national data for lumbar surgery in Medicare recipients in 1985. Excluded were those on Medicare for renal failure or those on Social Security Disability. Among the factors analyzed were cost and complication rate. Data were available on 27,111 patients, of whom 1524 (5.6%) underwent fusion. Comparison was made, retrospectively, between patients who underwent fusion and those who did not. Mean hospital costs were $10,091 for those who underwent fusion compared with $6754 for those who did not ($p < .0005$, chi-squared test). Using logistic regression for multiple variables, the relative risk of complication was 1.9 (95% confidence interval [CI], 1.6–2.2) for the fusion group compared with the nonfusion group.

Katz el al[6] reported on 272 patients with lumbar stenosis who underwent surgery over a 4-year period. Surgical treatment included decompression ($n = 194$), decompression with fusion ($n = 37$), and decompression with fusion and fixation ($n = 41$). The rate of fusion varied greatly by surgery (relative risk 10-fold). Mean hospital costs were calculated as follows: $12,615 for decompression alone, $18,495 for decompression with fusion, and $25,914 for decompression with fusion and fixation.

Not unexpectedly, each of the studies above details increased cost associated with lumbar fusion and fixation. However, several issues need to be addressed. Most importantly, none of these studies addresses patient selection or efficacy. If patients are selected for fusion based on clinical criteria (for example, disabling back pain and claudication with regional kyphosis), then it is inappropriate to compare the costs associated with treating these patients to those associated with treating patients without that clinical characteristic (neurogenic claudication without back pain or deformity). Other methodologic issues decrease the ability to draw conclusions from these studies. The study by Katz et al[6] was skewed by the fact that the decision for fusion was surgeon dependent. Also, the greatest functional improvement in this study was observed in those patients who had decompression with fusion and fixation. The data analyses of Malter et al[3] and Deyo et al[4,5] were post hoc and did not review the indications for surgery or the clinical outcomes from surgery, nor did they determine whether fusion and nonfusion patients were eligible for either treatment.

Cost-Effectiveness and Quality of Life

Cost-effectiveness is rapidly becoming the paramount factor for assessing the utility of spinal surgery. Scientifically assessing cost patterns and their effectiveness remains considerably elusive. One common theme observed in the studies reviewed here is that the more society is willing to pay for a given benefit, the greater likelihood that the surgery will prove beneficial **(Fig. 19.1)**. This sort of analysis refers to the cost-effectiveness of surgery prior to factoring in any financial productivity gains from the patient returning to work.

Soegaard and colleagues[7] reported on a group of 136 patients with a history of segmental instability due to isthmic spondylolisthesis (grades I and II), primary disk degeneration, or secondary disk degeneration. Patients underwent fusion without fixation ($n = 17$), fusion with fixation ($n = 74$), or circumferential fusion with fixation ($n = 45$). Clinical follow-up was available in 83% of patients at 2 years. Evaluation of cost was available in 100%, and cost was assessed in Danish kroner (DKK). The group undergoing circumferential fusion had a preponderantly younger age ($p < .001$). All groups demonstrated significant improvement on the Dallas Pain Questionnaire (DPQ, $p < .05$).

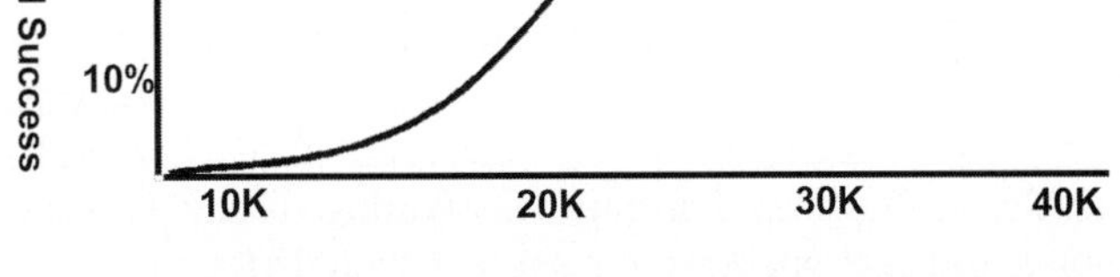

Fig. 19.1 A hypothetical acceptability curve for lumbar fusion or any surgical procedure. As society increases the amount it is willing to pay for a unit of improvement such as a quality-adjusted-life-year (QALY), the probability that surgery will be cost-effective increases. If society is willing to pay $40,000 per QALY, the probability that surgery would be cost-effective is much higher than if society is only willing to pay $15,000.

As expected, costs rose with complexity of the fusion surgery and with the addition of the fixation; significant differences were observed in surgical minutes and the costs of the implants ($p < .0001$). For the uninstrumented fusion, the total cost was DKK 88,285. For the fusion with fixation, the cost was DKK 94,396. For the circumferential fusion/fixation group, the cost was DKK 120,759.[7]

Comparing procedures, the authors found that fusion with fixation was as effective as fusion alone but more costly. Circumferential fusion with fixation was slightly more effective than simple fusion with fixation but at a significant cost. In comparing costs with incremental improvement on the DPQ, this study found the incremental cost of circumferential fusion/fixation to be DKK 28,000 and that of fusion/fixation to be DKK 4,684. These data may be viewed from the point of acceptability curves. If society was willing to pay DKK 8000 per unit of improvement on the DPQ, then there is an 80% probability that surgery would benefit the work, leisure, and daily activities scales of the DPQ. There is also a 50% probability that surgery would benefit the anxiety-depression and social life scales of the DPQ; if society is willing to pay only DKK 2000 per unit of improvement, the probabilities for surgical success diminish to 20% and 10%, respectively, for these two scales. Appropriately, these authors concluded that practitioners should focus on the determinants for cost-effectiveness rather than the surgical technique itself.[7]

Fritzell et al[8] undertook a cost analysis following a prospective study of spinal fusion in 294 patients. The study utilized 26 surgeons in 19 departments. Four groups of patients were studied: group I ($n = 73$) underwent posterolateral fusion, group II ($n = 74$) underwent posterolateral fusion/fixation, group III ($n = 75$) underwent circumferential fusion, and group IV ($n = 72$) underwent nonoperative therapy. Follow-up was over 2 years and was available in more than 80% of each group, except for group IV (69%). Assessed were overall improvement (self-rating of success), return-to-work status, and function as quantified using the Oswestry Disability Index (ODI).

Costs were evaluated in Swedish kroner (SEK). Total inpatient and outpatient costs were as follows: group I, SEK 87,000; group II, SEK 136,000; and group III, SEK 168,000.[8] These same surgical groups were prospectively compared with conservative therapy in a previous report using the clinical outcome measures described above.[9] In this report, those patients who underwent surgical fusion compared favorably to those patients who did not undergo surgery. Therefore, Fritzell and colleagues[8] performed an incremental cost-effectiveness evaluation in these patients. The incremental cost for overall, self-assessed improvement was SEK 2600, and that for functional improvement on the ODI was SEK 11,300. For return-to-work, the cost of incremental improvement was SEK 4100.

These authors also analyzed acceptability. Specifically, their study examined the rates at which the probability of surgery would be 95% effective. For self-assessed improvement, the price per incremental improvement would be SEK 5100. For incremental improvement on the ODI, the price would be SEK 36,500. For return-to-work status, the price would be SEK 14,400. Accordingly, if society was willing to pay these prices, surgery would have a 95% probability for effectiveness.[8]

Kuntz and colleagues[10] constructed a cost-effectiveness model for spinal surgery and applied it to large groups of patients culled from other studies. These authors studied lumbar decompression, decompression with fusion, and decompression with fusion/fixation. Follow-up evaluations were undertaken in the perioperative period, 6 months after surgery, and at last follow-up. Their model involved quality-of-life adjustments (QAL) and quality-adjusted-life years (QALY). Adjustments were made for short-term and long-term complications and negative outcomes. Short-term adjustments were for deep infection, nerve root injury, dural tear, and medical complications. Long-term adjustments were for chronic sequelae of short-term complications and persistent back pain.

In U.S. dollars, costs were $21,025 for decompression, $26,965 for decompression and fusion, and $35,669 for decompression with fusion and fixation. In QALY, the cost-effectiveness ratios were $56,500 for fusion and $3,112,800 for fusion with fixation. However, if relief from fusion with fixation was hypothetically 10% greater, then the cost-effectiveness ratio diminished to $82,400 per QALY. For a 15% improvement, the ratio diminished to $54,400. The authors also reflected on the biases inherent in their models. In terms of cost, when their model was biased against fusion, the cost-effectiveness ratio was fourfold greater than when biased toward fusion. In terms of the cost of symptom relief, when the model was biased against fusion, the cost was 20-fold greater than when biased toward fusion.[10]

This study did not initially account for lost productivity due to illness. In addition to improving functional outcome and increasing the number of patients who returned to work, a successful intervention would be expected to increase productivity. When factoring lost productivity into the problem, the authors found that every $1000 in lost productivity diminished the cost-effectiveness ratio by $5827. In essence, as the cost of lost productivity rises, any intervention that improves functional outcome and increases productivity becomes more cost-effective. These authors reported that an annual cost of lost productivity above $9700 would change the economics of spine fusion. In this scenario, if spine fusion improves function more effectively than decompression alone, then the added cost of fusion would be more than offset over a 10-year period. In essence, spinal fusion would be the cheaper alternative.[10] These authors appropriately concluded that every patient needs to contrast the increases in short-term complications after fusion with surgery with any purported long-term improvements.

Similar to the work by Fritzell et al, Rivero-Arias and colleagues[11] undertook a cost analysis of lumbar spinal fusion after completing a prospective study regarding its clinical efficacy versus intensive rehabilitation. In their study, patients were randomized to spinal fusion ($n = 176$) or intensive rehabilitation ($n = 173$). In those randomized to spinal fusion surgery, 139 patients elected to undergo surgery (circumferential fusion, $n = 57$; posterolateral fusion, $n = 57$; Graf fusion, $n = 25$), whereas 37 chose not to undergo surgery. In the rehabilitation group, 153 patients undertook rehabilitation and 22 chose not to do rehabilitation. The study detected a slight clinical improvement in the ODI in patients who underwent spinal fusion compared with those who underwent intensive rehabilitation.[12]

Costs were calculated in pounds sterling for 2002 to 2003. The initial cost for spinal fusion was £6041 compared with £1410 for a course of intensive rehabilitation. Eleven of the spinal fusion patients required revision surgery (£451) and 14 spinal fusion patients underwent unplanned rehabilitation (£162). In contrast, 48 rehabilitation patients crossed over to surgery (10 instead of rehabilitation and 38 in addition to rehabilitation)—a cost of £2128 per patient. The total costs of each arm of the study were £7830 for spinal fusion and £4526 for intensive rehabilitation. The study reported an insignificant difference in mean QALY over the trial period of 1.004 for spinal fusion compared with 0.936 for rehabilitation. These authors noted no difference in return-to-work rates, time to return, hours worked, and earnings between groups.[11]

Based on the differences in QALY and the costs, the authors performed an incremental cost analysis. The cost-effectiveness of spinal fusion was £48,588 per QALY. When the less expensive alternative of posterolateral fusion was reviewed, the cost-effectiveness reduced to £35,388. It increased when circumferential fusion only was analyzed (£60,765). If the 2-year QALY gains observed with spinal fusion were maintained over 4-years, the cost-effectiveness would drop to £25,398 for spinal fusion. These authors also noted that 45 patients undertook both therapies (38 rehabilitation patients crossed over and seven surgical patients underwent rehabilitation). If the same rates of dual therapy occurred over a 5-year period compared with a 2-year period, the cost-effectiveness of spinal fusion would drop to £31,838.[11]

These authors also completed an acceptability analysis. They concluded that spinal fusion would have a 20% probability for success if society was willing to pay £30,000 for a QALY. Probability for success would rise to 50% at a rate of £55,000 per QALY. This study concluded that spinal fusion is not cost-effective as a first-line therapy for lower back pain. These authors also noted that spinal fusion might be more cost-effective if more rehabilitation patients need subsequent surgery. Appropriately, they conceded that longer follow-up is necessary.[11]

Even in the realm of nonoperative therapy, controversy abounds as to the optimal level of treatment. In contrast to the study of Rivero-Arias et al, Skouen and colleagues[13] reported findings that extensive rehabilitation may not be more efficacious than expectant management or light rehabilitation. These authors analyzed 195 patients with chronic lower back pain who underwent expectant management ($n = 86$), light rehabilitation ($n = 52$), or extensive rehabilitation ($n = 57$). Patients were a subgroup of a larger study on musculoskeletal pain. Costs were measured in 1996 Norwegian Kroner (NoK). The average cost per patient across all treatments was NoK 9023 ($1120). The benefit was return-to-work and was based on an annual average salary of NoK 238,700 ($28,000).

These authors found that light rehabilitation proved more effective than intensive rehabilitation in returning patients to work. When each treatment was compared with expectant management, only light rehabilitation proved significantly better. The aggregate cost savings over 2 years for the 57 patients in the light rehabilitation was NoK 7,240,900 or NoK 127,033 per patient. This translates to a savings of approximately $15,000 per patient.[13]

■ Conclusion

The appropriate assessment of cost-effectiveness for lumbar surgery remains in its incipient phases.[14] The studies reviewed above have differing conclusions, with some showing a more discernible benefit at a reasonable cost than others. Some problems encountered during this review include the fact that the criteria for patient selection for comparative procedures have generally not been provided and that return to employment data, a factor that has great importance, has not been reported. One conclusion that almost all authors agree upon is that the more society is willing to pay for a given benefit, the greater likelihood that surgery will prove beneficial (**Fig. 19.1**). It also appears evident that practitioners need to focus less on specific surgical technique and more on determining which patients will benefit from a given surgical intervention. Accordingly, if the costs of an intervention are fixed, then the greater the benefit provided, the greater the cost-effectiveness.

References

1. Cowan JA, Dimick JB, Wainess R, Upchurch GR, Chandler WF, La Marca F. Changes in the utilization of spinal fusion in the United States. Neurosurgery 2006;59:15–20
2. Deyo RA, Gray DT, Kreuter W, Mirza S, Martin BI. United States trends in lumbar fusion surgery for degenerative conditions. Spine 2005;30:1441–1447
3. Malter AD, McNeney B, Loeser JD, Deyo RA. 5-year reoperation rates after different types of lumbar spine surgery. Spine 1998;23:814–820
4. Deyo RA, Cherkin DC, Loeser JD, Bigos SJ, Ciol MA. Morbidity and mortality in association with operations on the lumbar spine. The influence of age, diagnosis, and procedure. J Bone Joint Surg Am 1992;74:536–543
5. Deyo RA, Ciol MA, Cherkin DC, Loeser JD, Bigos SJ. Lumbar spinal fusion. A cohort study of complications, reoperations, and resource use in the Medicare population. Spine 1993;18:1463–1470
6. Katz JN, Lipson SJ, Lew RA, et al. Lumbar laminectomy alone or with instrumented or noninstrumented arthrodesis in degenerative lumbar spinal stenosis. Patient selection, costs, and surgical outcomes. Spine 1997;22:1123–1131
7. Soegaard R, Christensen FB, Christiansen T, Bunger C. Costs and effects in lumbar spinal fusion. A follow-up study in 136 consecutive patients with chronic low back pain. Eur Spine J 2007;16:657–668
8. Fritzell P, Hagg O, Jonsson D, Nordwall A. Cost-effectiveness of lumbar fusion and nonsurgical treatment for chronic low back pain in the Swedish Lumbar Spine Study: a multicenter, randomized, controlled trial from the Swedish Lumbar Spine Study Group. Spine 2004;29:421–434
9. Fritzell P, Hagg O, Wessberg P, Nordwall A. 2001 Volvo Award Winner in Clinical Studies: Lumbar fusion versus nonsurgical treatment for chronic low back pain: a multicenter randomized controlled trial from the Swedish Lumbar Spine Study Group. Spine 2001;26:2521–2534
10. Kuntz KM, Snider RK, Weinstein JN, Pope MH, Katz JN. Cost-effectiveness of fusion with and without instrumentation for patients with degenerative spondylolisthesis and spinal stenosis. Spine 2000;25:1132–1139
11. Rivero-Arias O, Campbell H, Gray A, Fairbank J, Frost H, Wilson-MacDonald J. Surgical stabilisation of the spine compared with a programme of intensive rehabilitation for the management of patients with chronic low back pain: cost utility analysis based on a randomised controlled trial. BMJ 2005;330:1239–1243
12. Fairbank J, Frost H, Wilson-MacDonald J, Yu LM, Barker K, Collins R. Randomised controlled trial to compare surgical stabilisation of the lumbar spine with an intensive rehabilitation programme for patients with chronic low back pain: the MRC spine stabilisation trial. BMJ 2005;330:1233–1239
13. Skouen JS, Grasdal AL, Haldorsen EM, Ursin H. Relative cost-effectiveness of extensive and light multidisciplinary treatment programs versus treatment as usual for patients with chronic low back pain on long-term sick leave: randomized controlled study. Spine 2002;27:901–910
14. Fenwick E, O'Brien BJ, Briggs A. Cost-effectiveness acceptability curves–facts, fallacies and frequently asked questions. Health Econ 2004;13:405–415

20 Intradiskal Electrothermal Therapy

Richard Derby, Ray M. Baker, and Paul A. Anderson

The use of heat energy to treat chronic low back pain is an alternative to standard surgical procedures. A common technique is application of heat using an intradiskal electrothermy (IDET). The IDET procedure is done primarily for discogenic low back pain, and it remains controversial. Although complications are rare, efficacy has not been established. Furthermore, basic science investigations were largely performed after the introduction of the procedure. Results from these studies often do not provide fundamental support for the procedure or are conflicting.

This chapter discusses the scientific basis for the IDET procedure. The technique is described and clinical results are reviewed. The results are assessed on the basis of the strength of evidence.

■ Basic Science Principles

The goals of thermal disk treatments are to remove unwanted tissue such as herniated disks, create a seal to limit expression of matrix components, shrink collagen tissue, and to destroy nociceptors. Although intradiskal heating can be accomplished through a variety of means, including electrocautery, thermal cautery, laser, and radiofrequency energy (RFE), most current intradiskal thermal treatments are performed using RFE.

Radiofrequency energy may be applied with unipolar or bipolar probes. Similar to electrocautery, with unipolar RFE, currents pass through the probe to the body and to a grounding pad. The bipolar probe allows energy to pass through positive and negative poles on the probe, theoretically decreasing collateral damage. The bipolar devices have the potential to create greater control of heating, thereby allowing greater focus of heat energy. A modification of the bipolar probe has been termed "coblation," which has been claimed to generate a plasma of high-energy ionized particles in the tissues surrounding the probe rather than a traditional heat lesion. The plasma can disrupt organic bonds, thus allowing debridement and effective heat treatment of soft tissues.

Neural Applications of Radiofrequency Energy

In addition to the use of radiofrequency energy to cauterize or vaporize tissue, RFE has been used for neural ablation. In 1976 Sweet[1] described the use of radiofrequency thermocoagulation to destroy the trigeminal nerve fibers within the gasserian ganglion. This technique proved safer and more effective than both chemical and open surgical lesioning, and within several years radiofrequency neurotomy became the standard method for the ablation of small nerves. In particular, radiofrequency neurotomy became the standard method to ablate the medial branch nerves of the dorsal ramus in an attempt to reduce pain caused by the posterior elements of the spine.[2–4]

Originally, the heat created by RFE adjacent to a nerve was thought to cause selective destruction of smaller pain conducting nerve fibers and to spare larger afferent and motor fibers.[5] Frohling et al,[6] however, showed that following controlled thermocoagulation of rabbit sciatic nerve at temperatures above 50°C for 45 seconds, histologic sections and electron micrographs at various intervals after the lesion showed generalized and not selective destruction.[6] At 90°C, most of the myelinated fibers of all calibers were destroyed, with survival only of Schwann cells. The regeneration process began within several days, and by 12 days the site of the lesion was covered by regenerating, partly remyelinated fibers of all calibers. The observation of early regeneration is consistent with the duration of pain relief between 6 and 12 months following medial branch neurotomies.[7]

Collagen Modifying Applications of Radiofrequency Energy

The rationale for heating disks was strongly influenced by animal and clinical investigations testing the ability of heat to stabilize joints by modifying collagen. Since 1994 thermal capsulorrhaphy has been used alone or in combination with traditional surgical treatments to treat shoulder instabilities. Typically, the shoulder capsule is visualized through an arthroscope, and either laser or radiofrequency heating devices are used to denature the collagen of the shoulder capsule causing capsular shrinkage.[8]

Like the outer disk annulus, type I collagen in the shoulder capsule has a triple-helical configuration that is responsible for the molecule's ability to resist tensile forces. Heating first disrupts the weaker intramolecular bonds, unraveling and denaturing the triple helix. The stronger nonreducible intermolecular cross-links remain intact and thus the amount of collagen is unchanged. This "melting" into an amorphous state causes the observed tissue shrinkage and is a phase transition from a highly ordered crystalline structure to a random coil state. The effect plateaus at temperatures above 75°C, but higher temperatures eventually cause tissue destruction. Because temperatures above 45°C cause cell necrosis, cells are assumed to be destroyed after treatment. By 2 weeks, animal experiments show an enhanced healing response with the proliferation of cells and capillary sprouting. However, the treated ligaments are two to three more times susceptible to cyclic and static creep strains, and in one study two of eight treated ligaments experienced partial failure during creep testing.[9]

The biologic effects of laser thermal modification were investigated by Hayashi et al.[10,11] Using a yttrium-aluminum-garnet (YAG) laser, 250 joules were applied to the glenohumeral and patellofemoral joint capsules. Joint capsule thickness immediately increased but normalized by 60 days. Laser-treated capsules had immediately decreased stiffness and strength compared with sham controls, but they normalized by 30 days. Histologically, collagen hyalinization and cell death occurred. The surrounding untreated tissue was normal. An active reparative process commenced with fibroblast migration and neovascularization. By 60 days the tissue appeared normal, and no inflammatory changes were present at any time. Biochemical analysis revealed that the laser treatment denatured collagen by disrupting α bands, resulting in unwinding of the triple helix.

Animal data and direct arthroscopic observation show that collagen can be made to contract by applying heat, but it is also clear that the initial effects are deleterious and recovery is dependent on a healing response. Even though cartilaginous tissue may regain most of its preinjury strength, the tissue remains weaker during creep strains. This repair process is dependent on inflammation followed by repair, and thus is dependent on the migration of blood vessels and cells to the area of injury.

Treatment Effect

Electron microscopy of cadaver disks following standardized IDET have shown extensive collagen disorganization, decreased quantity of collagen, collagen fibril shrinkage, and chondrocyte damage when compared with a control.[12] Despite these and numerous other in vivo and in vitro studies using human and animal models, the precise pain relieving mechanism of intradiskal heating is unclear. The following subsections offer theoretic explanations of its mechanism of action as well as a review of the basic science literature supporting intradiskal heating.

Changes in Disk Biomechanics

Although postheating changes in disk compliance could lead to alterations in the biomechanical properties of a vertebral segment, studies have not provided clear evidence that this occurs. Pre- and posttesting of human cadaver disks following a standardized IDET treatment of 65° to 90°C over 17 minutes with a 6-cm active tip thermal-resistive coil resulted in a minor decreased compliance and increased motion in all planes but greatest in lateral bending.[13] The amount of increased motion did not, however, approach clinical significance, and the authors concluded that IDET did not adversely affect stability. Similarly, Wang et al[14] heated bovine disk core samples consisting of the vertebrae and disk nucleus in a water bath and found no significant difference in either stiffness ($p = .182$) or failure strength ($p = .998$) after heating. All failures occurred in midsubstance of the specimen.

In contrast, Kleinstueck et al[15] in a larger series of disks found that heating cadaver intervertebral disks with a standardized IDET protocol placed 10 to 15 mm from the outer annulus resulted in a significant (6 to 12%) decrease in stiffness even though temperatures greater than 65°C were seen only within a 2-mm radius of the catheter. To achieve a more uniform heating, Bass et al[16] heated their human cadaver segments in a water bath. They found that when the annulus was heated to 75°C, it was more compliant at higher applied stresses.

Annular Contraction

A decrease in disk herniation size secondary to contraction of collagen in the annulus might lead to decreased pain. Indeed, when bovine annular tissue was placed in a tube and heated, Schaufele and Huckle[17] measured a 2% decrease in mass, 15% decrease in volume, and a 3% decrease in diameter. In addition, they reported two anecdotal cases where before-and-after magnetic resonance imaging (MRI) scans showed a reduction in herniation size following clinical application of heat using a thermal-resistive coil. Just the opposite, however, occurred in Cohen et al's[18] retrospective case series. They reported that two of 79 patients undergoing IDET later had an apparent new disk herniation. They postulated that the usual slow recovery post-IDET and the observed results were more consistent with a mechanism of collagen modulation rather than reduced nociception. Additionally, Bass et al[16] showed that, unlike the shoulder capsule that will shrink 60 to 80%, the annulus will only shrink 7.5% after heating to 85°C. Further shrinkage is likely retarded by the attachment of the annulus to the bony end plates.

Thermally Induced Healing Response

Although there is a loss of cell viability using live/dead staining after IDET treatment, IDET treated disks maintained in cell culture conditions have demonstrated the ability to recover cell viability in the treated areas over 2 to 4 weeks.[19] The authors demonstrated thermal modification of collagen following IDET treatment, observing changes in both histologic and scanning electron microscopy (SEM) collagen morphology. The authors concluded that their findings were consistent with other studies showing that shoulder capsular tissues regain biomechanical integrity after thermal treatment. In contrast, an in vitro ovine study by Freeman et al found that IDET did not modulate the healing response in any way at various time intervals up to 12 weeks. Both the treated and the untreated disks showed similar degrees of degeneration, and the sheep disks in which an annular incision was made showed the most pronounced degenerative changes. At 12 weeks there was pronounced granulation tissue accompanied by small nerves up to the outer three layers.

Bass et al[20] confirmed these findings by heating ovine cervical disks. They hypothesized that a low-temperature heating protocol would stimulate repair. At serial harvesting up to 3 months postprocedure, the disks were examined and underwent biomechanical testing. There was no indication that thermal treatment led to increased stability and every indication that high temperatures delivered to large regions of the disk had no discernible therapeutic benefit, and the authors postulated that the effect would be deleterious. In support, Derby et al[21] found that in clinical practice, higher temperatures and larger total heating doses during IDET procedures with catheters placed in the outer annulus increased the duration of postprocedure pain flare-ups and led to less favorable outcomes at 8-month follow-up. The long-term outcomes at 16 months, however, were unaffected by these heating variables.

Sealing of Annular Tears

Several authors have postulated that IDET might "seal" annular tears, leading to decreased pain. No clinical data support this contention. In fact, Narvani et al obtained MRI scans before and at an average of 6 months after performing a standard IDET procedure in patients with discogenic pain, a positive diskogram, and postdiskogram computed tomography (CT) showing a least one grade 3 annular tear. Six of ten patients had a preoperative MRI scan showing a HIZ in the outer posterior annulus. All six patients had an unchanged HIZ in the outer posterior annulus in the follow-up MRI scan.

Annular Denervation

A heating element placed in close proximity to the outer annulus and heated according to protocol will most likely achieve temperatures greater than 45°C within 5 to 9 mm from the catheter.[22–24] Because most current techniques involve catheters placed in the outer annulus, denervation is theoretically possible. Bono et al[25] showed that a zone of potential denervation occurred at distances 12 to 14 mm from the catheter, with temperatures of 42°C achieved at distances up to 14 mm. Using an IDET catheter placed close to the area of pathology, Wright et al[24] measured mean outer annular temperatures of $43.9° \pm 2.3°C$ and concluded that these temperatures are sufficient to coagulate nociceptors.

Although a catheter placed within 5 mm of the outer annulus will achieve temperatures toxic to nociceptors within outer and middle annular fibers,[25] it is unclear if this mechanism correlates with clinical recovery following IDET or intradiskal radiation therapy (IDRT). At issue is the duration of pain flare-up. Similar to medial branch neurotomies, one may expect several days to a week of flare due to tissue trauma followed by clinical improvement. Few published studies comment on the frequency and duration of post-intradiskal heating flare-up.[26] Derby et al[26] showed that in a series of 32 patients, all reported a flare-up lasting an average of 5 days. If patients having no flare or minimal (<1 week) flare achieved a significantly better outcome, these data would be consistent with the theory that intradiskal heating reduces pain by destroying nociceptor input.

A potential benefit would result if pain originated partially from the ingrowth of nociceptive fibers into the inner annular layers that were eliminated during healing with fibrous tissue.[27] However, in an in vitro sheep study, Freeman et al were unable to show any difference in the number of nerve fibers observed in the anterior sheep annulus in a control annular incision with or without the IDET procedure, and in fact the ingrowth of granulation tissue in both control and IDET specimens were accompanied by small never fibers.

Decreased Intradiskal Pressure

Using a recently introduced shorter electrothermal IDET catheter (SpineCATH® intradiskal catheter, Smith & Nephew, London, UK) the controlled intradiskal application of thermal energy on bovine disk material resulted in a 15% decrease in volume, 2% decrease in mass, and a 3% decrease in disk diameter.[28] The authors postulated that this mechanism might provide an explanation for observed improvements in radicular symptoms in patients with lumbar herniated nucleus pulposus (HNP). In the same study Podhajsky et al[28] found pressure reductions approximating 30 to 50% in sheep nucleus pulposus following IDET treatment using a 1.5 cm electrothermal device (Decompression® catheter, Smith & Nephew). The authors also found that the hydrophilic property of nucleus pulposus is temperature dependent, and that increasing the treatment temperature resulted in a decreasing ability of the nucleus to absorb water. Such pressure reduction might account for a more significant reduction in referred leg symptoms than back pain following IDET procedure in one retrospective study.[29]

■ Outcomes

Observational Studies

As with many other newly introduced treatments, early IDET outcome studies reported optimistic results. The initial prospective case series by the cofounders of Oratec Interventions, Saal et al, reported a positive response rate of 80%, and Derby et al's[26] initial patient audit reported positive response rates of 73% when the catheter position was optimal and 16.5% in patients with a fair catheter placement. Saal et al[30,31] also reported decreases in the Short Form (SF)-36 reports of body pain of 59 to 78% and average decreases in VA scores of 62 to 72%. Despite early published results similar to the Saal's, Derby was quoted in the *Back Letter*[32] as stating that approximately one third of his IDET-treated patients were much better, one third were slightly better, and one third were the same or worse. In addition, his patients had on average only a 1.84/10 (18%) average decrease in VA score.

Since then, prospective and retrospective case series studies report a dichotomy of results. Four studies reported overall poor results,[33–36] with an average decrease in VA score of approximately 20%[33,34] and reporting 30% of the patients with the same amount or pain and 30% of the patients with more pain at 1 year post-IDET.[35] The worst results are reported by the Davis study that was conducted by surgeons uninvolved with the IDET procedure who called the patients post-IDET. They retrospectively reported a 13% decrease in the number of patients employed and a 37% satisfaction rate 1 year postprocedure.[35] The other retrospective study conducted by the Liberty Mutual Center reported on narcotic use, spine surgery, and epidural injections following IDET performed on 142 patients in 23 states. They found that 68% of the cases did not meet the published criteria, 37% had at least one injection post-IDET, 55% had at least two narcotic prescriptions, 23% had spinal surgery, and 20% returned to work.[36]

On the other hand, not counting the original Saal and Derby studies, there was an approximate 50% decrease in visual analogue scale (VAS) score in the five published case series studies having different population groups.[18,37–40] Interestingly, the only study with institutional review board (IRB) approval, and therefore a validated study design prior to inception, was a retrospective case audit series.[18] The other four prospective case series should perhaps be classified as retrospective audits with prospectively obtained information. The best reported outcome scores were from a recent study by Mekhail et al, who compared the results in 42 patients randomized to either IDET or IDRT. From months 3 to 12 the IDET group had significantly lower mean pain scores than the IDRT group. VAS pain scores decreased from 6.6 ± 2.0 before to 4.4 ± 2.4 at 1 year after IDRT ($p = .001$), whereas in the IDET group the average VAS pain score decreased from 7.4 ± 1.9 before IDTA to 1.4 ± 1.9 at 1-year follow-up. Similarly, the PDI scores in the IDET group had a significantly larger improvement than those for patients who received IDRT.

There were two prospective practice audits without IRBs that used a case-control group.[41–43] Both centers used a convenience control group of patients who were offered IDET but could either not afford the procedure or failed to obtain authorization from their insurance companies. Although the results are criticized because the denial of care introduced a potential selection bias and probably immediate patient dissatisfaction in the control population,[44] both studies were confined by the realities of private practice.

The Karasek and Bogduk[41] study included a group of 17 patients who were denied insurance authorization and were reported to have continued a conservative treatment protocol identical to 36 patients receiving IDET. The patient selection included only patients with well-hydrated disks in which annular disruption was limited to two quadrants or less. At 1 year, with the exception of one patient, none of the control group had any significant relief of pain. In the IDET group the VA score was decreased by 63%. Sixty percent of the patients had ≥50% pain relief, with 23% obtaining complete relief of pain. All 18 patients who were working before IDET were able to return to work, and eight of the 15 who were not working returned to work after IDET. At the 2-year follow-up, 54% of the patients continued to have at least a 50% reduction in pain.[42] At 1 year post-IDET, with the exception of one patient, the control group continued to have no significant relief.[42] In a more recent but similar case-controlled series, Finch et al[43] performed IDRT on the posterior annulus using a flexible radiofrequency electrode (discTRODE™ RF catheter, Radionics®) in 46 patients with single-level painful disks. They compared the outcome in 17 patients who were unable to obtain funding for the procedure. The VAS decreased 37% in treated patients at 12 months follow-up compared with an increase of 3% in control subjects.

Randomized Controlled Trials

Intradiskal electrothermy is one of the few interventional spinal procedures to have two published and one aborted randomized blinded controlled studies. The Pauza et al[45] study is a double-blind, placebo-controlled trial in carefully selected patients with painful disk disruption identified with carefully performed pressure-controlled lumbar diskography The patients were in general only mildly disabled, with pretreatment SF-36 pain scores of 56. The disk heights were maintained and protrusions were ≤4 mm. In addition, the patients had neither litigation nor compensation issues. The IDET procedures were performed by two experienced clinicians. The catheters were navigated circumferentially to both the lateral and posterior annulus on both sides of the disk. Catheter insertions from both sides of the midline were performed when necessary to provide complete coverage of the outer annulus. After randomization, 37 were assigned to undergo IDET and 27 were assigned to a sham treatment. Those undergoing a control procedure had a sham treatment in which the introducer needle was inserted to the lateral margin of the disk. Although there was no statistical difference in the SF-36 bodily pain outcome measure between groups (a decrease in 17 versus 9), there was a statistical difference in the VA scores

7.4 to 5.0 (36%) in the IDET group versus 8.1 to 5.2 (17%) in the sham control group. In addition, 33% of the control group worsened compared with only 6% of the IDET group, and 22% of the patients in the IDET group had $\geq$75% relief of pain compared with 4% of the control group. Although there was no difference in SF-36 physical functioning (a decrease in 15 versus 11) there was a statistical 11% improvement in the Oswestry Disability Scale compared with a 4% in the control group. The data also showed that IDET was significantly more effective for patients with pain scores less than 70 and for patients with poor function or greater disability.

Both groups exhibited significant improvements in pain scores, and at 6-month follow-up there was an average difference of 1.3 in the VA score between the IDET and control groups, with a calculated p value of .045.[45] A similar pattern of improvement occurred in the bodily pain scores on the SF-36 but was not significantly different between the two groups ($p = .086$).

Freeman et al[46] performed a randomized double-blind controlled IDET efficacy study in which patients were selected on the basis of one- or two- level symptomatic disk degeneration with posterior or posterolateral annular tears as determined by provocative CT/diskography. Patients were excluded if there was >50% loss of disk height or previous back surgery. The study did not demonstrate a significant benefit from IDET over placebo. No subject in either treatment group showed improvement of >7 points in low back outcome score or specified domains of the SF-36. The study has been criticized because some felt the patients were improperly selected and included patients with multilevel disk disease and patients on workers' compensation, and the study did not state the weight of the patients, the significantly reduced disk heights, and the long histories of pain and disability. In addition, all of the commentators, including the authors, were surprised that even the control group did not report any significant improvement. Nonetheless, the authors' results are perhaps more consistent with reality given the fact that patient selection criteria are usually less stringent in clinical practice than in a randomized control trial.

Bogduk presented, but did not publish, the results of an aborted randomized controlled IDET study by Lau et al[47] at the 2004 International Spinal Injection Society (ISIS) annual scientific meeting. Patients with single-level painful disk disruption were identified by a positive diskogram using ISIS criteria. The study included six patients randomized to the control sham group, 11 patients randomized to the IDET group, and a benchmark group of patients who initially refused the requirements of enrollment randomization but had IDET performed after obtaining approval from their insurance company. Similar to the Pauza et al[45] study, there was an average of 2.5 (7.0 to 4.5) decrease in the VA score at 12 months in the 11 patients in the IDET group. Although the benchmark group showed less favorable outcome, there was no statistical difference in the groups at 12 months. Fifty percent of the randomized IDET cases achieved 50% or greater pain relief. The control IDET group, however, included six patients, and five of the six patients were somewhat better at 3 months. One control patient was pain free at 3 months and remained pain free at 1-year follow-up. Because of this one patient in the control group, the calculated number of patients needed to show a statistical difference between the active and sham group was about 100, and the study was stopped. Bogduk concluded that IDET was too weak a treatment to prove conclusively against a placebo without a large number of patients.

Meta-Analyses and Systematic Reviews

Appleby et al[48] recently published a meta-analysis of IDET outcomes based on the following: pain intensity measured by a numerical pain rating scale, a VAS, or bodily pain (BP) on the SF-36; and physical function (PF) measured by the Oswestry Disability Index (ODI) or the SF-36. Seventeen studies included follow-up of between 6 months and 2 years, and contained one or more of these validated outcome measures. The pooled analysis from these studies found a mean decrease in the VAS of 2.9 (CI, 2.5–3.4), a mean decrease in PF statistic of 21.1 (CI 13.4–28.8), a mean decrease in BP of 18 (CI, 11.9–24.1), a mean decrease in ODI of 7.0 (CI, 2.0–11.9). All of the above statistics were significant. The Appleby meta-analysis (funded by Smith and Nephew) concluded, "Published studies provide compelling evidence of the relative efficacy and safety of the IDET procedure."

A final study by Gunner Andersson et al[49] compared validated outcome measurements of 18 IDET studies with the same outcome measurements reported by 33 fusion studies performed for degenerative disk disease. Pain severity was measured by either the VAS or numerical pain scores, functional improvement was measured by the ODI, and quality of life was measured by either the PF statistic or physical component summary (PCS) score of the SF-36. Outcome was summarized by percentage improvement in each type of study stratified into randomized controlled trials, non–randomized-controlled trials, before and after cohorts, and case series. Interestingly, the overall median decrease in pain reported following IDET was very similar to those following spinal fusion. For example, in eight before-and-after studies, there was a mean 61% decrease in VA score in the surgery patients compared with a mean 50% decrease following IDET, but a 63% drop in the VA score in the two nonrandomized control IDET studies compared with one surgery study that did not report VAS improvement. On the other hand, the back-specific impairment as measured by the ODI showed a median 40% drop in eight spinal fusion randomized controlled trials compared with a 20% median decrease in two IDET randomized controlled trials. The quality of life as measured by the physical component summary score or PF statistic also showed an

Table 20.1 Summary of Percentage Improvement in Outcomes by Study Design for Each Treatment Type: Spinal Fusion Data from Previous Study

Procedure		Pain Severity*				Back-Specific Impairment				Quality of Life			
		RCT	NCT	BA	CS	RCT	NCT	BA	CS	RCT	NCT	BA	CS
Spinal fusion	No. of 33	6	1	8	11	8	1	2	6	5	0	0	0
	%	36	NA	61	53	40	NA	NA	42	43	NA	110	NA
	Median (range)	(30–77)	(37–52)	(42–75)	(24–62)	(17–73)	(39–54)	(58–77)	(17–49)	(21–123)			
IDET	No. of 29	3	3	12	2	3	1	2	0	3	0	7	0
	(patients)	(129)	(148)	(548)	(115)	(129)	(53)	(47)		(149)		(292)	
	%	14	63	46	29	4	41	45		4		47	
	Median (range)	(−9–36)	(63–81)	(22–71)	(29)	(−6–35)	(41)	(14–75)		(−16–35)		(22–69)	
	%	14	69	46	29	11	41	45		11		50	
	Mean (range)	(−9–36)	(63–81)	(22–71)	(29)	(−6–35)	(41)	(14–75)		(−6–35)		(22–69)	
	>50%	19	60	67	32								
	Median (range)	(0.08–38)	(57–81)	(50–70)	(16–48)								
	>50%	19	66	62	32								
	Mean (range)	(0.08–38)	(57–81)	(50–70)	(16–48)								

Abbreviation: NA, not applicable.
*Categorized by study design: RCT, randomized control trial; NCT, nonrandomized control trial; BA, prospective before-and-after trial; CS, retrospective case series.
Source: Andersson GB, Mekhail NA, Block JE. Treatment of intractable discogenic low back pain. a systematic review of spinal fusion and intradiscal electrothermal therapy (IDET). Pain Physician 2006;9(3):237–248.

approximately two to three times improvement for surgery compared with IDET.

In contrast to the Appleby paper, a meta-analysis by Freeman[50] reached an entirely different conclusion after reviewing the same studies. This review reports a stronger 3.4 mean improvement in VAS scores (compared with Appleby's 2.9), and only slightly lower mean ODI improvement of 5.2 (compared with 7.0 in the Appleby study). In addition, only 13 to 23% of the patients went on to have surgery. Despite this, Freeman concludes, "The evidence for efficacy of IDET remains weak and has not passed the standard of scientific proof."

Although mean and median improvement in VAS score is informative, a better measurement of clinical relevance is the percentage of patients who achieve 50% or greater improvement. There are six IDET studies containing enough data to calculate the percentage of patients obtaining 50% or more pain relief as measured by the VAS or a numerical pain score **(Table 20.1)**. The studies include one randomized controlled trial,[51] one nonrandomized controlled trial,[41,42] and four before-and-after case series.[30,52–55] Between 38% and 94% (average 71%) of patients reported 50% or more pain relief at between 6 months and 2 years following an IDET procedure.

Surgical Technique

Intradiskal Electrothermal Treatment

The IDET procedure utilizes a navigable intradiskal catheter with a thermal resistive coil. The procedure can be performed under conscious sedation. Using a standard posterolateral diskogram technique, a 30-cm catheter

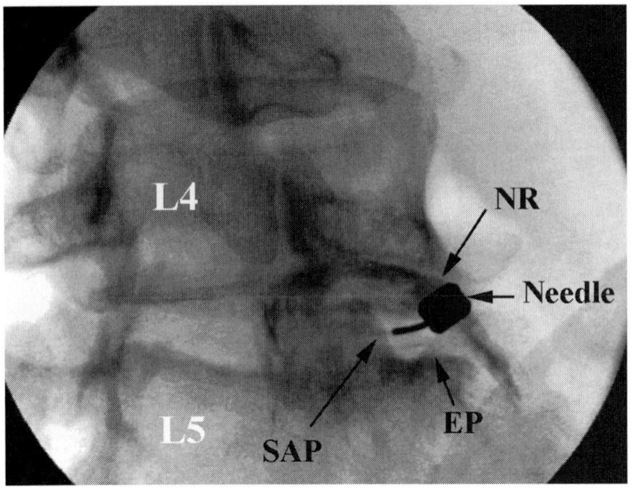

Fig. 20.1 The introducer needle is usually advanced parallel to the fluoroscopic beam on the oblique fluoroscope view in which the zygapophyseal joint space is located midway between the anterior and posterior vertebral margins. In this view, the borders of the safe triangle include the nerve root (NR) for the superior tangential border, the vertebral end plate (EP) of the target disk for inferior border, and the lateral margin of the

(Spine-CATH intradiskal catheter or decompression catheter, Smith & Nephew) with a 5-cm or 1.5-cm active electrothermal tip is inserted through a 17-gauge introducer needle and advanced circuitously to the posterior annulus **(Figs. 20.1, 20.2, 20.3, 20.4,** and **20.5).** Usually one catheter is enough, but in some cases a bilateral deployment is required to cover the entire posterior annular wall.[56]

Catheter position is important.[26,56] Ideally, the active length of the catheter should cross the "symptomatic" annular fissure and lie close enough (approximately 5 mm) to the outer annulus to allow spread of sufficient heat to both the outer and inner annulus **(Fig. 20.6).**[41] Interestingly, the original Oratec Company brochure showed the catheter lying within the nuclear-annular junction, and many of the original studies on inadequate spread of heat to the outer annular fibers were based on this catheter position. In clinical practice, however, the electrode tip inevitably ends up in the outer annular fibers. Although one may try multiple attempts and use a formed hockey-stick bend on the outer catheter, ideal positioning 5 mm from the outer annulus is seldom achieved. Furthermore, frequent passage and multiple catheter removals could theoretically increase the risk of infection and often results in irrevocably damaging an expensive disposable device. In many cases the catheter is in the outer annular fibers of the contralateral posterior lateral annulus and then passes more anterior **(Fig. 20.2).** The second bold mark on the catheter must be placed beyond the introducer needle hub. Before heating, the position of catheter should be confirmed and documented by anteroposterior (AP) and lateral views. The catheter should not be placed outside of the annulus of the disk.

Heating Protocol

The original 5-cm active heating element catheter introduced by Oratec has the temperature electrode placed within the catheter and it measured catheter temperatures that were on average 13°C higher than the adjacent disk tissue. The standard empirically derived protocol begins heating at 65°C with incremental increases of 1°C every 30 seconds to achieve a final temperature of between 80° and 90°C. The final temperature was maintained for 5 minutes for a total treatment time of 13.5 to 16.5 minutes.[22] Some advocated heating to higher temperatures, but there was no standard method for determining final temperatures. Analyzing the study results using the 5-cm catheter, Derby et al[21] could not show a correlation between higher temperatures and improved outcome at either 8 months or 16 months postprocedure. In fact, when catheter positions were less than 5 mm from the outer annulus, higher thermal dosage was associated with longer flare-up durations postprocedure. The authors proposed an alternative protocol in which temperatures are incrementally increased to an 80°C measured temperature, but the final temperature and duration were determined by the

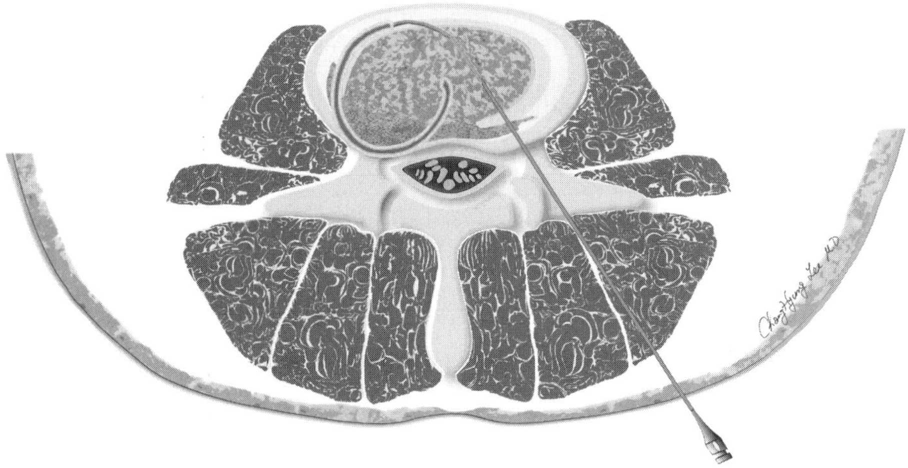

Fig. 20.2 A SpineCATH® intradiskal catheter (Smith & Nephew) with a 5-cm active electrothermal tip is placed circuitously to the posterior annulus and turns back anteriorly. The distance the catheter is placed from the outer annulus depends on the degree and location of the preexisting annular disruption. Once the catheter crosses to within 4 to 5 mm of the opposite midline, it often turns back anteriorly.

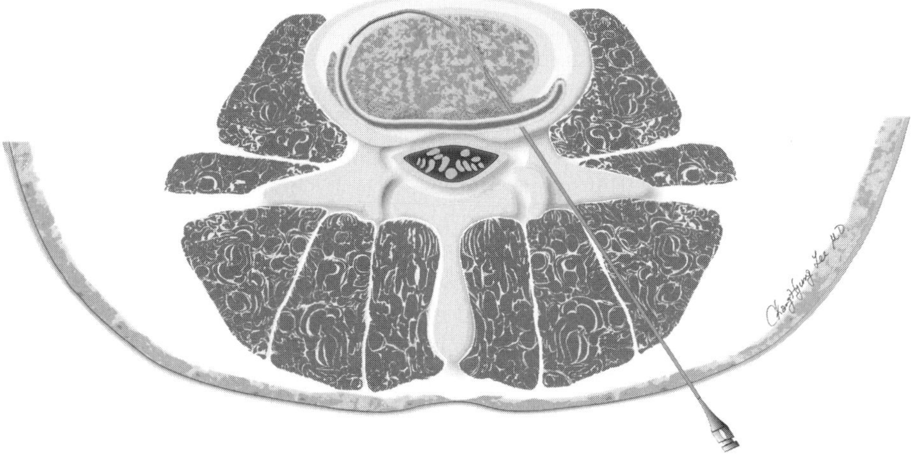

Fig. 20.3 A SpineCATH intradiskal catheter is placed circuitously in the outer posterior annulus. In cases with a more extensive posterior annular disruption, the catheter tip will stay in the outer annulus as it crosses the midline.

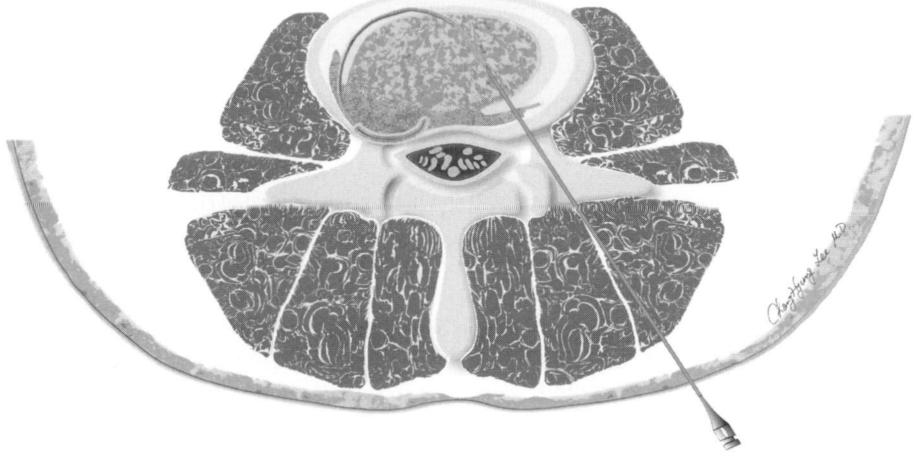

Fig. 20.4 Using a standard posterolateral diskogram technique a decompression catheter (Smith & Nephew) with a 1.5-cm active electrothermal tip is inserted through a 17-gauge introducer needle and advanced circuitously to the posterior annulus. Most of the active heating tip remains in the outer annulus on the opposite side. The very outer part of the catheter is usually within 2 mm of the outer annulus.

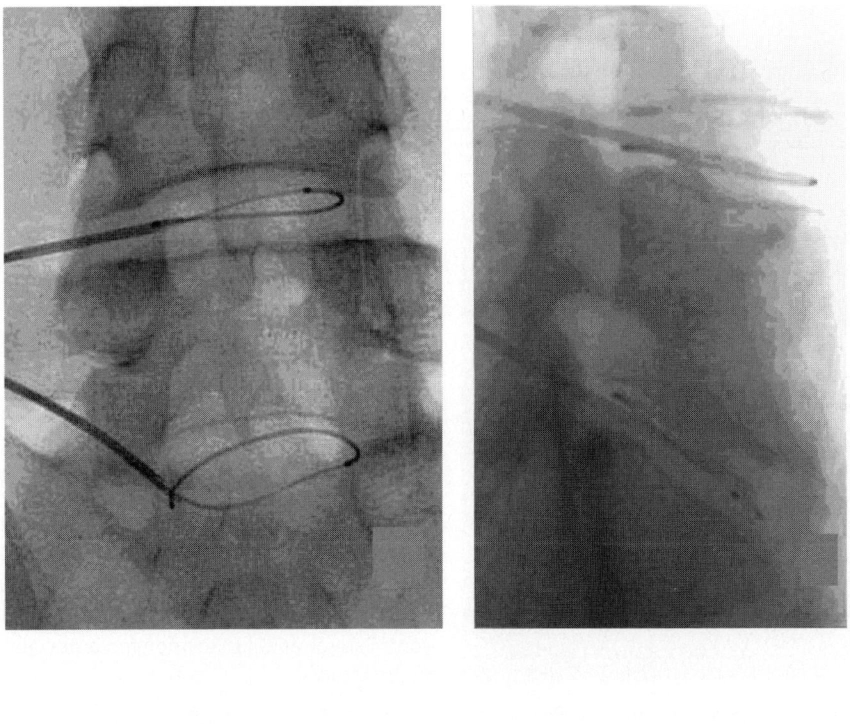

A B

Fig. 20.5 Fluoroscopy image of the IDET procedure. The intradiskal electrothermal catheter electrode (SpineCATH intradiskal catheter, Smith & Nephew) is placed within the L4-L5 and L5-S1 disks.

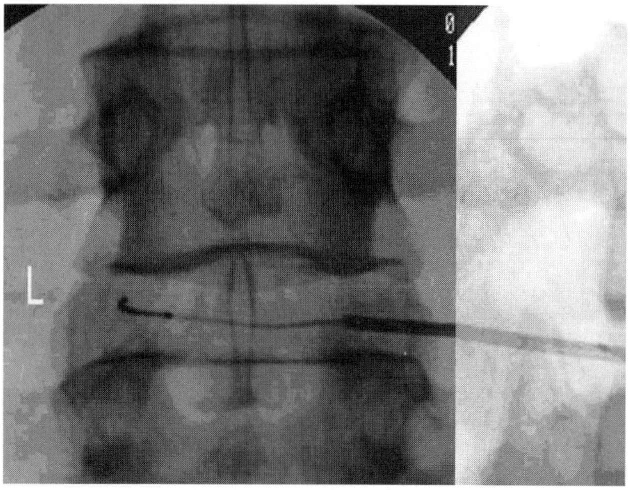

Fig. 20.6 Fluoroscopy image of the IDET procedure. The shorter 1.5 cm electrothermal wire (decompression catheter, Smith & Nephew) has been positioned within the torn outer posterior annulus of the L4-L5 disk. After thermal heating, the patient was injected the fibrin sealant (Tisseel VH®, Baxter Healthcare, Deerfield, IL) into the disk to help "seal" the painful torn annulus.

patient's pain response from baseline. Depending on the patient's pain tolerance and degree of sedation, incremental increases in temperature are stopped when the patient reports pain of greater than a 6 to 8 on a 10-point scale, based on their baseline pain. The temperature is then maintained for up to 4 minutes as long as the patient's back pain remains below an intensity of 8.

The new shorter catheter (decompression catheter, Smith & Nephew) uses a shorter 1.5 cm heating element, which may help limit destruction of normal disk annulus (**Figs. 20.4** and **20.6**). The temperature electrode is placed on the outside of the catheter, and therefore measured temperatures reflect the adjacent tissue temperatures. The heating protocol still incrementally increases temperatures to 90°C and then maintains them for 6 minutes, but in effect this temperature is 13° to 15° higher than that of the 5-cm catheter. More heat is reaching a shorter segment of the annulus, nucleus, or both, but because the catheter length is shorter the total heat dose is probably less. Some practitioner's initial impressions suggest improved outcomes with shorter duration flare-ups and some feel that patients tolerate higher temperatures before complaining of excessive pain.

Intradiskal Radiofrequency Treatment

The approach to the intervertebral disk is similar to the description above, but rather than passing the introducer needle into the disk nucleus, the needle tip is directed into the outer posterior lateral annulus and the active electrode is advanced across the posterior annulus (**Fig. 20.7**). The discTRODE device includes a sensor that measures tissue resistance, and the higher resistance of the disk annulus can be detected with both sound and digital readings. By passing the needle tip slightly more posterior and medially in the disk annulus, an asymmetric opening in the needle tip helps direct the active electrode across the posterior disk annulus. The setup also includes a temperature-monitoring needle that can be placed into the outer posterior outer annulus, and one can monitor the increase in outer annular temperatures as the electrode is heated (**Fig. 20.7**).

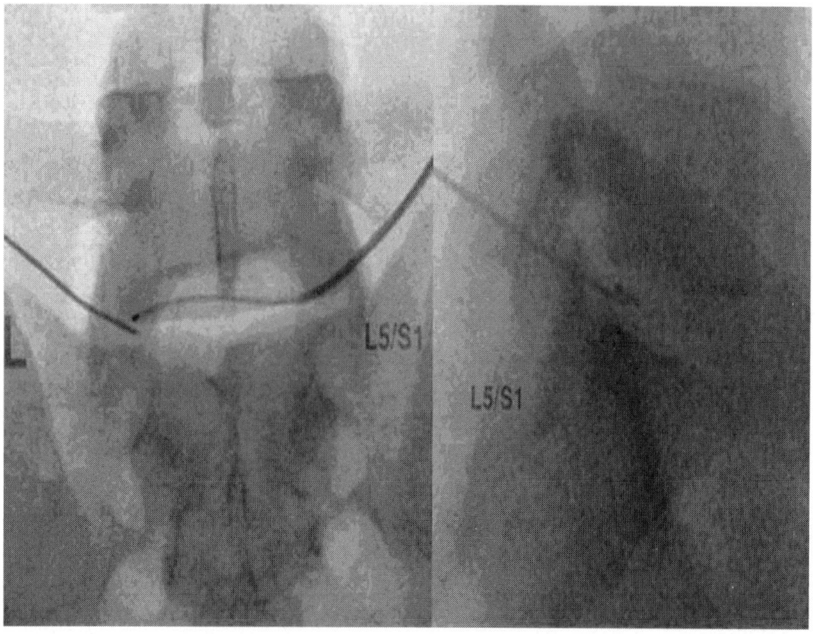

Fig. 20.7 Fluoroscopy image of the intradiskal radiation therapy (IDRT) procedure. An introducer needle is placed into the outer posterior lateral annulus and the active tip is then advanced across the posterior annulus. A separate needle with a temperature electrode is placed into the outer contralateral annulus to monitor outer annular temperatures.

A graduated temperature protocol beginning at 65°C is used, but the final temperature is determined by measuring the temperatures in the contralateral annulus using the temperature-monitoring needle inserted into the contralateral outer annulus. When the temperature measured in the outer annulus by the temperature-monitoring needle reaches 45°C, the final temperature is maintained for 4 minutes. Although a seemingly more accurate method of determining final temperature, the distance of the measuring electrode from the radiofrequency electrode is variable.

Postprocedure Care

The patient is monitored in the recovery room for 1 to 3 hours postprocedure and is discharged the same day.[26] The patient is warned to expect a significant increase in the baseline pain and is told that the usual flare-up lasts 2 to 7 days, but infrequently can last for an indefinite period of time.

Patients are typically braced for several weeks to several months after the procedure. During the initial several months, the outer annulus is rehealing, and there is probably an increased risk of reinjury from excessive disk loading. Activities such as walking and exercise in a swimming pool are encouraged, but aggressive physical therapy is usually begun only after 1 to 2 months postprocedure.[54] Most patients have reached maximal improvement by 3 months, but a minority may take 3 to 6 months.[30,41,42,54] Several studies have documented stable and enduring pain relief in 2-year follow-up.[30,41,42,54]

Complications

Complications are infrequent. One retrospective study[31] reviewed the complications of 1675 IDET procedures performed at five spine centers and analyzed data of 35,000 SpineCATH intradiskal catheters reported by the medical device reports (MDRs) of the U.S. Food and Drug Administration (FDA). A total of six nerve root injuries were reported, all but one of which occurred during insertion of the introducer needle. Five of the six completely resolved and one case was resolving. No cases of diskitis were reported. Six cases of post-IDET disk herniation were reported at the treated level 2 to 12 months after treatment. Four resolved with nonoperative care, and two required disk excision. Nineteen cases of catheter breakage were reported. All were associated with repeated catheter manipulation that resulted in kinking. In 16 cases the catheter was uneventfully left within the disk. Eight cases of superficial skin burn at the needle puncture site were reported. One case of post-IDET bladder dysfunction was reported.

Although few, other complications have been reported, including disk infections and neural injury.[57] Passing a catheter through the outer annulus and into the epidural space can occur, and is easily identified on a lateral fluoroscopic image. If this occurs, withdrawing the catheter back into the disk and redirecting it prevents injury. Heating an epidural catheter should cause the patient to complain of the almost immediate onset of leg pain. Thus performing IDET in a heavily sedated or anesthetized patient is not a good idea. Likewise, patient complaints of excessive early-onset pain (especially if the pain is in the leg) should be investigated.

Although transient increases in leg pain are not uncommon following IDET, prolonged increases in previous leg pain or occurrence of new leg pain is uncommon but may be underreported. When the catheter is in the outer disk periphery and lies within a few millimeters of the traversing or exiting nerve root, the roots and dorsal root ganglions may be vulnerable.[58] Temperatures >45°C applied for an extended period of time might cause transient or prolonged leg pain. One case of cauda equina syndrome was reported post–L4-L5 IDET.[44] The report, however, suggests that the injury was caused directly by the introducer needle or catheter rather than by the transfer of heat through the disk, and the authors later confirmed this impression in a reply to Wetzel, who suggested the same etiology.[59]

End-plate heat injury is another possible complication. Although cadaver studies have not demonstrated significantly elevated end-plate temperatures,[60] it is difficult to determine the proximity of the catheter to the end plates with fluoroscopy, and in some instances a portion of the catheter may contact an adjoining end plate. Scholl et al[61] reported one case of possible end-plate necrosis occurring after an IDET procedure.

Accelerated disk degeneration has been mentioned as a concern by some and as a goal by others. In the short term, however, there seems to be little change in the MRI reading pre- and post-IDET. Ho et al[62] reported no change in the MRI scans of 72 patients at 12 months post-IDET.

Conclusion

The IDET procedure is a minimally invasive technique designed to treat discogenic low back pain. The procedure provides only modest improvement. Functional improvement appears less often than pain relief. Therefore, for patients with less functional impairment, relatively well-maintained disk heights, and discogenic pain caused by annular tears or protrusions of less than 3 to 4 mm, IDET may be a reasonable first option if patients are unwilling to tolerate their pain and disability. As a treatment option, one should not expect IDET to return patients to a job requiring significant manual labor. As with spinal fusion or arthroplasty, even a technically satisfying procedure will not prevent a significant number of patients from reporting that they have worsening of pain from a variety of different factors.

References

1. Sweet WH. Controlled thermocoagulation of trigeminal ganglion and rootlets for differential destruction of pain fibers: facial pain other than trigeminal neuralgia. Clin Neurosurg 1976;23:96–102
2. Lord SM, Barnsley L, Wallis BJ, McDonald GJ, Bogduk N. Percutaneous radio-frequency neurotomy for chronic cervical zygapophyseal-joint pain. N Engl J Med 1996;335:1721–1726
3. McDonald GJ, Lord SM, Bogduk N. Long-term follow-up of patients treated with cervical radiofrequency neurotomy for chronic neck pain. Neurosurgery 1999;45:61–67 discussion 67–8
4. Dreyfuss P, Halbrook B, Pauza K, et al. Efficacy and validity of radiofrequency neurotomy for chronic lumbar zygapophysial joint pain. Spine 2000;25:1270–1277
5. Letcher FS, Goldring S. The effect of radiofrequency current and heat on peripheral nerve action potential in the cat. J Neurosurg 1968;29:42–47
6. Frohling MA, Schlote W, Wolburg-Buchholz K. Nonselective nerve fibre damage in peripheral nerves after experimental thermocoagulation. Acta Neurochir (Wien) 1998;140:1297–1302
7. Schofferman J, Kine G. Effectiveness of repeated radiofrequency neurotomy for lumbar facet pain. Spine 2004;29:2471–2473
8. Hecht P, Hayashi K, Lu Y, et al. Monopolar radiofrequency energy effects on joint capsular tissue: potential treatment for joint instability. An in vivo mechanical, morphological, and biochemical study using an ovine model. Am J Sports Med 1999;27:761–771
9. Wallace AL, Hollinshead RM, Frank CB. Creep behavior of a rabbit model of ligament laxity after electrothermal shrinkage in vivo. Am J Sports Med 2002;30:98–102
10. Hayashi K, Massa KL, Thabit G, et al. Histologic evaluation of the glenohumeral joint capsule after the laser-assisted capsular shift procedure for glenohumeral instability. Am J Sports Med 1999;27:162–167
11. Hayashi K, Thabit G, Massa KL, et al. The effect of thermal heating on the length and histologic properties of the glenohumeral joint capsule. Am J Sports Med 1997;25:107–112
12. Shah RV, Lutz GE, Lee J, Doty SB, Rodeo S. Intradiskal electrothermal therapy: a preliminary histologic study. Arch Phys Med Rehabil 2001;82:1230–1237
13. Lee J, Lutz GE, Campbell D, Rodeo SA, Wright T. Stability of the lumbar spine after intradiscal electrothermal therapy. Arch Phys Med Rehabil 2001;82:120–122
14. Wang JC, Kabo JM, Tsou PM, Halevi L, Shamie AN. The effect of uniform heating on the biomechanical properties of the intervertebral disc in a porcine model. Spine J 2005;5:64–70
15. Kleinstueck FS, Diederich CJ, Nau WH, et al. Acute biomechanical and histological effects of intradiscal electrothermal therapy on human lumbar discs. Spine 2001;26:2198–2207
16. Bass EC, Wistrom EV, Diederich CJ, et al. Heat-induced changes in porcine annulus fibrosus biomechanics. J Biomech 2004;37:233–240
17. Schaufele MAN, Huckle J. Volumetric reduction of bovine intervertebral discs with the use of an intradiscal decompression catheter. Presented at the International Spinal Injection Society (ISIS) annual meeting, 1994, Maui, Hawaii
18. Cohen SP, Larkin T, Abdi S, Chang A, Stojanovic M. Risk factors for failure and complications of intradiscal electrothermal therapy: a pilot study. Spine 2003;28:1142–1147
19. Andersson G, Andrews N, Huckle J. Alteration of the collagen and cell viability within the disc following intradiscal electrothermal therapy. Presented at the ISIS annual meeting, 1994, Maui, Hawaii
20. Bass EC, Nau WH, Diederich CJ, et al. Intradiscal thermal therapy does not stimulate biologic remodeling in an in vivo sheep model. Spine 2006;31:139–145
21. Derby R, Seo KS, Kazala K, et al. A factor analysis of lumbar intradiscal electrothermal annuloplasty outcomes. Spine J 2005;5:256–261 discussion 262
22. Kleinstueck FS, Diederich CJ, Nau WH, et al. Temperature and thermal dose distributions during intradiscal electrothermal therapy in the cadaveric lumbar spine. Spine 2003;28:1700–1708
23. Freeman BJ, Walters RM, Moore RJ, Fraser RD. Does intradiscal electrothermal therapy denervate and repair experimentally induced posterolateral annular tears in an animal model? Spine 2003;28:2602–2608
24. Wright RE, et al. Precise in vivo measurement of peak intra-annular temperatures obtained during intradiscal electrothermal therapy. Presented at the 13th annual meeting of IITS, Williamsburg, VA, June 8–10, 2000
25. Bono C, Garfin S, Iki K, Jalota A, Dawson K. Temperatures within the lumbar disc and endplates during intradiscal electrothermal therapy: formulation of a predictive temperature map in relation to distance from the catheter. Presented at the ISIS 10th annual scientific meeting, 2002, Austin, TX
26. Derby REB, Chen Y, O' Neill C, Ryan D. Intradiscal electrothermal annuloplasty: a novel approach for treating chronic discogenic back pain. Neuromodulation 2000;3:82–88
27. Freemont AJ, Peacock TE, Goupille P, et al. Nerve ingrowth into diseased intervertebral disc in chronic back pain. Lancet 1997;350:178–181
28. Podhajsky R, Belous A. The effects of temperature on nucleus pulposus; intervertebral pressure and hydrokinetics. Presented at the ISIS 12th annual scientific meeting, 2004, Maui, Hawaii
29. Derby R, Lee S-H, Seo KS, et al. Efficacy of IDET for Relief of Leg Pain Associated with Discogenic Low Back Pain. Pain Pract 2004;4:281–285
30. Saal JA, Saal JS. Intradiscal electrothermal treatment for chronic discogenic low back pain: prospective outcome study with a minimum 2-year follow-up. Spine 2002;27:966–973 discussion 973–974
31. Saal JASJ, Wetzel FT. IDET related complications: a multi-center study of 1675 treated patients with a review of the FDA MDR data base. Presented at the 16th annual meeting of the North American Spine Society, 2001, Seattle
32. Two recent studies of thermal disc therapy. The Back Letter 1999;14:
33. Spruit M, Jacobs WC. Pain and function after intradiscal electrothermal treatment (IDET) for symptomatic lumbar disc degeneration. Eur Spine J 2002;11:589–593
34. Ercelen O, Bulutcu E, Oktenoglu T, et al. Radiofrequency lesioning using two different time modalities for the treatment of lumbar discogenic pain: a randomized trial. Spine 2003;28:1922–1927
35. Davis TT, Delamarter RB, Sra P, Goldstein TB. The IDET procedure for chronic discogenic low back pain. Spine 2004;29:752–756
36. Webster BS, Verma S, Pransky GS. Outcomes of workers' compensation claimants with low back pain undergoing intradiscal electrothermal therapy. Spine 2004;29:435–441
37. Lutz C, Lutz GE, Cooke PM. Treatment of chronic lumbar diskogenic pain with intradiskal electrothermal therapy: a prospective outcome study. Arch Phys Med Rehabil 2003;84:23–28
38. Kapural L, Hayek S, Malak O, Arrigain S, Mekhail N. Intradiscal thermal annuloplasty versus intradiscal radiofrequency ablation

for the treatment of discogenic pain: a prospective matched control trial. Pain Med 2005;6:425–431
39. Park SY, Moon SH, Park MS, et al. Intradiscal electrothermal treatment for chronic lower back pain patients with internal disc disruption. Yonsei Med J 2005;46:539–545
40. Derby R, Lee SH, Seo KS, et al. Efficacy of IDET for relief of leg pain associated with discogenic low back pain. Pain Pract 2004;4:281–285
41. Karasek M, Bogduk N. Twelve-month follow-up of a controlled trial of intradiscal thermal anuloplasty for back pain due to internal disc disruption. Spine 2000;25:2601–2607
42. Bogduk N, Karasek M. Two-year follow-up of a controlled trial of intradiscal electrothermal anuloplasty for chronic low back pain resulting from internal disc disruption. Spine J 2002;2:343–350
43. Finch PM, Price LM, Drummond PD. Radiofrequency heating of painful annular disruptions: one-year outcomes. J Spinal Disord Tech 2005;18:6–13
44. Hsia AW, Isaac K, Katz JS. Cauda equina syndrome from intradiscal electrothermal therapy. Neurology 2000;55:320
45. Pauza KJ, Howell S, Dreyfuss P, et al. A randomized, placebo-controlled trial of intradiscal electrothermal therapy for the treatment of discogenic low back pain. Spine J 2004;4:27–35
46. Freeman B, Fraser R, Cain C, Hall D. A randomized, double-blind controlled efficacy study: intradiscal electrothermal therapy (IDET) versus placebo. Presented at the International Society for the Study of the Lumbar Spine, 30th annual meeting, Vancouver, Canada, May 13–17, 2003
47. Lau P, Mercer S, Govind J, Bogduk N. The surgical anatomy of lumbar medial branch neurotomy (facet denervation). Pain Med 2004;5:289–298
48. Appleby D, Andersson G, Totta M. Meta-analysis of the efficacy and safety of intradiscal electrothermal therapy (IDET). Pain Med 2006;7:308–316
49. Andersson GB, Mekhail NA, Block JE. Treatment of intractable discogenic low back pain. a systematic review of spinal fusion and intradiscal electrothermal therapy (IDET). Pain Physician 2006;9:237–248
50. Freeman BA. IDET: a critical appraisal of the evidence. Eur Spine J 2006;15(suppl 3):S448–457
51. Pauza K, Howell S, Dreyfuss P, Peloza J, Park K. A randomized, double-blind, placebo controlled trial evaluating the efficacy of intradiscal electrothermal anuloplasty for the treatment of chronic discogenic low back pain: 6-month outcomes. Presented at the International Spinal Injection Society, 10th annual scientific meeting, Austin, TX, September 7, 2002
52. Lutz C, Lutz G, Cooke P. Treatment of chronic lumbar diskogenic pain with intradiskal electrothermal therapy: a prospective outcome study. Arch Phys Med Rehabil 2003;84:23–28
53. Lee MS, Cooper G, Lutz GE, Lutz C, Hong HM. Intradiscal electrothermal therapy (IDET) for treatment of chronic lumbar discogenic pain: a minimum 2-year clinical outcome study. Pain Physician 2003;6:443–448
54. Saal JA, Saal JS. Intradiscal electrothermal treatment for chronic discogenic low back pain: a prospective outcome study with minimum 1-year follow-up. Spine 2000;25:2622–2627
55. Maurer P, Squillante D, Dawson K. Is IDET effective treatment for discogenic low back pain? A prospective cohort outcome study (1–2 year follow-up) Identifying successful patient selection criteria. Presented at the 9th annual scientific meeting of the International Spinal Injection Society, 2002, Austin, TX
56. Saal JA, Saal JS. Intradiscal electrothermal therapy for the treatment of chronic discogenic low back pain. Clin Sports Med 2002;21:167–187
57. Thomas PS. Image-Guided Pain Management. Philadelphia: Lippincott-Raven, 1997
58. Konno S, Olmarker K, Byrod G, et al. The European Spine Society AcroMed Prize 1994. Acute thermal nerve root injury. Eur Spine J 1994;3:299–302
59. Hsia AW, Isaac K, Katz JS. Cauda equina syndrome from intradiscal electrothermal therapy. Neurology 2000;55:320
60. Yetkinler DN, Nau WH, Brandt LL. Disc temperature measurements during nucleoplasty and IDET procedures. Presented at the 6th International Congress on Spinal Surgery, September 4–7, 2002, Ankara, Turkey
61. Scholl BM, Theiss SM, Lopez-Ben R, Kraft M. Vertebral osteonecrosis related to intradiscal electrothermal therapy: a case report. Spine 2003;28:E161–E164
62. Ho C, Kaiser J, Saal J, Saal J. Does IDET cause advancement of disc degeneration? A one year MRI follow-up study of 72 patients. Presented at the 16th annual meeting of the North American Spine Society, October 31 to November 3, 2001, Seattle, WA
63. Freeman BJ, Fraser RD, Cain CM, Hall DJ, Chapple DC. A randomized, double-blind, controlled trial: intradiscal electrothermal therapy versus placebo for the treatment of chronic discogenic low back pain. Spine 2005;30:2369–2377 discussion 2378
64. Barendse GA, van Den Berg SG, Kessels AH, Weber WE, van Kleef M. Randomized controlled trial of percutaneous intradiscal radiofrequency thermocoagulation for chronic discogenic back pain: lack of effect from a 90-second 70 C lesion. Spine 2001;26:287–292

21 Radiofrequency Nuclear Decompression Nucleoplasty

Richard Derby, Ray M. Baker, and Paul A. Anderson

In the last decade there has been a shift toward less invasive treatments for treating discogenic pain. Beginning with chymopapain, and progressing through automated percutaneous disk decompression and laser nuclear decompressions, these technologies continue to evolve. In the last chapter we reviewed thermal treatment of the disk using intradiskal heating by electrothermal and radiofrequency devices that directly affect the disk nucleus and annulus. Laser and bipolar radiofrequency heat are used to decompress the disk nucleus. This chapter covers the scientific rationale and evidence-based outcome results for nuclear decompression using a bipolar radiofrequency device; however, the concept of minimally invasive nuclear decompression for the treatment of axial and referred leg pain applies to all minimally invasive nuclear decompression techniques.

■ Concept Validity of Nuclear Decompression

Percutaneous removal of nuclear tissue by thermal energy is thought to lower nuclear pressure, thereby reducing nerve root tension and allowing a protrusion to implode inward. Although the inflammatory response is likely to be the most important cause of pain, contact pressure between a protruding disk and the nerve root may be a primary cause of radicular pain. However, few studies have established this mechanical etiology.

Takahashi et al[1] measured the contact pressure between the nerve and annulus in patients under general anesthesia in a prone position before and after removing a herniated disk. They found pressures that varied between 7 and 256 mm Hg (average, 54.2) before diskectomy and 0 mm after. The pressure directly correlated with the amount of trunk list and degree of neurologic deficits prior to the operation. Because nerve edema can be induced by compression at 50 mm for 2 minutes, and the pressure in the patient's nerve roots was probably higher when awake and in a loaded position, compression likely did contribute to the patient's pain.[2] Thus, although one might conclude that percutaneously removing a herniated nucleus with either an inside-out or outside-in approach would likewise relieve pressure on a nerve root, the effect of lowering nuclear pressure by removing a small amount of nucleus from the center of the disk is conceptually harder to understand. It is even harder to understand if the desired effect is to lower annular tension for the purpose of decreasing axial pain.

■ Pressure Theory

The concept of removing a small amount of nuclear material to lower the intradiskal pressure was postulated by surgeons to justify nuclear decompression using laser heat ablation. Case et al[3] measured a rapid rise in the pressure of cadaver disks while slowly infusing normal saline into the disk nucleus. Their data supported the concept that the nucleus, surrounded by a relatively inelastic annulus and solid vertebral end plates, acts like a tight hydraulic space where large pressure increases occur with a small increase in volume. They then assumed that the opposite must be true: small decreases in volume must lead to large decreases in intradiskal pressure. In a follow-up study, using 1000 joules (J) from a neodymium:yttrium-aluminum-garnet (Nd:YAG), 1.32-μm laser delivered through a quartz fiber they lowered the mean intradiskal pressure in cadaver disks by 43%.[4,5] Likewise, using 350 J of laser energy delivered by a Nd:YAG laser, Yonezawa[6] vaporized central nuclear tissue in rabbit disks, creating a hole in the nucleus that over an 8-week period gradually filled with fibrous tissue. The immediate effect was to lower the vertically measured disk pressure by about 50%. Removing even less nuclear material by creating six channels in the nucleus of cadaver disks, Chen and Lee showed a 100% drop in pressure in normal disks in young cadavers, but a negligible drop in pressure in degenerated disks.

In addition to direct pressure measurements in animal models, Hellinger et al[7] indirectly studied disk pressure changes in 21 patients by comparing the disk densities in computed tomography (CT) scans before and after nonendoscopic Nd:YAG laser nuclear ablation. The measured decreased density of tissue within disk protrusions showed a statistical difference of 66.3 Hounsfield units, corresponding to a 20% postoperative density reduction. He attributed his "excellent" therapeutic results secondary to reduced improved flow of venous and cerebrospinal fluid due to this indirect measurement of intradiskal pressure.

Although these studies show that nuclear pressure is lowered immediately after ablating central nuclear tissue, no studies have specifically measured the tensional forces in the outer annulus following nuclear ablation or determined whether the pressure drop was lasting. However, increasing nuclear pressure by injecting the disk with fluid is reflected as a proportional increase in the outer annular pressure when radial annular tears extend to the outer annulus.[8] One might speculate that this artificially increased pressure is analogous to compressing a well-hydrated nucleus and transmitting horizontal forces through hydrated nuclear material to the outer annulus, and therefore one might reasonably conclude that lowering the fluid pressure would decrease the annular tension.

Several surgical studies have indirectly shown that removing less tissue may be preferable to removing more. In a 10-year longitudinal study, Mochida et al[9] between 1983 and 1988 performed percutaneous diskectomies on 47 young patients (27.3 average age) with herniations causing radicular pain. Before 1986, surgery was performed in 25 patients with instruments that allowed removal of tissue in front of the scope, and an average of 3.8 g of tissue was removed. Afterward, the authors used special forceps that were able to "get around the corner," and an average of 1 g of tissue was removed from the posterior protrusion. Although the shorter term 2-year favorable outcomes were comparable at approximately 70%, the 10-year results were 71% in the group that had less tissue removed from behind the protrusions compared with a 36% success rate in those having more tissue removed only from the central nucleus. More importantly, the poor outcome was attributed to low back pain resulting from a greater than 30% disk space collapse in 57% of their earlier group that had more tissue removed compared with 20% of the targeted group that had less tissue removed. A decrease in disk herniation size did not correlate with outcome. Further supporting these findings, the authors later showed that in elite athletes a more extensive arthroscopic removal of tissue was associated with an acute worsening of symptoms and a delayed return to sports activity.[10]

Similarly, Carragee et al[11] had better outcomes following open surgical removal of herniated disks when less nuclear material was removed. Comparing removal of all the free fragments through an annulotomy incision with a more limited removal of the herniated mass alone, Carragee et al found that even though the recurrent herniation rate was higher, a considerably better outcome (although not necessarily long-term) as reflected in satisfaction, pain, and function was seen in the group that had less nuclear material removed.

Although removing nuclear tissue decreases disk pressure, most of the effect occurs in the inner and middle annular fibers, with little effect on the outer and more commonly innervated collagenous layers.[12] In addition, during creep loading the reduced nuclear tension allows the inner layers to bulge inward, reducing height, reducing the compressive strength, and potentially leading to lateral segmental instability.[13]

Reduced nuclear pressure causes loads to be shifted to the relatively thin outer annulus.[13–15] The resulting increased compressive load on the outer annulus causes high, irregular stress concentrations within the outer annular fibers and adjoining end plates, which could directly or indirectly cause pain.[13,16] In addition, the lowered pressure in the nucleus and the elevated pressures in the annulus will suppress chondrocyte metabolism, leading to further disk dehydration and reduction of osmotic forces.[17,18] Wognum et al[19] showed that decreased osmotic pressure exposes the tips of annular tears to increased stress concentrations, causing cracks to open and potentially increasing the risk of herniation.

In addition, a drop in nuclear pressure will cause disk space narrowing and disk bulging. In hydrated cadaver disks, Brinckmann et al showed a significant drop of pressure when up to 3 g of nuclear material was removed. However, for every gram of tissue removed from the nucleus, the disk height collapsed by an average of 0.8 mm and the disk bulge by 0.02 mm. In support, Castro et al[20] showed that removal of 4.6 g of nuclear material using automated percutaneous lumbar diskectomy (APLD) narrowed the disk space by 1.42 mm and increased the disk bulge by 0.45 mm.

Finally, perhaps the most difficult justification for rapidly lowering the intranuclear pressure with the removal of large amounts of nucleus is that the majority of disks selected for this procedure may already have lowered nuclear pressures. Both end-plate injury and disk herniation cause the nuclear pressures to fall either because of an increased nuclear volume due to end-plate bulging or loss of nuclear volume secondary to herniation through the end plates or into an annular fissure. With the nucleus already decompressed, making a few channels in the nucleus or removing a few grams of nuclear material would not seem to be of any positive consequence. However, removing less would perhaps cause less harm than removing more. Interestingly, there are finite element studies supported by in vivo measurements that predict elevated nuclear pressures if an annular tear without herniation occurred in a healthy hydrated nucleus.[12] The elevated nuclear pressures increase the risk of nuclear disruption, but also depress chondrocyte metabolism, which should eventually decrease nuclear pressure.[21]

Even though excessive and rapid nuclear decompression has theoretical disadvantages, nuclear compression is a natural occurrence in response to injury. Any disk injury, including an end-plate fracture, an annular tear with herniation, an outer rim lesion, or a concentric annular tear, initiates a progressive deterioration that includes disk decompression.[22,23] One might therefore conclude that there may be an evolutionary advantage if decompression is controlled and accompanied by compensatory solidification of the nucleus and annulus. Perhaps in some well-hydrated disks in young patients, after an injury the nuclear pressure remains high and only slowly falls. One might

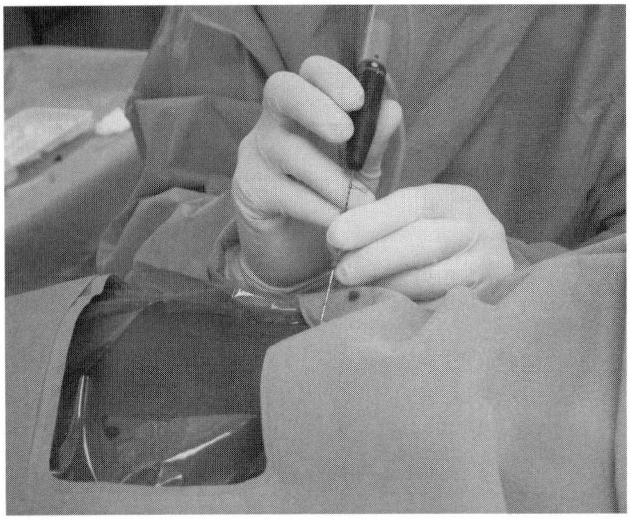

A

Fig. 21.1 Lumbar Nucleoplasty. **(A)** Nucleoplasty procedure. **(B)** Lateral view with needle purposely placed posteriorly to achieve decompression behind the central disk protrusion. **(C)** Anteroposterior (AP) view.

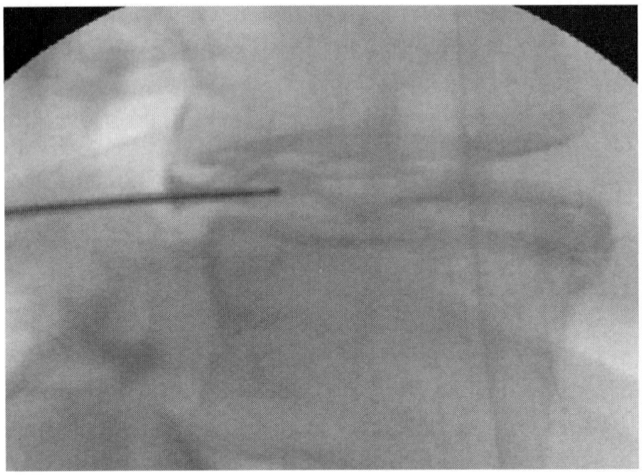

B

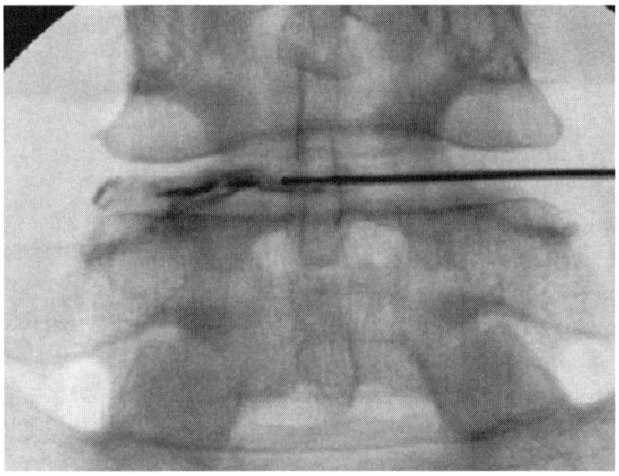

C

accelerate the natural history by ablating a minimal amount of nuclear material. It would be a very easy process to measure opening pressures during diskography to validate continued nuclear hydration. In fact the standard is to do exactly this, and it is surprising that although nucleoplasty is justified based on lowering nuclear pressure, no studies considered or reported on whether the nuclear pressure was in fact low, normal, or high prior to the procedure.

■ Implosion Theory

The other most often stated goal of central nuclear decompression is to lower nuclear pressures (or create a hole) and allow room for the herniated fragment to implode inward. The implosion theory postulates that intact outer annular fibers will be able to contract enough to reduce the tension on both the nerve root and annulus. However, there is little proof that implosion actually occurs. In fact, Delamarter et al[24] reviewed the magnetic resonance imaging (MRI) scans of 33 patients with radicular pain due to a disk herniation before and after APLD decompression, and saw no measurable changes at 6 weeks. Still, if the instruments and technique would allow for more targeted removal of tissue behind or within the protrusion, conceptually there should be a reduction of focal annular stress (like removing a pebble in one's shoe), and perhaps more importantly, one would remove the source of inflammation. At the L4-L5 level and above, a more lateral approach enables a more posterior needle placement[25] and facilitates more targeted tissue removal **(Fig. 21.1)**.

■ Chemical Theory

Lastly, perhaps the application of heat beneficially enhances the chemical environment. Cultured disk cells subjected to "coblation" (coagulation-ablation) within the culture medium[26] show differing responses depending on whether there was exposure to interleukin-1 (IL-1) and depending on the cell phenotype. Although treatment increased inflammatory mediators in normal nuclear and annular cells, there was a decrease in inflammatory mediators in abnormal nuclear cells.

■ Nucleoplasty Procedure

Smaller protrusions are postulated to cause both axial and referred extremity pain, due to neural inflammation, and axial pain, due to a combination of a sensitized outer annulus and increased outer annular tension.[27] During percutaneous endoscopic diskectomies, surgeons often see an inflamed outer annulus adjacent to the disk protrusion.[28] Directly removing the herniated disk within the protrusion should remove the source of inflammation and pressure on the innervated outer annulus and adjacent posterior longitudinal ligament and nerve roots. Percutaneous techniques using medium and smaller diameter cannulae were not, however, designed to remove nucleus directly behind the protrusion, and unless the protrusion lies in the path of the posterolateral approach, the source of inflammation is typically not removed.

Unlike larger 3- to 5-mm outer diameter cannulae used for surgical percutaneous disk decompression, decompressions performed though smaller 2.5- to 3-mm cannulae (APLD, Laser, SpineJet, MicroResector) and even small 1.5-mm diameter cannulae (Nucleoplasty™ and Dekompressor) provide easy access only to the disk nucleus and not to the herniated nucleus within posterior annular fissures and protrusions **(Fig. 21.1)**. These techniques primarily remove tissue by cutting and aspirating, screwing out, or vaporizing nucleus within the center of the disk, and do not necessarily remove nuclear material within the protrusion unless the protrusion is located along its access path.

A minimally invasive bipolar radiofrequency device for vaporizing disk nucleus was introduced by ArthroCare (Sunnyvale, CA). The technique, called disk Nucleoplasty™, was patterned after ArthroCare's existing devices used for knee debridement, and was marketed as a percutaneous technique to ablate nuclear tissue by creating channels within the nucleus (**Fig. 21.1**). A "wand" is introduced through a 17-gauge needle placed into the annular-nuclear junction using standard posterolateral access techniques. During the advancing phase, nuclear tissue is ablated by high voltage (typically 100 to 300 V depending on operator settings) delivered at a frequency of 120 KHz using bipolar radiofrequency energy. In hydrated tissue conductive medium containing normal saline, the high-voltage radiofrequency current creates a plasma field approximately 75 μm thick that is composed of highly ionized particles with sufficient energy to break organic molecular bonds and thus vaporize tissue. By advancing the Perc-DL Spine Wand™ (Arthrocare Corp., Sunnyvale, CA) in ablation mode and retracting the probe while delivering a bipolar RF coagulation, 1-mm channels are created. Histologic examination following channel "coblation" in harvested sheep disks validated that 1-mm channels are indeed created and, more importantly, that there was no evidence of collateral tissue or cell destruction.[29]

Technique

Nucleoplasty is performed by an interventionalist in a sterile surgical suit with the patient under conscious sedation (**Fig. 21.1A**). A 17-gauge introducer needle is advanced from approximately 8 cm lateral to the midline using an oblique fluoroscopic projection. The needle is aimed at the Kambin safe triangle, and the exiting nerve can be outlined to help avoid injury. The 17-gauge introducer needle is advanced through the annulus to the annular-nuclear junction and can often be felt by a slight loss of resistance. In this position, the "wand" can be advanced through the introducer needle and diagonally across the nucleus from the posterior to the anterior annulus. The path is checked in anteroposterior (AP) and lateral fluoroscopy views, and a series of six passes is recommended. The slight distal curve on the tip of the wand was designed to cause the wand to pass in different paths when rotated between passes. It is difficult, however, to tell whether the catheter is in fact creating new channels or just repeatedly passing into the same channel. The wand is first advanced at 5 mm beyond the cannulae tip to ensure that the active portion of the wand is within the nucleus and behind the needle hub. Depth markers can be used to delineate the length of the path. The wand is advanced at 0.5 cm per second in ablation mode and retracted at the same speed using coagulation. Typically six channels are made at the 12, 2, 4, 6, 8, and 10 o'clock positions. Care must be taken not to lodge the tip of the wand within normal nucleus because it will dislodge. Although there is no reason to believe that a tiny inert tip would cause any harm, the tip can be seen on the fluoroscopy image.

Some interventionalists try to achieve a more posterior placement when the protrusion has a broad base. In this case a more lateral approach to the disk is made to allow the introducer needle to lie more posterior in the disk (**Fig. 21.1B,C**). The distal curve may be gently placed on the wand to further facilitate posterior travel and help ensure that the wand will advance in separate channels. The wand is typically advanced approximately 0.5 cm or less, and one tries to create a larger cone of tissue removal without injuring the end plates or vaporizing healthy annulus.

■ Morbidity

Performed by an experienced interventionalist, Nucleoplasty™ is relatively safe. One can expect the same low incidence of infection and nerve root injury inherent in any disk access procedure, but the use of intradiskal and preoperative intravenous antibiotics should significantly reduce the incidence of infection. Because the introducer

Table 21.1 Study Design and Demographics: Prospective or Case-Control Series

Author, Year Journal	Study Design[a]	Sample Size[b] (Final)	Follow-Up Period	Pain Duration	Pain Indication[c]	Performed by[d]	Workers' Compensation/ Litigation[e]
Nardi et al, 2005[42] (cervical disc study), Acta Neurochir	NCT	N: 50 CM: 20	2 months	NR	Cervical disks: contained, <3 mm protrusion, cervical or arm pain	S	NR
Marin, 2005,[43] Acta Neurochir	NCT	N: 64 (60) CAM: 13	12 months	1.3 year	CLBP w/wo RP	S	NR
Derby, Lee et al, 2006, current study	PCS	N: 92 I: 63	12.7 months 14.9 months	37.5 months	Discogenic, w/wo leg pain	I	WC & LT: N: 79.8% I :73.9%
Gerszten et al, 2006,[40] J Neurosurg Spine	PCS	67	6 months	NR	More leg, contained, discogenic	S	NR
Bhagia et al, 2006,[31] Am J Phys Med Rehabil	PCS	53	2 weeks	NR	Contained, discogenic or leg pain	S	NR
Alexandre et al, 2005,[33] Acta Neurochir	PCS	64	1 year	>3 months	CLBP w/wo RP, discogenic	NR	NR
Singh, 2004,[44] Pain Physician	PCS	47 (37)	12 months	6.3 years	Discogenic	I	EX
Singh, Piryani et al, 2003,[38] Pain Physician	PCS	80 (69)	12 months	5.5 years	Discogenic or leg pain, small herniation	I	EX
Singh Piryani et al, 2002,[37] Pain Physician	PCS	67	12 months	5.4 years	Contained, discogenic, or leg pain	I	EX
Sharps and Issac, 2002,[31] Pain Physician	PCS	49 (13)	12 months	38 months	More leg, contained, discogenic	S	NR
Slipman et al, 2002,[45] IITS meeting	PCS	14	NR	58.4 months	CFP	I	NR

[a]Study design: NCT, nonrandomized control trial; PCS, prospective case series.
[b]Sample size: CAM, coblation-assisted microdiscectomy; CM, conservative management; I, IDET; N, Nucleoplasty.
[c]Pain indication: contained indicates contained disc herniation; more leg, patient has more leg pain than back pain; discogenic, discogenic low back pain confirmed with provocative diskography, which is elicitation of concordant pain with control disk; CLBP w/wo RP, chronic low back pain with or without radicular pain; CFP, central focal protrusion; Leg, pain referred to leg ; radicular, radicular symptom with leg pain greater than back pain.
[d]Performed by: I, interventionalist; S, surgeon.
[e]Workers' compensation and litigation: EX, excluded; LT, litigation; NR, not reported; WC, worker's compensation.

needle is only 17 gauge and the patient is awake, prolonged nerve root injury should also be uncommon. Common to any procedure that uses heat within the intervertebral disk, there is the risk of end-plate damage and neural injury. Nau and Diederich[30] measured temperature maximums and thermal doses along the channels created in cadaver human disks. Their data showed transient peak temperatures of 80° to 90°C along the cannel paths and temperatures greater than 65°C at radial distances of 3 to 4 mm from the channels and thermal doses of >250 minutes up to 6 mm from the probes. Because operators cannot always guarantee the exact path of the advancing wand in relation to its transient proximity to the end plate, end-plate damage is possible, and if the probe were to be passed outside the disk, injury to neural structures could occur.

Bhagia et al[31,32] recorded the short-term side effects and complications in a series of 53 patients following percutaneous disk decompression using Nucleoplasty. The most common side effects were soreness at the needle insertion site (76%), new numbness and tingling (26%), increased intensity of preprocedure back pain (15%), and new areas of back pain (15%). These symptoms resolved over 2 weeks, except for a 15% incidence of new numbness and tingling and a 4% incidence of increased intensity of preprocedure back pain.

Probably the most significant risk that would be difficult to recognize is the inadvertent destruction of normal annulus. Typically the advancing probe does not penetrate normal annulus, but if one is trying to achieve a more posterior placement closer to the protrusion and because the probe will be advanced roughly perpendicular to the annular tear, there would be a risk that one would create channels in normal annulus on either side of the annular tear.

■ Nucleoplasty Outcome Studies

No randomized controlled or cohort studies are available evaluating the therapeutic value of nucleoplasty. There are many case series providing level-3 evidence, but most have small study size and incomplete or short-term follow-up data, and none has a validated control group. Furthermore, the lack of acceptable evidence is demonstrated by wide variation in published success rates ranging from 80% in 1300 patients reported by two Italian neurosurgeons[33] to 20% in several small American case series on average pain relief[34–36] (**Tables 21.1, 21.2, 21.3,** and **21.4**).

In 2001, Sharps's group[31] was the first to report a case series of before and after outcomes following Nucleoplasty. Their preliminary results included 49 patients with 1 month of follow-up, 41 patients with 3 months, 24 patients with 6 months, and 13 patients with 12 months. Inclusion criteria included patients with back pain with or without leg pain, and excluded patients who had protrusions greater than one-third the sagittal canal diameter. The patients (average age 38) had an average of 38 months of symptoms. The procedure was performed as recommended by the manufacturer. The 1-month through 12-month outcomes based on visual analogue scale (VAS) showed a relatively consistent drop in the VAS pain score of between 4.3 (54%) and 3.6 (45%) from a preoperative average of 7.9. Interestingly, despite the reported near 50% drop in VAS pain score, as judged by a 5-point patient satisfaction scoring system (0 = unsatisfactory to 4 = excellent), the mean postprocedural satisfaction score was only 2.14. Nonetheless, the authors reported a 79% success rate based on a patient satisfaction of greater than 1 in a group of patients with relatively severe pain secondary to small disk protrusions in which no other

Table 21.2 Study Design and Demographics: Retrospective Series

Author, Year Journal	Study Design[a]	Sample Size[b] (Final)	Follow-Up Period	Pain Duration	Pain Indication[c]	Performed by[d]	Workers' Compensation/ Litigation[e]
Cohen et al, 2005,[41] J Spinal Disord Tech	RA	N: 7 N + I: 9	9 months	7.2 years 3.8 years	More leg, small herniation, radicular, discogenic	I	MMC
Reddy et al, 2005,[39] Pain Physician	RA	49	>1 year	5 years	More leg, discogenic, contained	S	NR

[a] Study design: RA, retrospective analysis.
[b] Sample size: I, intradiskal electrothermy (IDET); N, Nucleoplasty.
[c] Pain indication: contained indicates contained disc herniation; more leg, patient has more leg pain then back pain; discogenic, discogenic low back pain confirmed with provocative diskography, which is elicitation of concordant pain with control disk; radicular, radicular symptom with leg pain greater than back pain.
[d] Performed by: I, interventionalist; S, surgeon.
[e] Workers' compensation and litigation: MMC, military medical compensation; NR, not reported.

Table 21.3 Outcome Measurement: Prospective or Case-Control Studies

	Pain							Function	
Author, Year	**Overall Any Pain Improvement[a]**		**Index[b]**	**Initial Follow-Up[c]**		**Percent**	**>50% VAS**	**Index[d]**	**Initial: Follow-Up[e]**
Nardi et al, 2005	N	80%	VAS		NR		NR	NR	NR
	C	20%							
	M								
Marin et al, 2005	80%		VAS	At 12 months	78% improved (compared with baseline)		NR	Walking Standing Sitting	N: >75% CAM: no conclusion
Derby, Lee, et al, 2006	N	80.4% (>10% VAS)	VAS	N	7.45 ± 1.44→5.02 ± 2.21	33	25%	NR	NR
				I	7.60 ± 1.78→6.06 ± 2.08	20			
			BPI	N		27.59			
				I		7.62			
	I	55.5% (>10% VAS)	LPI	N		30.24			
				I		17.86			
			SAT	N		68.2			
						44.4			
Gerszten et al, 2006	NR		VAS		0.63→0.5 (3 mo) →0.48 (6 mo)	24	NR	NR	NR
			SF-36 PCS		33→37 (3 mo) →41 (6 mo)	24			
			Eq. 5D		0.2→0.4 (3 mo) →0.6 (6 mo)	200			
Bhagia et al, 2006.	NR		VAS	Back	6.74→4.27	37	NR	NR	NR
				Right leg	5.14→3.59	30			
				Left leg	6.63→4.01	40			
Alexandre et al, 2005	51.5%: excellent		JOA	Excellent		55.8	NR	NR	NR
				Good		24.9			
	31.5%: good (6 months)			Scanty		12.4			
				None		6.9			
Singh Piryania, Liao et al, 2004	NR		VAS		6.7 ± 1.1→4.4 ± 2.3	34	53%	Sitting	11–32%
								Standing	13–30%
								Walking	15–35%
Singh Piryani et al, 2003	75% (1 year)		VAS	At 12 months	6.8→ 4.5	34	54%	Sitting	54%
				At 6 months	4.2	38		Standing	44%
								Walking	49%
Singh Piryani et al, 2002	80%		VAS		6.8 ± 1.1→4.1 ± 2.5	40	56%	Sitting	62%
								Standing	59%
								Walking	60%

(continued)

Table 21.3 (Continued)

		Pain				Function	
Author, Year	**Overall Any Pain Improvement[a]**	**Index[b]**	**Initial Follow-Up[c]**	**Percent**	**>50% VAS**	**Index[d]**	**Initial: Follow-Up[e]**
Sharps and Issac, 2002	79% (OP: 67%, NoOP: 82%)	VAS	7.9 ± 1.3→4.3 ± 2.8	46	56%	NR	NR
Slipman et al, 2002	64.3% (w/o CFP: 30%)	VAS	NR	NR	NR	NR	

[a]Overall: N, Nucleoplasty ;CM, conservative management; OP, group that had previous surgery; NoOP, no previous surgery; w/o CFP, without central focal protrusion group (axial LBP); NR, not reported; I, intradiskal electrothermy (IDET).
[b]Pain index: SF-36 PCS, Short Form–36 physical component summary scale; VAS, visual analogue pain scale; SAT, satisfaction; JOA, JOA score scale; BPI, back pain index; LPI, leg pain index; Eq. 5D, EuroQol 5D.
[c]Pain, initial: follow-up: N, Nucleoplasty; I, IDET; back, pain on back; right leg, pain on right leg; left leg, pain on left leg.
[d]Function index: sitting, standing, walking indicate functional improvement of sitting, standing, walking abilities; NR, not reported.
[e]Function, initial follow-up: N, Nucleoplasty; CAM, coblation-assisted microdisk.

Table 21.4 Outcome Measurement: Retrospective Series

		Pain					Function		
Author, Year	**Overall Any Pain Improvement[a]**	**Index[b]**		**Initial Follow-Up[c]**	**%**	**>50% VAS**	**Index[d]**	**Initial: Follow-up**	**Medication**
Cohen et al, 2005	NR	VAS	N	6.0 ± 2.0→4.8 ± 1.8	20	20% N: 1/5 N+I: 0/9	Return	N: 83%	86%→ 71%
			N+I	7.2 ± 0.8→6.3± 1.0	13			N+I:86%	34%→34%
Reddy et al, 2005	NR	VAS		8.08 →4.41	45	NR	Work impairment	1. 3.9→2.7 2. 3.7→2.2 3. 4.2→3	1. 3.8→2.7 2. 3.2→2 3. 3.7→2.4
			<6 months	8.1→4.5	56.4				
			6 mo to approximately 1 yr	8→3.9	64.6				
			>1 year	7.1→5.4	45				
		SAT	<6 months		75				
			6 mo to approximately 1 yr		73				
			>1 year		91				

[a]Overall any pain improvement: NR, not reported.
[b]Pain index: VAS, visual analogue pain scale; SAT, satisfaction.
[c]Pain initial follow-up: N, Nucleoplasty; N+I, Nucleoplasty + IDET.
[d]Function index: Return, percentage of the patients return to work; work impairment, level of work impairment.

surgical or interventional therapy has proven to be consistently successful.

In the following year, Singh et al[37] similarly reported a practice audit of before-and-after results on a group of 67 patients with back and leg pain of long duration (5.4 ± 5.6 years). They reported outcomes in 61 patients at 6 months and 41 patients at 12 months. There was an average decrease in pain score of 38% from a preoperative average score of 6.80. In addition to this modest average improvement, the authors also reported a 59% at 6 months and 56% at 12 months numerical pain score decrease of 50% or more. Although improvement is difficult to quantify, the authors also reported improvement in patients' self-reported sitting and standing duration tolerance. The same group published results of a consecutive series of 84 patients with back pain with or without leg pain. The patients presumably include the original 67 patients and 17 additional patients.[38] Although not specifically stated in their first published report, the second study excluded any patient with secondary-gain issues and therefore left open to the authors' discretion which patients would be included in the consecutive series. At 12-month follow-up in 77% of the patients, there was 34% decrease in the numerical pain score. Only 15% of the patients unemployed prior to Nucleoplasty were able to work after it.

In 2005 Reddy et al[39] reported on the outcome of 67 patients undergoing Nucleoplasty for back and leg pain with various follow-up intervals: 16 patients at 3 months, 22 patients at 6 months, and 11 patients at 12 months. The authors reported small but statistically significant improvements in a 5-point impairment score for work and leisure activities. They also reported that 56%, 64%, and 45% of patients achieved 50% or more relief in pain at their respective 3-, 6-, and 12-month follow-up. However, despite the authors' enthusiastic interpretation, there was only a 15% (7.1 to 5.2) decrease in NRS reported by the 11 patients who were followed for 12 months. This score would be roughly consistent with five responders having 50% relief and six nonresponders having no relief.

Gerszten et al[40] performed a prospective nonrandomized longitudinal cohort study and reported outcomes in 2002 in patients who presented with contained disk protrusions with primarily radicular pain rather than back pain. Follow-up at 6 months was available in only 23 patients. No significant improvement was seen in the VAS pain score of 5.4 preoperative to 4.8 at follow-up (11% decrease). Although the authors reported significant improvement in several quality-of-life outcome instruments, the reported success was based on only 20 of the 67 patients, and the authors did not comment on what happened to the missing information.

Cohen et al[41] reported before-and-after outcomes in a case series of 16 active-duty soldiers with long-standing back and leg pain of an average of 5.6 years. Seven had Nucleoplasty alone and nine had intradiskal electrothermy (IDET) followed by Nucleoplasty at the same level. The average decrease in VAS pain score was 16%, with only one patient having greater than 50% relief of pain. There was no significant difference in outcome between the two groups.

Derby[35,36] reported outcome on a nonrandomized before-and-after initial case series of 67 patients undergoing IDET compared with a later series of 92 patients undergoing Nucleoplasty. Both patient series included similar inclusion and exclusion criteria. The series included a large percentage of workers' compensation and litigation cases. Most patients had approximately 60 to 70% back pain and 30 to 40% leg pain. At an average 1-year follow-up, the numerical pain score showed a statistical decrease of 17% (7.6 to 6.06) in the IDET group and 33% (7.45 to 5.02) in the Nucleoplasty group. An index rating improvement in back and leg pain showed approximately equal improvement in back and leg pain in the Nucleoplasty group. Patient satisfaction was based a standard four-item questionnaire; 44% of the IDET group and 68.2% of the Nucleoplasty group indicated that the procedure met expectations or that they would repeat the procedure for the same outcome.

■ Conclusion

Despite Nucleoplasty's variable results, the procedure is appealing because it is simple and relatively safe, and it destroys minimal tissue. Because little tissue is ablated, disk height should be maintained or at least should collapse more slowly and allow the body time to adapt. In addition, the 17-gauge introducer needle should cause significantly less collateral damage to the normal annulus compared with surgical arthroscopic decompression techniques that remove herniations from inside the disk.

Performed in an outpatient surgery center with a relatively inexpensive disposable apparatus, the facility and physician expense in time, labor, equipment, and facility overhead is between five and 10 times less than a comparable fusion or arthroplasty. Because surgical decompression outcome for small protrusions causing axial pain is inconsistent and patients often would like fusion or arthroplasty to be the last resort, nuclear decompression using a minimally invasive technique may be a reasonable next option for hydrated disks with relatively well-maintained disk heights. For patients with back and referred leg pain, outcomes are comparable to those with IDET. The average mean percentage relief following Nucleoplasty is 45% in prospective before-and-after series **(Table 21.2)** and 43% in retrospective case series **(Table 21.1).** Despite the data that show that intradiskal heating has somewhat better average reported outcomes, in the only unpublished study that specifically compared outcome between the two procedures, Nucleoplasty had better patient satisfaction and somewhat better pain relief.[35] Nucleoplasty, however, was designed and marketed for treating leg pain. Relief of back pain is commonly less than 50%.

Outcomes based on before-and-after case series reporting VAS pain score show an average decrease in 6-month pain score of between 20% and 46%. There does, however, appear to be a subset of patients who have significant relief of pain. Both Singh and Sharps, in series of patients without secondary gain, reported 50% or more relief in pain in 50% and 60% of their respective cases series studies. On the other hand, when patients with secondary gain comprise the majority, Derby reported 25% and Cohen reported 20% of patients with 50% or greater pain relief.

The current nuclear decompression devices are a first iteration. Targeted removal of herniated nucleus behind a protrusion is a more logical strategy for achieving the desired effect of removing the source of inflammation and relieving tension on the adjacent irritated annulus. It is hoped that future designs will allow better navigation into the protrusions and will incorporate enhanced methods to safely remove herniated nuclear material. Indeed, early favorable reports of good outcome following Nucleoplasty for small cervical disk protrusions support the better access strategy.[32,42] Using the anterior approach, coblation can be done directly behind a protrusion and, in addition, the smaller size of the cervical disk might accentuate the potential beneficial effects of transiently increased temperatures.

References

1. Takahashi K, Shima I, Porter RW. Nerve root pressure in lumbar disc herniation. Spine 1999;24:2003–2006
2. Olmarker K, Rydevik B, Holm S, et al. Effects of experimental graded compression on blood flow in spinal nerve roots. A vital microscopic study on the porcine cauda equina. J Orthop Res 1989;7:817–823
3. Case RB, Choy DS, Altman P. Change of intradisc pressure versus volume change. J Clin Laser Med Surg 1995;13:143–147
4. Choy DS, Diwan S. In vitro and in vivo fall of intradiscal pressure with laser disc decompression. J Clin Laser Med Surg 1992;10:435–437
5. Maroon JC. Current concepts in minimally invasive discectomy. Neurosurgery 2002;51(suppl):S137–S145
6. Yonezawa T, Onomura T, Kosaka R, et al. The system and procedures of percutaneous intradiscal laser nucleotomy. Spine 1990;15:1175–1185
7. Hellinger J, Linke R, Heller H. A biophysical explanation for Nd:YAG percutaneous laser disc decompression success. J Clin Laser Med Surg 2001;19:235–238
8. Lee SH, Derby R, Chen Y, et al. In vitro measurement of pressure in intervertebral discs and annulus fibrosus with and without annular tears during discography. Spine J 2004;4:614–618
9. Mochida J, Toh E, Nomura T, et al. The risks and benefits of percutaneous nucleotomy for lumbar disc herniation. A 10-year longitudinal study. J Bone Joint Surg Br 2001;83:501–505
10. Mochida J, Nishimura K, Okuma M, et al. Percutaneous nucleotomy in elite athletes. J Spinal Disord 2001;14:159–164
11. Carragee EJ, Han MY, Suen PW, Kim D. Clinical outcomes after lumbar discectomy for sciatica: the effects of fragment type and anular competence. J Bone Joint Surg Am 2003;85-A:102–108
12. Martinez JB, Oloyede VO, Broom ND. Biomechanics of load-bearing of the intervertebral disc: an experimental and finite element model. Med Eng Phys 1997;19:145–156
13. Adams MA, McNally DS, Dolan P. "Stress" distributions inside intervertebral discs. The effects of age and degeneration. J Bone Joint Surg Br 1996;78:965–972
14. Adams MA, McMillan DW, Green TP, Dolan P. Sustained loading generates stress concentrations in lumbar intervertebral discs. Spine 1996;21:434–438
15. Edwards WT, Ordway NR, Zheng Y, et al. Peak stresses observed in the posterior lateral anulus. Spine 2001;26:1753–1759
16. McNally DS, Adams MA. Internal intervertebral disc mechanics as revealed by stress profilometry. Spine 1992;17:66–73
17. Hutton WC, Elmer WA, Bryce LM, et al. Do the intervertebral disc cells respond to different levels of hydrostatic pressure? Clin Biomech (Bristol, Avon) 2001;16:728–734
18. Hutton WC, Elmer WA, Boden SD, et al. The effect of hydrostatic pressure on intervertebral disc metabolism. Spine 1999;24:1507–1515
19. Wognum S, Huyghe JM, Baaijens FP. Influence of osmotic pressure changes on the opening of existing cracks in 2 intervertebral disc models. Spine 2006;31:1783–1788
20. Castro WH, Halm H, Rondhuis J. The influence of automated percutaneous lumbar discectomy (APLD) on the biomechanics of the lumbar intervertebral disc. An experimental study. Acta Orthop Belg 1992;58:400–405
21. Simunic DI, Robertson PA, Broom ND. Mechanically induced disruption of the healthy bovine intervertebral disc. Spine 2004;29:972–978
22. Osti OL, Vernon-Roberts B, Moore R, et al. Annular tears and disc degeneration in the lumbar spine. A post-mortem study of 135 discs. J Bone Joint Surg Br 1992;74:678–682
23. Osti OL, Vernon-Roberts B, Fraser RD. 1990 Volvo Award in experimental studies. Anulus tears and intervertebral disc degeneration. An experimental study using an animal model. Spine 1990;15:762–767
24. Delamarter RB, Howard MW, Goldstein T, et al. Percutaneous lumbar discectomy. Preoperative and postoperative magnetic resonance imaging. J Bone Joint Surg Am 1995;77:578–584
25. Derby R. Percutaneous disc decompression. Presented at the International Spine Intervention Society 13th annual scientific meeting, 2005, New York
26. O'Neill CW, Liu JJ, Leibenberg E, et al. Percutaneous plasma decompression alters cytokine expression in injured porcine intervertebral discs. Spine J 2004;4:88–98
27. O'Neill CW, Kurgansky ME, Derby R, et al. Disc stimulation and patterns of referred pain. Spine 2002;27:2776–2781
28. Yeung AT, Tsou PM. Posterolateral endoscopic excision for lumbar disc herniation: surgical technique, outcome, and complications in 307 consecutive cases. Spine 2002;27:722–731
29. Lee MS, Cooper G, Lutz GE, Doty SB. Histologic characterization of coblation nucleoplasty performed on sheep intervertebral discs. Pain Physician 2003;6:439–442
30. Nau WH, Diederich CJ. Evaluation of temperature distributions in cadaveric lumbar spine during nucleoplasty. Phys Med Biol 2004;49:1583–1594

31. Bhagia SM, Slipman CW, Nirschl M, et al. Side effects and complications after percutaneous disc decompression using coblation technology. Am J Phys Med Rehabil 2006;85:6–13
32. Slipman CW, Bhagia SM, Abd OE, Garvin C. Nucleoplasty procedure for cervical radicular pain-initial case series. Presented at the Interventional Spinal Injection Society, 2003, Orlando, FL
33. Alexandre A, Coro L, Azuelos A, Pellone M. Percutaneous nucleoplasty for discoradicular conflict. Acta Neurochir Suppl (Wien) 2005;92:83–86
34. Freedman BA, Cohen SP, Kuklo TR, et al. Intradiscal electrothermal therapy (IDET) for chronic low back pain in active-duty soldiers: 2-year follow-up. Spine J 2003;3:502–509
35. Derby R. Outcome comparison between IDET, combined IDET nucleoplasty and biochemical injection treatment. Presented at the International Spinal Injection Society, 10th annual scientific meeting, September 7, 2002, Austin, TX
36. Derby R. Comparison between IDET and nucleoplasty outcome in patients with discogenic pain. Presented at the ISIS annual scientific conference, 2006, Salt Lake City, UT
37. Singh V, Piryani C, Liao K. Percutaneous disc decompression in the treatment of chronic discogenic pain. Pain Physician 2002;5:250–259
38. Singh V, Piryani C, Liao K. Evaluation of percutaneous disc decompression using coblation in chronic back pain with or without leg pain. Pain Physician 2003;6:273–280
39. Reddy AS, Loh S, Cutts J, et al. New approach to the management of acute disc herniation. Pain Physician 2005;8:385–389
40. Gerszten PC, Welch WC, McGrath PM, Willis SL. A prospective outcomes study of patients undergoing intradiscal electrothermy (IDET) for chronic low back pain. Pain Physician 2002;5:360–364
41. Cohen SP, Williams S, Kurihara C, et al. Nucleoplasty with or without intradiscal electrothermal therapy (IDET) as a treatment for lumbar herniated disc. J Spinal Disord Tech 2005;18(suppl):S119–S124
42. Nardi PV, Cabezas D, Cesaroni A. Percutaneous cervical nucleoplasty using coblation technology. Clinical results in fifty consecutive cases. Acta Neurochir Suppl (Wien) 2005;92:73–78
43. Marin FZ. CAM versus nucleoplasty. Acta Neurochir Suppl (Wien) 2005;92:111–114
44. Singh V. Percutaneous disc decompression for the treatment of chronic atypical cervical discogenic pain. Pain Physician 2004;7:115–118
45. Slipman C, Isaac Z, Gilchrist R. Preliminary outcomes of percutaneous nucleoplasty for treatment of axial low back pain: a comparison of patients with versus without an associated central focal protrusion. Presented at the International Intradiscal Therapy Society (IITS) 15th annual meeting, 2002, Seoul, Korea

22 Disk Arthroplasty: Basic Principles, Rationale, and Overview

David H. Kim and Howard S. An

Lumbar disk arthroplasty represents a relatively new option for surgical treatment of degenerative disk disease. In principle, disk arthroplasty has the potential for providing low back pain relief comparable to that achieved through fusion surgery, while preserving lumbar spinal motion and possibly reducing the risk of adjacent segment degeneration. The first widely available commercially produced implant, the Charité III, was introduced in Europe in 1987. Since then, several different implant designs have been developed and are in various stages of study or clinical application. Overall, the number of arthroplasty cases performed has increased rapidly in Europe and at a somewhat more modest pace in the United States. At this time, two arthroplasty designs have been approved by the United States Food and Drug Administration (FDA) for use in the treatment of patients with degenerative disk disease meeting specific indications: the Charité III (Depuy Spine, Raynham, MA) and ProDisc-L (Synthes, Paoli, IL) devices. Short-term follow-up data have demonstrated clinical results in terms of pain reduction and functional restoration that are at least equivalent to those achieved through various lumbar spinal fusion procedures. Prospective intermediate- and long-term data as well as detailed information regarding associated complications of these devices remains largely unknown.

■ History

Although lumbar disk arthroplasty is generally regarded as a novel treatment option, the history of spinal disk replacement surgery is nearly as long as that of joint replacement surgery, and published reports of early devices date back to the 1950s, the decade in which Charnley introduced his total hip arthroplasty. Initial disk replacement procedures represented an attempt to utilize a functional spacer to prevent progressive disk space collapse following en bloc diskectomy. Early strategies were first reported in the 1950s and included injection of methyl acrylic into the disk space as well as insertion of Lucite pegs. Fernström is widely credited with performing the first reported disk arthroplasty procedures in human patients. Although good early results were reported, the implants tended to subside into the adjacent vertebral bodies with time, and this procedure was eventually abandoned. Since the 1970s there have been an increasing number of reported disk arthroplasty designs and concepts, the vast majority of which have never undergone human implantation.[1]

The AcroFlex (Depuy Spine) disk was designed by Steffee and consisted of a rubber core sandwiched between titanium metal end plates **(Fig. 22.1)**. Porous coating of the end plates was used to promote bone ingrowth. In 1990, the FDA expressed concern regarding the potential carcinogenicity of the benzene-based solvents used during vulcanization of the polyolefin rubber core, and clinical trials of this device were suspended. The manufacturing process was revised and implantation of the device was resumed beginning in 1998. Unfortunately, 1- to 2-year follow-up evaluation revealed a relatively high rate of core failure, and implantation of the device was halted.

The first design to undergo successful clinical trials was developed by Schellnack and Büttner-Janz at the Charité Hospital in East Berlin in the former German Democratic Republic and was based on the low-friction principle successfully established in hip and knee arthroplasty.[2] The prototype SB Charité I was first implanted in 1984 and consisted of stainless steel end plates and an ultrahigh molecular weight polyethylene sliding core. Early subsidence of the implant into the adjacent vertebral bodies resulted in a design modification in 1985, and the SB Charité II included bilateral wing extensions of the metal end plates. A problem with device end-plate fracture and insufficient instrumentation for implantation led to collaboration with the Waldemar Link company and a redesigned LINK SB Charité III device in 1987 **(Fig. 22.2)**. With a few minor modifications, this version is essentially the same as the one in current usage and consists of cobalt chrome metal end plates with anterior and posterior teeth to prevent early migration, and plasma-sprayed titanium and hydroxyapatite coating to promote bony ingrowth. The concept of a biconvex mobile sliding polyethylene core has been retained through all models. The early European experience with the Charité III was favorable, with multiple series reporting good to excellent results in the vast majority of treated patients. These results supported initiation of an FDA Investigational Device Exemption (IDE) trial of the device in the U.S. in 2000. The first total disk arthroplasty in the U.S. was performed in March 2000. The FDA trial was closed in 2001, and favorable 2-year results led to FDA approval of the Charité III in November 2004. In August 2006, the FDA approved a second commercial design for a lumbar disk arthroplasty device, the ProDisc-L.

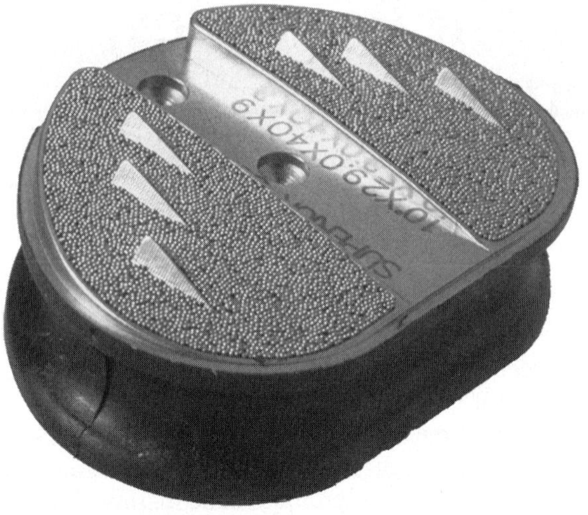

Fig. 22.1 The AcroFlex disk.

■ Principles of Disk Arthroplasty Design

Lumbar disk arthroplasty is intended to relieve low back pain from degenerative disk disease by removing the purported pain generator, that is, the degenerated disk, and replacing it with a device that preserves near-normal lumbar spinal segmental motion. The device must provide adequate initial stability to allow early patient mobilization, and it must remain stable over the long term in the setting of repetitive cycling with physiologic loads as well as occasional exposure to supraphysiologic loads. Given the relatively young age of patients undergoing surgical treatment for degenerative disk disease, the component materials must be sufficiently durable in the biomechanical and biologic environment of the human spinal column to allow consistent function for decades.

Biomechanics

The kinematics of normal lumbar spine segmental motion remain crudely understood and are challenging to preserve following subtotal diskectomy. The spinal segment is considered a three-joint complex consisting of the anterior diskovertebral joint and two posterolateral facet joints. Although the entire lumbar spine normally provides a significant amount of global motion, segmental motion at any given lumbar level is relatively limited and normally allows for 5.0 to 9.1 degrees of flexion, 2.6 to 5.3 degrees of extension, 4.2 to 4.8 degrees of lateral bend to either side, and 1.1 to 2.2 degrees of axial rotation to either side.[3] Rotation and translation occur along three axes. The instantaneous axis of rotation migrates with both flexion-extension and lateral bending to describe an ellipse localized in the posterior half to posterior third of the disk space at the level of the inferior end plate.[4–6] Age-related degeneration of the motion segment results in expansion of the range of instantaneous axes of rotation and in load shifting to the facet joints. To minimize distortion of normally occurring forces and loads, an arthroplasty device should reproduce as closely as possible the natural range of axes of rotation while considering the potential for age-related changes in motion and load distribution. In general, values for range of motion and axes of rotation have been obtained from cadaveric models using simplified and somewhat arbitrary loads. As a result, the figures may not accurately reflect true values in vivo. For example, although high-precision measurements using cadaveric models have suggested that the axis of rotation during extension is anterior to the axis of rotation during flexion, radiographic evaluation of living subjects has indicated that the reverse is true.[5,7,8]

The neutral zone and lax zone are biomechanical concepts representing subsets of a joint's global range of motion and are a reflection of joint laxity. The neutral zone represents the range of motion that occurs with only frictional resistance. The lax zone represents the range of motion that occurs without substantial ligamentous resistance.[9] For the average lumbar motion segment, the neutral zone represents 13% of global range of motion, whereas the lax zone represents 46%.[9] Neither the neutral zone nor the lax zone can be measured in living subjects, which limits their usefulness in assessing clinical performance of implanted devices. However, whether disk arthroplasty should reproduce normal neutral zone and lax zone values remains unclear.

The normal lumbar spine demonstrates coupled motion due to sloping of the facet joints. For example, right axial rotation is associated with right lateral bending. It has been suggested that this coupled motion should be accounted for in disk arthroplasty design to avoid unnatural forces on local tissues and the potential for accelerated facet joint degeneration or osteophyte formation.[8]

Compressive failure strength of cancellous vertebral bone has been reported to be between 1.6 and 4.6 MPa. With 20 degrees of flexion in the upright posture, load on the lumbar disk is approximately 1200 N, with 80% transmitted through the vertebral bodies and disks and 20% transmitted through the facet joints. Arthroplasty designs

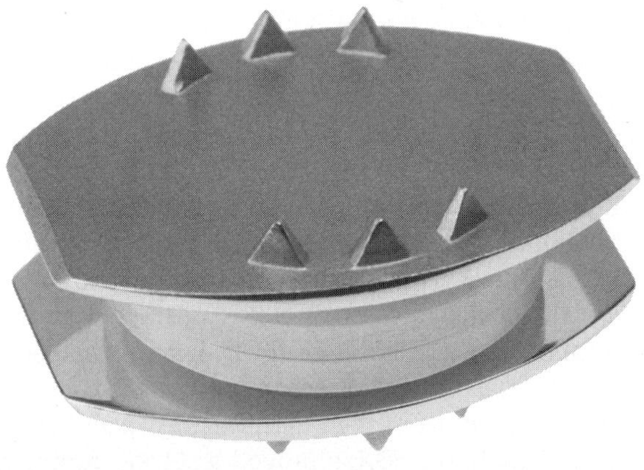

Fig. 22.2 The Charité disk.

must be able to withstand up to a million loading cycles of up to three times body weight per year. The loading rate is comparable to that experienced by the hip joint (2 million cycles per year times two to four times body weight), but most disk arthroplasty devices are implanted in patients decades younger than typical hip arthroplasty recipients, and the marked decrease in vertebral bone strength that commonly occurs with aging as well as the frequent occurrence of osteoporotic vertebral compression fractures in elderly patients is of concern when considering disk arthroplasty.

On the other hand, an advantage of disk arthroplasty devices may be a more biomechanically favorable environment for osseointegration. A 56% surface area ingrowth of bone with porous coated titanium disk end plates has been demonstrated at 12 months in a baboon model.[10] This figure is considerably better than the 12 to 33% rates observed with cementless acetabular and femoral components, respectively.[11,12]

Proponents of disk arthroplasty have suggested that a potential advantage of motion preservation is possible decreased risk of adjacent segment degeneration compared with fusion surgery. Biomechanical studies of cadaveric specimens and finite element analysis have suggested that stress and motion may be increased at levels adjacent to a fused spinal segment.[13–16] Clinical studies, however, have failed to demonstrate convincing evidence that fusion surgery accelerates the rate of adjacent segment degeneration beyond that which might occur with natural history in the absence of surgery.[17–20]

Materials

Current disk arthroplasty designs have borrowed heavily from principles previously established for hip and knee arthroplasty. Use of cobalt chrome alloys and ultrahigh molecular weight polyethylene (UHMWPE) is a direct result of the success of these materials in hip and knee prostheses. Cobalt-chrome-molybdenum demonstrates excellent wear resistance and performs well as a prosthetic joint surface. By comparison, titanium has the advantages of greater magnetic resonance imaging (MRI) compatibility and less susceptibility to bacterial colonization than cobalt chrome. Unfortunately, poor wear characteristics and decreased hardness have so far limited its use in disk arthroplasty to porous coating of the nonarticulating vertebral surface of device end plates.

Careful study of the lessons learned during development of hip and knee arthroplasty has saved time and effort but has also resulted in uncertainty regarding the relevance of specific concerns such as the relevance of osteolysis to lumbar disk arthroplasty. Although osteolysis is the most common cause of delayed prosthesis loosening in hip arthroplasty, no unequivocal case of osteolytic device loosening has been reported following disk arthroplasty. For metal-on-metal devices, generation of wear particles have been measured at 1 mm^3 per million cycles, an order of magnitude less than that observed with polyethylene-on-metal prostheses. However, material-related toxicity may be more of a concern with metal-on-metal devices. Whether osteolysis or metal toxicity is the greater concern for disk arthroplasty remains unknown. The disk space is certainly a different biomechanical and biologic environment compared with the hip joint and is likely to place unique demands on arthroplasty devices.

■ Specific Arthroplasty Designs

Nucleoplasty

The earliest disk arthroplasty device, the Fernström ball, was essentially a nucleoplasty device that sought to replace only the nucleus pulposus component of the intervertebral disk. As previously described, problems with implant subsidence led to early clinical failure and eventual abandonment of the technique. However, the strategy of partial disk replacement through nucleoplasty persisted, and several more sophisticated nucleoplasty designs are currently undergoing evaluation.

The device with the largest clinical experience is the Raymedica PDN (Prosthetic Disc Nucleus; Raymedica, Inc., Minneapolis, MN) or PDN-SOLO (**Fig. 22.3**). This implant is composed of a hydrogel core contained within a flexible inelastic woven polyethylene jacket. The core is designed to undergo cyclical hydrodynamic swelling and shrinking depending on loading conditions. The device has been implanted in several thousand patients in Europe, and initial short-term results appeared favorable. However, an FDA-IDE study that began in 2002 failed. Although 1-year clinical results of the PDN were encouraging, there were multiple cases of device extrusion into the spinal canal. Subsequently, the insertion technique was modified from the original posterolateral approach to a direct lateral

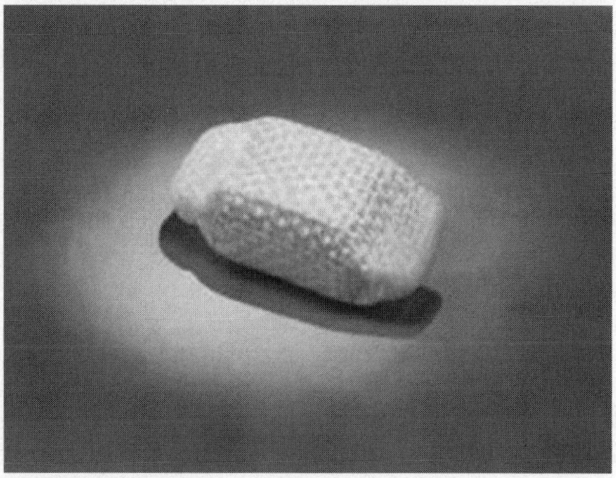

Fig. 22.3 The PDN-SOLO device.

approach to retain an intact posterior annular layer. Persistent problems with implant migration and subsidence eventually led to failure of the trial. The device has been redesigned with a larger footprint to resist migration and a softer hydrogel material to resist subsidence and is currently in early clinical trials. Other nucleoplasty designs, the NeuDisc (Replication Medical, Inc., New Brunswick, NJ), Newcleus (Zimmer Spine, Warsaw, IN), and Aquarelle (Stryker Corp., Kalamazoo, MI), are in much earlier stages of evaluation and clinical testing.

Total Disk Arthroplasty

Total disk arthroplasty represents a conceptual evolution from nucleoplasty. Device migration is prevented by incorporation of rigid end plates fixed to adjacent vertebrae, and articulation occurs between separate device component surfaces. As previously noted, implant materials and design principles have largely been borrowed from hip and knee arthroplasty devices. Currently available devices have been classified according to degree of motion constraint demonstrated, such as unconstrained, semiconstrained, or fully constrained, and the type of motion bearing surface, such as metal-on-polyethylene or metal-on-metal.

Unconstrained designs provide independent rotation and translation about three axes. Point stress within the device is significantly reduced compared with more constrained designs. However, it has been proposed that segmental instability contributes to development of disk degeneration and that the presence of abnormal motion patterns must be addressed in disk arthroplasty design. This opinion has led to development of semiconstrained and fully constrained devices that provide intrinsic limits to range of motion and more controlled articulation. Although shear forces external to the device, such as within the facet joints, are reduced, internal stress within the device is increased, and stress is concentrated at the device–bone interface, resulting in potentially increased risk of implant loosening. For example, biomechanical study of hip and knee implants has demonstrated a similar trade-off between constrained and unconstrained devices in which constrained devices provide greater initial joint stability but at a cost of increased stress on fixation of the implant and an increased risk of delayed loosening. Biomechanical testing of ball-and-socket disk arthroplasty devices has also revealed that performance is more sensitive to device positioning. Which of these design strategies provides the greatest potential for long-term clinical success in disk arthroplasty has yet to be determined.

The ideal material for the articulating surfaces of disk arthroplasty devices is also unknown. Metal-on-metal disk prostheses have been marketed as the third generation of disk replacement technology following nuclear replacements and modular metal-on-plastic designs. However, this label is misleading given the lack of sufficient mid- and long-term outcome data from second-generation disk designs. Sequential generations of implant designs in hip and knee prostheses have been developed over the course of decades, with each design generation representing a paradigm shift in arthroplasty principles based on careful data collection and analysis of failures from the preceding generation. Such information is currently unavailable for total disk arthroplasty. Although generation of polyethylene wear debris and osteolysis have been a major source of implant loosening and failure of total hip prostheses, the same problems have not been demonstrated to contribute to significant rates of clinical failure following disk arthroplasty.

It has been estimated that the lumbar spine is exposed to 2 million nonsignificant motions and 125,000 significant bends per year.[21] A significant bend through the lumbar spine generates 10 times the wear debris of a single walking cycle.[22] Metal-on-polyethylene hip devices generate 43 to 135 mm^3 volumetric wear debris per year compared with 5 mm^3 per year for metal-on-metal designs.[22] Although polyethylene wear and osteolysis have not been proven to be significant clinical issues with disk arthroplasty, the long-term effects of polyethylene particles on regional tissues are unknown and some authors have expressed concern regarding the potential for epidural fibrosis and pathologic effects on neural tissue.

Metal-on-metal devices simplify engineering by eliminating a material (polyethylene) that was borrowed directly from hip and knee designs but that may not be required for long-term function of implants in the spine. Although the disk undergoes greater cycling than either the hip or knee, the translation experienced by disk arthroplasty surfaces is considerably more limited. Moreover, the vast majority of loading forces experienced in the intervertebral environment approximate one-tenth those typically encountered in the hip joint.

Charité III

The Charité artificial disk (DePuy Spine, Raynham, MA) consists of a sliding ultrahigh molecular weight polyethylene disk core sandwiched between cobalt chrome metal end plates. The core and end plates are not directly attached, and there is no device-related limit on range of motion, so this is considered an unconstrained device. The core polyethylene is moderately cross-linked by gamma irradiation and has a calculated wear rate of 0.15 mm/year based on the experience in metal-backed acetabular cups.[23] To minimize the risk of core fracture, minimal recommended thickness for the core is 7.5 mm.[24] The perimeter contains a radiopaque ring for radiographic localization. Core extrusion is prevented by the complementary concave end-plate surfaces and biconvex lens-shaped core. During flexion and extension the core translates posteriorly and anteriorly, respectively, providing a variable axis of rotation that more closely resembles that occurring in the normal lumbar spine. However, critics have noted that the average center of rotation for this device remains relatively more anterior than the naturally occurring axis of rotation, which as noted varies in position around the junction of the middle and posterior thirds of the disk space. Immediate fixation is achieved through six small peripheral spikes, three anterior and three posterior. Delayed fixation occurs through bony ingrowth of the end plates, which have a titanium porous coating followed by a layer of hydroxyapatite calcium phosphate. Histologic evaluation of a limited number of retrieved specimens has demonstrated excellent ingrowth of bone.[2] Following favorable results of an FDA-IDE trial, the Charité was approved by the FDA in 2004.

ProDisc-L

The ProDisc (Synthes, Inc., Paoli, PA) was initially developed in the late 1980s by Thierry Marnay. Like the Charité device, the ProDisc consists of cobalt chrome metal end plates and a polyethylene core **(Fig. 22.4)**. Unlike the Charité, however, the core is snap-fit to the inferior end plate, resulting in a semiconstrained spherical articulating interface between the concave superior end plate and the convex superior core surface. The center of rotation is fixed and located within the inferior vertebral body below the disk space. Immediate fixation is provided by a midline keel and two spikes. Delayed fixation occurs through bony ingrowth of the titanium porous coating. Concern has been expressed regarding sacrifice of bone stock in preparation for the midline keel, and the potential need for corpectomy if the device is removed during revision surgery.

The semiconstrained design prevents extrusion of the polyethylene core but results in a fixed nonanatomic axis of rotation located slightly anterior in the caudad vertebral body. With the device in place, a degree of anterior-posterior translation of the cephalad vertebral body occurs during flexion and extension through the operated segment and has raised concerns regarding the potential for damaging forces to the facet joints as well as dynamic foraminal stenosis. An FDA-IDE study yielded favorable results, and the ProDisc was approved by the FDA in August 2006.

Maverick Total Disk Replacement

The Maverick disk (Medtronic Sofamor Danek, Memphis, TN) is a semiconstrained device developed by Mathews in the 1990s that consists of directly articulating highly polished cobalt-chrome metal end plates **(Fig. 22.5)**. Like the ProDisc, immediate bone fixation is achieved by way of a large midline sagittal fin, and delayed fixation is accomplished through bony ingrowth into the hydroxyapatite-coated end plates. The complementary ball-and-socket articulating surfaces are not perfectly congruent with the convex inferior component, demonstrating a slightly smaller radius of curvature compared with the concave superior component. This arrangement allows for 1.5 mm of translation in any axial direction. The center of rotation is nonanatomic and fixed posterior to the middle of the inferior vertebral body. This design has been proposed to limit shear forces experienced by the facet joints, but biomechanical testing has also suggested that performance of the device is very sensitive to positioning. The biomechanical profile appears similar to the ProDisc.[25] In contrast to the Charité and ProDisc, the device is assembled outside the disk space and inserted as a single piece. The Maverick disk was first implanted in Europe in January 2002, and the first U.S. implantation was performed in 2003. A randomized FDA-IDE clinical trial began enrollment in May 2003 and is comparing the Maverick disk to anterior lumbar interbody fusion utilizing a lumbar tapered (LT) cage (Medtronic Sofamor Danek) with Infuse recombinant bone morphogenetic protein (Medtronic Sofamor Danek).

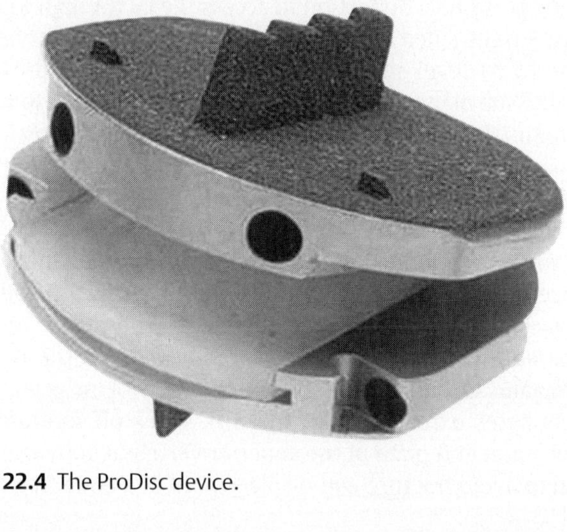

Fig. 22.4 The ProDisc device.

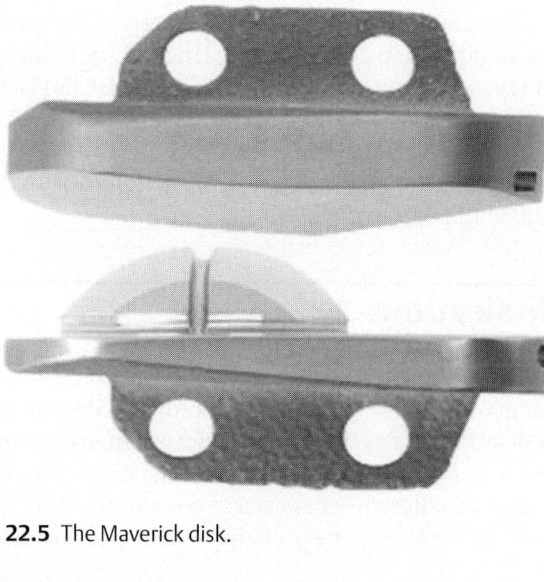

Fig. 22.5 The Maverick disk.

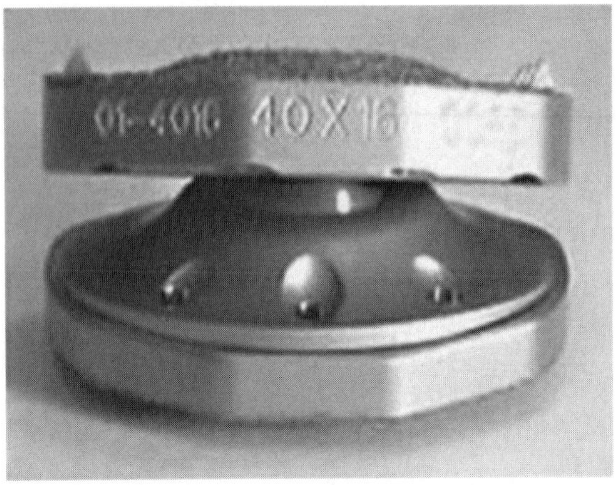

Fig. 22.6 The Flexicore disk.

Flexicore

The Flexicore intervertebral disk (Stryker Howmedica Osteonics, Allendale, NJ) is a fully constrained metal-on-metal device **(Fig. 22.6)**. The design incorporates four separate cobalt chrome parts that are snap-fit together prior to insertion. Immediate fixation is achieved through multiple end plate spikes, whereas delayed fixation is enhanced through a titanium plasma spray to promote bone on-growth. The highly polished ball-and-socket articulation yields a fixed axis of rotation that is positioned centrally between the end plates.

The press-fit design resists separation of the device once assembled, thereby providing constraint against axial distraction forces. A rotational stop limits rotation to 5 degrees in either direction and is meant to offload the facet joints in conditions of hypermobility that might otherwise contribute to accelerated arthropathy. Flexion, extension, and lateral bend are also limited to 15 degrees, making the device fully constrained. Concern has been raised that such constraint results in increased stress absorbed by the implant, which may in turn lead to increased rates of wear and loosening over time. Instrumentation is designed to allow implantation anterolaterally if necessary. A randomized FDA-IDE study began in the U.S. in August 2003 and is enrolling patients with single-level degenerative disk disease between L1 and S1. Patients are being compared with a control group undergoing anterior-posterior instrumented fusion with pedicle screw fixation.

■ Indications

In general, lumbar disk arthroplasty is indicated for treatment of moderately to severely symptomatic degenerative disk disease that has failed a minimum of 6 months of organized nonoperative treatment. The diagnosis of surgically treatable degenerative disk disease remains ill-defined but should be supported by a characteristic clinical history, findings on MRI or computed tomography (CT) and possibly provocative diskography. Reasonable potential should exist for significant motion restoration at the operated level. General contraindications include osteoporosis, metabolic bone disease, significant facet joint degeneration, spondylolisthesis >3 mm, scoliosis >11 degrees, or significant instability, infection, or malignancy. Beyond these broad principles, there is currently little expert consensus regarding more explicit indications and contraindications for application of disk arthroplasty surgery. Explicit FDA-approved indications simply reflect the original criteria defining eligibility for participation in the original FDA-IDE trials and are established for only two devices, the Charité and ProDisc-L. The Charité device is FDA-approved for use in single-level disease at either the L4-L5 or L5-S1 levels. The ProDisc-L is FDA-approved for use at one level or two adjacent levels between L3-L4 and L5-S1. However, there is no clear evidence that the Charité produces less favorable clinical results compared with the ProDisc-L when utilized off-label at two levels. Treatment of three levels is not FDA-approved for either device but has been performed in some centers in the U.S. Clinical experience treating three or more levels is very limited, and such treatment should be undertaken with great caution.

There are no FDA-approved nuclear replacement devices, and these implants should be considered experimental in nature. The prevailing opinion is that this genre of devices is most appropriately considered in the setting of relatively early stages of disk degeneration. Disk height loss should not exceed 50%. However, nucleoplasty does not directly address deficiencies of the annulus or end plates, so functional integrity of these structures appears to be a reasonable requirement for consideration of these devices.

■ Technique

For all four disk arthroplasty designs discussed here, the surgical approach can be performed in similar fashion. The most commonly performed exposure involves a left-sided retroperitoneal dissection to access the L3 through S1 levels. A right-sided retroperitoneal approach is an option for the L5-S1 level and has the potential benefit of preserving tissue planes for a future right-sided approach to more proximal levels. A transperitoneal approach is also an option for revision procedures or in the setting of previous retroperitoneal surgery.

During removal of disk tissue, preservation of the anterolateral annulus to the extent possible enhances device stability. Complete removal of end-plate cartilage enhances bony ingrowth into the device end plates. Avoiding end-plate fracture or perforation reduces the risk of implant subsidence. Resection of posterior marginal osteophytes extending into the disk space off the inferior vertebral end plate of the superior vertebral body is helpful to avoid fracture and displacement of a bone fragment during device insertion and resulting neuroforaminal compromise and postoperative sciatica. Actual device assembly and insertion varies among the different implants and is not reviewed here.

The mechanical performance of disk arthroplasty devices is strongly position-dependent. The ideal position for the implants is a symmetric midline placement on an anteroposterior view and slightly posterior to the midvertebral body on a lateral view. The interpedicular midpoint may provide the most accurate estimate of the functional midline as opposed to the spinous process position on anteroposterior radiographic views.[26] End-plate coverage should be maximized without overhang into the spinal canal or neuroforamen. Often, a compromise must be made between matching the flatness or convexity of the vertebral end plate to maximize stability and bony ingrowth and burring or resection of peripheral bone, which may weaken the end plate and result in implant subsidence. Although preoperative templating has evolved to an art form in total hip and knee arthroplasty, insufficient experience with disk arthroplasty, particularly with respect to major device failure modes, limits the development of useful principles with which to perform sophisticated preoperative templating for disk arthroplasty. Similarly, soft tissue balancing is now recognized as an important principle for optimizing stability following hip and knee arthroplasty. An analogous approach in terms of annular tension is likely to apply for disk replacement surgery but has yet to be developed. We have observed one case of progressive scoliosis and premature device failure that may have been due to asymmetric annular release **(Fig. 22.7)**. We currently recommend gentle use of a laminar spreader to judge the degree of annular soft tissue release on the right and left sides of the disk space following disk space preparation and prior to placement of the final implant. With some disk arthroplasty designs, this step can also be repeated with a trial spacer in position to determine whether the remaining soft tissue tension appears symmetric on both sides.

■ Clinical Outcomes

The early failure of the AcroFlex device provided a few valuable lessons. Despite durable performance with preclinical laboratory testing, 1- to 2-year follow-up of 40 patients with CT demonstrated a high rate of failure of the core. This unanticipated failure may reflect an inability to completely model physiologic spinal loading in the laboratory setting and also suggests that cellular processes and the biologic environment of the spine may have significant effects on material performance of disk arthroplasty devices.[27] Osteolysis and granuloma formation were also observed in four AcroFlex cases and reported as potential contributing factors in early failure. Thin-section CT with a slice width of 0.25 mm was used to detect early wear particle generation and also revealed development of periannular ossification within 1 year of implantation in all cases. Concern has been expressed that such periannular ossification may

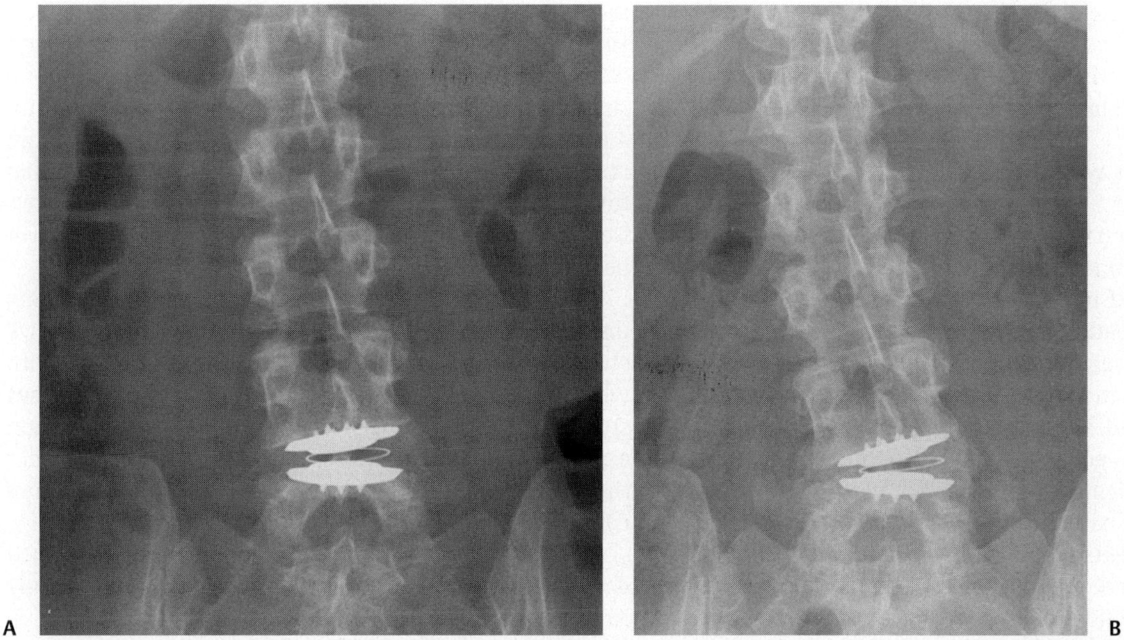

Fig. 22.7 A 45-year-old woman with L4-L5 single-level degenerative disk disease and discogenic pain confirmed on provocative discography. **(A)** Immediate postoperative radiograph showing asymmetric disk space release and lateral tilting of the implanted prosthesis. **(B)** Repeat radiograph 4 years after surgery shows significant worsening of the lateral tilt at the operated level. The patient experienced recurrent low back pain, and the patient was revised to a fusion.

contribute to loss of motion and eventual fusion of the disk space over time. As a result, many experts have recommended treating disk arthroplasty patients with steroids or nonsteroidal antiinflammatory medication in the early postoperative period.

The Charité has the longest available clinical follow-up and is currently the most widely implanted spinal arthroplasty device with over 7000 placed worldwide. In 1996, short-term 2-year follow-up for the Charité III was reported by Cinotti et al[28] with 69% good to excellent results in 46 patients. Average sagittal plane rotation was 9 degrees and complications included a 2% dislocation rate and 9% subsidence rate. Minimum 10-year follow-up data have been reported from Europe by Lemaire et al;[29] 100 patients underwent implantation at one to three levels with 62% excellent, 28% good, and 10% poor results. Mean flexion-extension motion was 10.3 degrees for all levels, 12.0 degrees at L3-L4, 9.6 degrees at L4-L5, and 9.2 degrees at L5-S1. Mean lateral bend motion was 5.4 degrees. There were no major device-related complications.

The best available clinical outcome data currently available are from the FDA-IDE study, a prospective randomized multicenter study comparing the Charité disk to anterior lumbar interbody fusion with Bagby and Kuslich (BAK) cages (Spine-Tech, Minneapolis, MN) and autologous bone graft.[30] Study inclusion criteria included age between 18 and 60 years, single-level degenerative disk disease at L4-L5 or L5-S1 confirmed by provocative diskography, a visual analogue scale (VAS) score ≥40, Oswestry Disability Index (ODI) score ≥30, and a minimum of 6 months of failed conservative management. A total of 304 patients were randomized 2:1, and yielded 205 arthroplasty patients and 99 fusion patients. Among patients undergoing disk arthroplasty, mean operative time was 110.8 minutes and mean blood loss was 205 mL; 70.2% of procedures occurred at the L5-S1 level.

Clinical success was defined as meeting all four of the following criteria: ≥25% improvement in ODI score at 24 months, no device failure, no major complication, and no neurologic deterioration. At 24 months, overall clinical success was achieved in 57.1% of arthroplasty patients and 46.5% of fusion patients. Mean reduction in ODI scores was 48.5% in arthroplasty patients and 42.4% in fusion patients. Mean reduction in VAS scores was 40.6% in arthroplasty patients and 34.1% in fusion patients. These results were statistically equivalent between the two groups. Among patients identified as having successful clinical outcomes, persistent narcotic usage was reported in 64.0% of arthroplasty patients and 80.4% of fusion patients. Complication rates were equivalent between the two groups. Overall, the study identified a trend toward earlier pain relief in patients undergoing arthroplasty and statistical equivalence in terms of pain relief and function between arthroplasty and fusion at 2 years.

Short-term radiographic data has been reported for the patients participating in the Charité FDA-IDE trial.[31] At 2 years, flexion-extension motion based on plain radiographs was increased by a mean of 13.6% compared with preoperative baseline. Mean flexion-extension range of motion exceeded 7 degrees. Both range of motion and clinical outcomes were significantly correlated with accuracy of implant positioning.

Reported clinical results for the ProDisc-L have been comparably favorable. Over a 3-year period from 1990 to 1993, Marnay's group[32] implanted their design in 64 patients. At mean follow-up of 8.7 years, of 55 patients with sufficient data, 60% experienced excellent, 15% good, and 25% poor results. There were no cases of subsidence or device-related failures. No difference in outcome was noted between one- and two-level cases. Observable motion of at least 2 degrees was demonstrated in 66% of implants, and among functioning implants, average motion was 7.5 degrees at L3-L4, 6.2 degrees at L4-L5, and 4.1 degrees at L5-S1.[33] The rate of radiographic junctional degeneration was 24%. Significantly less motion was observed in devices placed below a degenerated junctional disk (1.6 degrees) compared with those placed below a radiographically normal appearing disk (4.7 degrees).

Additional European data are available from a minimum 2-year follow-up study of 104 patients undergoing single level ProDisc implantation.[34] Mean Oswestry scores decreased from 53 preoperatively to 29 at 2-year follow-up. Mean VAS scores for low back pain decreased from 7.6 to 3 at 2 years; 96% of patients reported being satisfied or completely satisfied with their results at 2 years. No device related complications were reported.

The FDA-IDE study for the ProDisc-L included two separate arms for one-level and for two-adjacent-level surgery between L3 and S1. Implantation of the device was compared with anteroposterior fusion using femoral ring allograft anteriorly and pedicle screw fixation with autograft posteriorly. The 2-year follow-up results again revealed statistical equivalence between arthroplasty and fusion in terms of reported clinical outcome measures. Detailed analysis of the data from this study has not yet been made available.

One criticism of the published clinical data regarding disk arthroplasty, including data from the major FDA-IDE studies, is the absence of an explicit power analysis with which to judge the statistical conclusions of the relevant studies. Without reasonable justification for deciding upon a given study population size, it was distinctly possible that the studies were underpowered and that type II errors were committed.[35]

Another criticism is a lack of comprehensive published data regarding adverse outcomes and complications occurring in patients participating in the two major prospective FDA trials. A review of reoperations following placement of the Charité device has been reported and was based on a total of 589 patients undergoing disk arthroplasty as part of the FDA-IDE trial.[36] Overall, an 8.8% reoperation rate was identified with a mean time to reoperation of

9.7 months. There were 24 cases (4.1%) of device migration ≥3 mm; 22 (3.7%) of the devices were removed. In seven cases, another, typically smaller, device was reinserted. The remaining cases underwent anterior interbody fusion; 29 (4.9%) of patients underwent a posterior instrumented fusion at the arthroplasty level. A total of 14 patients (2.4%) underwent posterior fusion for persistent low back pain. Functional device survivorship was calculated as 93.9% at minimum 2-year follow-up. Fourteen patients (2.4%) experienced postoperative radicular leg pain, eight of whom underwent posterior surgical decompression with resolution of radicular symptoms. A significant majority of patients with postoperative radicular pain demonstrated left-sided symptoms, and the authors speculated that retractor injury of the left lumbosacral plexus during surgery may be a common cause.

Complications associated with the anterior surgical approach have been well described in other clinical series and include vascular injury, venous thrombosis, ureteral injury, ventral hernia, and retrograde ejaculation. In general, short-term device-related complications appear uncommon, and early catastrophic device failure appears to be a very rare occurrence. However, van Ooij et al[37] have reported a series of complications in 27 patients following placement of the Charité disk. In this small series, early complications consisted of two device migrations, four abdominal wall hematomas, and two cases of sexual dysfunction. Delayed complications included gradual device migration in two cases, one of which resulted in compression of iliac vessels and device subsidence in 16 patients. Recurrent or persistent back pain was attributed to a combination of adjacent segment degeneration in 14 patients and facet arthrosis in 11 patients, in addition to device subsidence. One case of significant polyethylene wear was reported 12 years following implantation. Salvage fusion surgery in 10 cases was associated with suboptimal results. Unfortunately, the significance of this report is difficult to determine without corresponding information regarding the original surgical patient population.

Because the Charité clinical experience is longer, there has been more analysis of device-related complications. End-plate fracture and device subsidence have been reported in patients with osteopenia.[38] Isolated case reports have also been published describing vertical split fractures of the vertebral body following ProDisc implantation as well as bilateral pedicle fractures following anterior dislocation of the ProDisc insert.[39,40]

In terms of the two major proposed advantages of disk arthroplasty over traditional fusion surgery, preservation of segmental motion appears to occur in a majority of patients over the short term, but prevention of adjacent segment degeneration has not been demonstrated. Reports of motion preservation based on lateral plain radiograph flexion-extension views should be interpreted with caution. Intraobserver and interobserver variability of disk arthroplasty motion based on this modality has been shown to be ±4.6 degrees and ±5.2 degrees, respectively.[41] Also, the occurrence of adjacent segment degeneration has been reported in several series of disk arthroplasty.[32,33,42] In terms of postoperative imaging with MRI, T1-weighted FLAIR (fluid-attenuated inversion recovery) sequences may provide improved and complementary visualization of adjacent levels when assessed with T2-weighted sequences.[43]

Published 2-year results are available only for the PDN nucleoplasty device. An international multicenter study of 243 patients found mean Oswestry scores improved from 52.7 preoperatively to 21 at 3-month follow-up, 12.6 at 1 year, and 9.0 at 2 years.[44] The VAS scores for low back pain improved from a mean of 7.1 preoperatively to 3.0 at 3 months, 2.5 at 1 year, and 1.8 at 2 years. Disk heights were evaluated for 218 patients and a sustained increase was observed from an average of 8.1 mm preoperatively to 10.5 mm at 3 months, 9.7 mm at 1 year, and 10.2 mm at 2 years. The most commonly reported complications included device migration, extrusion, end-plate reactions, and subsidence. With the original paired PDN design, complications rates of 25 to 53% were observed.[45] The redesigned PDN-SOLO device has been associated with a reduced complication rate of less than 10%.

■ Discussion

Proponents of disk replacement consistently suggest two potential advantages of disk arthroplasty over fusion: preservation of motion and prevention of adjacent segment degeneration. Unfortunately, neither of these issues is clear-cut.

An important but often unasked question is whether the amount of motion savings afforded by disk arthroplasty is functionally important to the patient. In contrast with hip or knee arthrodesis, spinal fusion typically does not result in significant functional loss. Given the segmental nature of spinal motion, the greater the number of levels fused, the greater the potential for functional loss and the larger the potential advantage of disk arthroplasty. However, the vast majority of disk replacements will be performed for one- or two-level degeneration. For three or more levels of degeneration, the appropriateness of surgical intervention in general remains unclear.

In terms of the second issue, a distinction must be made between adjacent segment degeneration and accelerated degeneration. Adjacent segment degeneration naturally occurs, but whether such degeneration occurs at a more rapid rate adjacent to a surgical fusion remains unknown. Suggestive evidence from crude biomechanical experiments has not been substantiated by strong clinical data. On the contrary, the best available clinical studies have demonstrated that it is surprisingly difficult to show that fusion leads to accelerated adjacent segment degeneration. Also, at least one finite element modeling study has suggested that disk arthroplasty may actually be associated with increased mobility of the adjacent untreated segment, as well as excessive forces on the capsular and interspinous ligaments and facet joint cartilage of the implanted level.[46] For a semiconstrained ball-and-socket type device with no rotational constraint, an increase in adverse forces was associated with more anterior position of the implant and a greater degree of anterior annular resection. The potential for segmental instability resulting from arthroplasty has also been suggested by the finding of a progressive increase in mean flexion/extension motion observed in the Charité FDA-IDE trial.[31] This increasing motion was observed out to 24 months without apparent plateau.

Conclusion

Perhaps the single greatest factor currently limiting success of disk arthroplasty surgery is lack of understanding regarding the very disorder it is designed to treat. There is no consensus regarding reliable diagnostic strategies or accepted indications for surgical treatment of patients with degenerative disk disease, and there are many experts who do not believe that disk degeneration even represents a distinct pathologic condition. Although widely practiced, fusion for back pain remains among the most controversial of indications for spinal surgery, yet back pain is the primary clinical indication for disk replacement surgery.

Available clinical data indicate that short-term results following lumbar disk arthroplasty are generally comparable to those observed following spinal fusion surgery with similar rates of pain reduction and functional improvement at 2 years in appropriately selected patients. A reduced initial perioperative hospital stay and more rapid recovery and return to functional activity may be short-term advantages of successful arthroplasty surgery. Early mechanical failure or migration of the device does not appear to be a major problem. Medium-term clinical data are limited but suggest that positive results are reasonably durable. Good-quality long-term outcome data are unavailable but are clearly critical in weighing the risks and benefits of arthroplasty versus fusion surgery.

References

1. Szpalski M, Gunzburg R, Mayer M. Spine arthroplasty: a historical review. Eur Spine J 2002;11(suppl 2):S65–S84
2. Link HD. History, design and biomechanics of the LINK SB Charite artificial disc. Eur Spine J 2002;11(suppl 2):S98–S105
3. Panjabi MM, Oxland TR, Yamamoto I, Crisco JJ. Mechanical behavior of the human lumbar and lumbosacral spine as shown by three-dimensional load-displacement curves. J Bone Joint Surg Am 1994;76:413–424
4. Gertzbein SD, Chan KH, Tile M, Seligman J, Kapasouri A. Moire patterns: an accurate technique for determination of the locus of the centres of rotation. J Biomech 1985;18:501–509
5. Pearcy MJ, Bogduk N. Instantaneous axes of rotation of the lumbar intervertebral joints. Spine 1988;13:1033–1041
6. Ogston NG, King GJ, Gertzbein SD, Tile M, Kapasouri A, Rubenstein JD. Centrode patterns in the lumbar spine: baseline studies in normal subjects. Spine 1986;11:591–595
7. Yoshioka T, Tsuji H, Hirano N, Sainoh S. Motion characteristic of the normal lumbar spine in young adults: instantaneous axis of rotation and vertebral center motion analyses. J Spinal Disord 1990;3:103–113
8. Crawford NR. Biomechanics of lumbar arthroplasty. Neurosurg Clin N Am 2005;16:595–602 v
9. Crawford NR, Peles JD, Dickman CA. The spinal lax zone and neutral zone: measurement techniques and parameter comparisons. J Spinal Disord 1998;11:416–429
10. Cunningham BW, Lowery GL, Serhan HA, et al. Total disc replacement arthroplasty using the AcroFlex lumbar disc: a non-human primate model. Eur Spine J 2002;11(suppl 2):S115–S123
11. Harvey EJ, Bobyn JD, Tanzer M, Stackpool GJ, Krygier JJ, Hacking SA. Effect of flexibility of the femoral stem on bone-remodeling and fixation of the stem in a canine total hip arthroplasty model without cement. J Bone Joint Surg Am 1999;81:93–107
12. Pidhorz LE, Urban RM, Jacobs JJ, Sumner DR, Galante JO. A quantitative study of bone and soft tissues in cementless porous-coated acetabular components retrieved at autopsy. J Arthroplasty 1993;8:213–225
13. Chosa E, Goto K, Totoribe K, Tajima N. Analysis of the effect of lumbar spine fusion on the superior adjacent intervertebral disk in the presence of disk degeneration, using the three-dimensional finite element method. J Spinal Disord Tech 2004;17:134–139
14. Weinhoffer SL, Guyer RD, Herbert M, Griffith SL. Intradiscal pressure measurements above an instrumented fusion. A cadaveric study. Spine 1995;20:526–531
15. Lee CK, Langrana NA. Lumbosacral spinal fusion. A biomechanical study. Spine 1984;9:574–581
16. Quinnell RC, Stockdale HR. Some experimental observations of the influence of a single lumbar floating fusion on the remaining lumbar spine. Spine 1981;6:263–267
17. Rinella A, Bridwell K, Kim Y, et al. Late complications of adult idiopathic scoliosis primary fusions to L4 and above: the effect of age and distal fusion level. Spine 2004;29:318–325
18. Seitsalo S, Schlenzka D, Poussa M, Osterman K. Disc degeneration in young patients with isthmic spondylolisthesis treated operatively or conservatively: a long-term follow-up. Eur Spine J 1997;6:393–397
19. Hambly MF, Wiltse LL, Raghavan N, Schneiderman G, Koenig C. The transition zone above a lumbosacral fusion. Spine 1998;23:1785–1792
20. Ghiselli G, Wang JC, Bhatia NN, Hsu WK, Dawson EG. Adjacent segment degeneration in the lumbar spine. J Bone Joint Surg Am 2004;86-A:1497–1503
21. Hedman TP, Kostuik JP, Fernie GR, Hellier WG. Design of an intervertebral disc prosthesis. Spine 1991;16(suppl):S256–S260
22. Mathews HH, Lehuec JC, Friesem T, Zdeblick T, Eisermann L. Design rationale and biomechanics of Maverick Total Disc arthroplasty with early clinical results. Spine J 2004;4(suppl):268S–275S
23. Devane PA, Robinson EJ, Bourne RB, Rorabeck CH, Nayak NN, Horne JG. Measurement of polyethylene wear in acetabular components

inserted with and without cement. A randomized trial. J Bone Joint Surg Am 1997;79:682–689
24. Guyer RD, McAfee PC, Hochschuler SH, et al. Prospective randomized study of the Charite artificial disc: data from two investigational centers. Spine J 2004;4:252S–259S
25. LeHuec JC, Kiaer T, Friesem T, Mathews H, Liu M, Eisermann L. Shock absorption in lumbar disc prosthesis: a preliminary mechanical study. J Spinal Disord Tech 2003;16:346–351
26. Mistry DN, Robertson PA. Radiologic landmark accuracy for optimum coronal placement of total disc arthroplasty in the lumbar spine. J Spinal Disord Tech 2006;19:231–236
27. Fraser RD, Ross RE, Lowery GL, Freeman BJ, Dolan M. AcroFlex design and results. Spine J 2004;4:245S–251S
28. Cinotti G, David T, Postacchini F. Results of disc prosthesis after a minimum follow-up period of 2 years. Spine 1996;21:995–1000
29. Lemaire JP, Carrier H, Sariali el H, Skalli W, Lavaste F. Clinical and radiological outcomes with the Charite artificial disc: a 10-year minimum follow-up. J Spinal Disord Tech 2005;18:353–359
30. Blumenthal S, McAfee PC, Guyer RD, et al. A prospective, randomized, multicenter Food and Drug Administration investigational device exemptions study of lumbar total disc replacement with the CHARITE artificial disc versus lumbar fusion: part I: evaluation of clinical outcomes. Spine 2005;30:1565–1575 discussion E1387–1591
31. McAfee PC, Cunningham B, Holsapple G, et al. A prospective, randomized, multicenter Food and Drug Administration investigational device exemption study of lumbar total disc replacement with the CHARITE artificial disc versus lumbar fusion: part II: evaluation of radiographic outcomes and correlation of surgical technique accuracy with clinical outcomes. Spine 2005;30:1576–1583 discussion E1388–1590
32. Tropiano P, Huang RC, Girardi FP, Cammisa FP, Marnay T. Lumbar total disc replacement. Seven to eleven-year follow-up. J Bone Joint Surg Am 2005;87:490–496
33. Huang RC, Girardi FP, Cammisa FP, Tropiano P, Marnay T. Long-term flexion-extension range of motion of the prodisc total disc replacement. J Spinal Disord Tech 2003;16:435–440
34. Bertagnoli R, Yue JJ, Shah RV, et al. The treatment of disabling single-level lumbar discogenic low back pain with total disc arthroplasty utilizing the Prodisc prosthesis: a prospective study with 2-year minimum follow-up. Spine 2005;30:2230–2236
35. German JW, Foley KT. Disc arthroplasty in the management of the painful lumbar motion segment. Spine 2005;30(suppl):S60–S67
36. McAfee PC, Geisler FH, Saiedy SS, et al. Revisability of the CHARITE artificial disc replacement: analysis of 688 patients enrolled in the U.S. IDE study of the CHARITE Artificial Disc. Spine 2006;31:1217–1226
37. van Ooij A, Oner FC, Verbout AJ. Complications of artificial disc replacement: a report of 27 patients with the SB Charite disc. J Spinal Disord Tech 2003;16:369–383
38. Tropiano P, Huang RC, Girardi FP, Marnay T. Lumbar disc replacement: preliminary results with ProDisc II after a minimum follow-up period of 1 year. J Spinal Disord Tech 2003;16:362–368
39. Shim CS, Lee S, Maeng DH, Lee SH. Vertical split fracture of the vertebral body following total disc replacement using ProDisc: report of two cases. J Spinal Disord Tech 2005;18:465–469
40. Mathew P, Blackman M, Redla S, Hussein AA. Bilateral pedicle fractures following anterior dislocation of the polyethylene inlay of a ProDisc artificial disc replacement: a case report of an unusual complication. Spine 2005;30:E311–E314
41. Lim MR, Loder RT, Huang RC, et al. Measurement error of lumbar total disc replacement range of motion. Spine 2006;31:E291–E297
42. Bertagnoli R, Kumar S. Indications for full prosthetic disc arthroplasty: a correlation of clinical outcome against a variety of indications. Eur Spine J 2002;11(suppl 2):S131–S136
43. Neal CJ, Rosner MK, Kuklo TR. Magnetic resonance imaging evaluation of adjacent segments after disc arthroplasty. J Neurosurg Spine 2005;3:342–347
44. Bertagnoli R, Schonmayr R. Surgical and clinical results with the PDN prosthetic disc-nucleus device. Eur Spine J 2002;11(suppl 2):S143–S148
45. Bertagnoli R, Karg A, Voigt S. Lumbar partial disc replacement. Orthop Clin North Am 2005;36:341–347
46. Denoziere G, Ku DN. Biomechanical comparison between fusion of two vertebrae and implantation of an artificial intervertebral disc. J Biomech 2006;39:766–775

23 The Charité Study of Disk Arthroplasty: What Does It Really Mean?

Richard D. Guyer and Raphael R. Roybal

On October 24, 2004, the Food and Drug Administration (FDA) approved the sale of the Charité Artificial Disk™ (Depuy Spine, Raynham, MA) implant for the treatment of back pain in the presence of degenerative disk disease (DDD) of the L4-L5 or L5-S1 spinal segment after the completion of an Investigative Device Exemption (IDE) level 1 study comparing total disk replacement to anterior lumbar interbody fusion (ALIF) using Bagby and Kuslich (BAK) cages (Spine-Tech, Minneapolis, MN).[1] In this landmark study evaluating six primary end points along with several clinical end points, the investigators concluded that the Charité total disk was at least as effective as BAK cage ALIF for the treatment of single-level DDD. This event ushered in a new age of motion-preserving treatment and reconstruction in degenerative spinal disease. Furthermore, the Charité FDA study provided a benchmark against which emerging similar devices will be compared. The use of the Charité over the last 8 years has emphasized the importance of strict adherence to inclusion and exclusion criteria. Moreover, the longer term data achieved from the study have shown that the patients do, indeed, rehabilitate faster, do return to work faster, and do return to function faster.[1,2] Motion is preserved, and as longer term data are accumulating abroad as well as in the United States, it is apparent that the adjacent segment disease is less than what has been reported for fusions.[3,4] Although preliminary studies show the cost-effectiveness of disk replacement compared with fusion (Guyer, 2007)[5], they do not take into account the societal costs, which show even greater benefit.

The intervertebral disks of the human spine coordinate the complicated functions of providing stability to the spine while simultaneously allowing motion and absorbing load transfer. These functions are made possible by the disk's morphology and histology. The natural history of the intervertebral disk involves age-related changes, which result in breakdown of hydrophilic molecules, accumulation of waste products, and the inevitable degeneration of the disk.[6] The resulting disk height loss, osteophyte formation, and pathologic motion through degenerative disks have often been associated with debilitating low back pain. The mainstay of surgical treatment following an appropriate and aggressive course of physical therapy has been arthrodesis of the degenerative segment[7] since Hibbs preformed the first spinal fusion in 1911. Fritzell et al[8] in 2001 demonstrated statistically superior results in patients with low back pain treated with spinal arthrodesis versus a similar population treated nonoperatively in terms of pain and disability. Subsequent studies positively correlated successful arthrodesis with superior long-term results.[9] However, this procedure can best be viewed as a reconstructive salvage procedure where normal motion, and kinematics are altered. With the technology of total disk arthroplasty, spine surgeons have begun to develop the concept of motion preservation and restoration of normal physiology and function of the spine.

■ Lumbar Arthrodesis

Although it is a proven surgical treatment for DDD of the lumbar spine, perhaps the most concerning challenge with lumbar arthrodesis is the concept of adjacent-level degeneration. Multiple studies have demonstrated a 5 to 18% rate of advanced breakdown in the spinal levels adjacent to a successful lumbar fusion. In a retrospective review of 78 homogeneous patients with DDD treated with fusion, Gillet[3] demonstrated a 41% rate of radiographic adjacent segment alterations with 20% of these patients requiring reoperation with fusion extension at 5-year follow-up. Risk factors for both increased rates of adjacent level degeneration and need for reoperation included length of original fusion and spinal imbalance. Ghiselli et al[4] reported retrospectively on 32 patients undergoing L4-L5 selective fusion specifically evaluating the fate of the L5-S1 segment. Only 3% of the population suffered symptomatic degeneration at 7.3-year follow-up, regardless of the initial degree of L5-S1 disk degeneration. Ghiselli et al,[10] however, later reported on 215 patients who had a 27.4% revision rate at 6.7 years with a predicted rate of 36.1% at 10 years. Also, in the lumbar tapered (LT) cage/Infuse IDE study, it was found that there was a 10.2% revision rate at 2 years and in LT cages with autograph it was 13.2% at 2 years.[11] Similarly, Rillardon et al[12] reported on 121 patients undergoing lumbar fusion at 10 years. Revision rate in this population was 10%. Meanwhile, numerous biomechanical studies have been conducted showing in vitro alteration of normal motion segment dynamics. As an example, one recent study in 2005 demonstrated single-level ALIF with threaded cages increased the range of motion of the caudal level by 12.5% while increasing intradiskal pressure by 21%.[13]

Theoretically, maintaining motion at the degenerative surgical level may protect the adjacent levels from abnormal physiologic loads.

■ History of Total Disk Arthroplasty

To directly address the issue of adjacent-level degeneration by maintaining physiologic motion, numerous authors pursued various technologies of intervertebral disk replacement. From 1955 through the 1960s, surgeons attempted various means of injecting artificial spacers into the disk space following diskectomy. Specifically, Fernström[14] in Sweden explored placing stainless steel ball bearings into the disk space. Although the ball bearings provided favorable results while limiting adjacent-level degeneration at 2.5 years, 4- to 8-year follow-up revealed significant subsidence of the ball bearing into the vertebral body, and the technology was abandoned.

The era of modern total disk arthroplasty began in 1982 with the initial developments of the Charité total disk implant at the Charité Hospital in Berlin, Germany. An Olympic champion gymnast and, at the time, an orthopedic surgery resident, Karin Buttner-Janz invented and supervised the revision of the current implant that consists of two metal end plates and a polyethylene core designed to duplicate the center of rotation of a native intervertebral disk. The Charité artificial disk is designed to closely resemble and function physiologically as a native human intervertebral disk. A sliding ultrahigh molecular weight polyethylene core is captured by two cobalt-chrome alloy end plates in a completely unconstrained manner.[15] Allowed to slide, the core moves anteriorly in extension and posteriorly in flexion, thereby replicating the center of rotation of a normal disk[16] (**Fig. 23.1**). Translation of the core within the implant's end plates allows for six-degree-of-freedom motion around three independent axes, theoretically encouraging increased range of motion.[17] However, this also theoretically allows increased anterior-posterior shear forces across the facet complexes at the operative level.

This concept, combined with the unfortunate reality that some patients did not improve with Charité total disk arthroplasty, caused concern among investigators about the integrity and history of the facet joint complexes after total disk replacement. Trouillier et al[18] in 2006 prospectively examined the preoperative versus postoperative loads of the facet joints at both the operative and adjacent levels of total disk arthroplasty by conducting computed tomography (CT) osteoabsorptiometry, examining the bone density changes and corresponding load across the facet complexes. This study did not reveal abnormal loads through the facets at any level after total disk arthroplasty. Furthermore, it did demonstrate an increase in disk space height by approximately 1.8 times, theoretically recreating normal and physiologic disk space height. Another recent cadaveric biomechanical study may imply a significant decrease in the overlap of facet complexes and subsequent facet joint subluxation after increasing disk space height with total disk arthroplasty.[19] Nonetheless, both the U.S. and European experience with the Charité total disk arthroplasty has been positive.

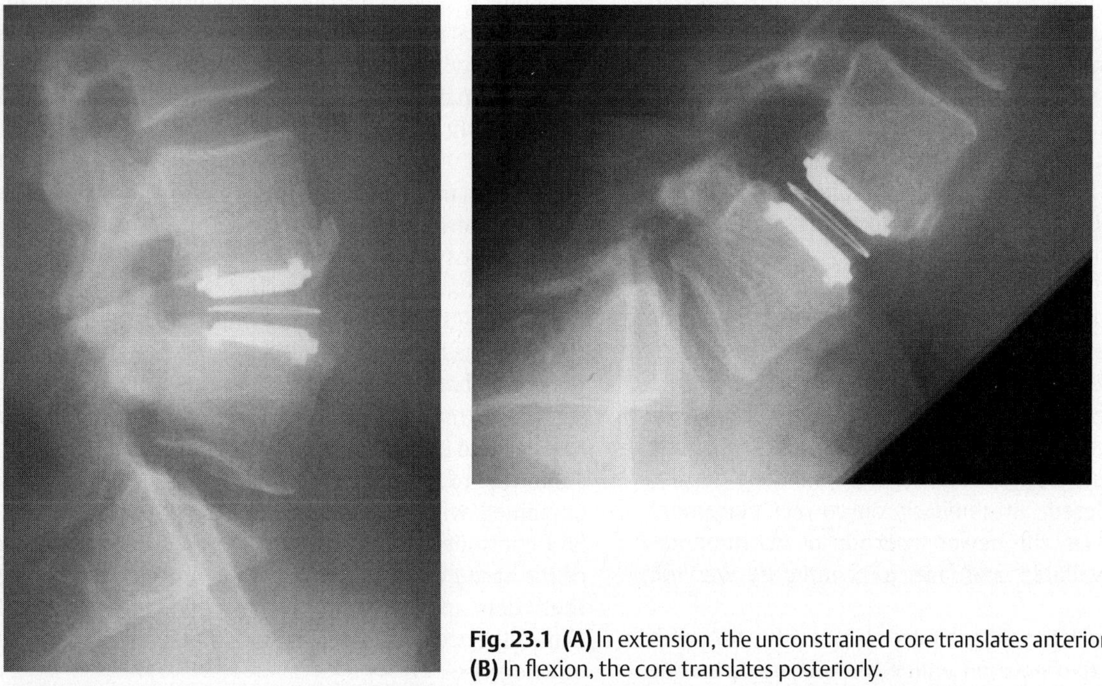

A B

Fig. 23.1 **(A)** In extension, the unconstrained core translates anteriorly. **(B)** In flexion, the core translates posteriorly.

European Experience with Charité

Since the initiation of the development of the Charité implant in 1982, numerous developments have been implemented that have improved the function and reduced the risk of subsidence. The currently used implant, available in Europe in 1987, was purchased by Depuy Spine in June 2002. Before the initiation of the FDA study, numerous studies had been published documenting the European experience with Charité at medium- to long-term follow-up.

In 2005, Lemaire et al[20] published their experience with the Charité total disk in 100 patients with a minimum of 10-year follow-up; 147 disks were successfully implanted, resulting in a mean range of motion of 10.3 degrees in flexion-extension and 5.4 degrees in lateral bending. Ninety-two percent of these patients returned to work, and only 3.3% of these cases were considered failures, all of which were treated with posterior fusion. Other important findings were that there was no statistical difference between single-level and multiple-level patients and that there were no complications of migration or spontaneous fusion.

In another study, David[21] reported at the North American Spine Society (NASS) annual meeting in 2000 his experience with 96 patients at 5-year follow-up. Although achieving excellent or good results in 75% of cases, he did report on various complications that included ossification around the implant, migration of the implant, and continued back/facet pain. Most recently, David[22] reported on 226 patients treated with Charité with a minimum of 10-year follow-up (range, 10–16). Presented in June 2006, the results included mobility in 87.4%, excellent or good clinical efficacy in 78.8%, return to work in 93.3%, and adjacent-level disease requiring reoperation in only 2.7%. In another paper published in 2003, van Ooij et al[23] reported on 27 patients treated at a neighboring European institution with Charité total disk with complications or unsatisfactory results. Fifteen of these patients required reoperation, and recurring complications included two patients with anterior dislocation, adjacent level degeneration in 14 patients, 16 patients with implant subsidence, and 11 patients with facet arthrosis. However, essential to interpreting this study is the fact that this subset of patients belongs to a population of about 500 patients treated by a single surgeon with the Charité implant. This represents a failed implant rate of only 5%. In addition, this study included many patients who had undersized prostheses, and furthermore the bone density was not considered, an emphasis on correct placement was not practiced, the newer insertion of instrumentation was not available, and facet joint integrity was not considered.

The European data have provided U.S. investigators with a plethora of experience on which to build upon for the effective and safe use of the Charité disk and total disk implants in general. Valuable lessons from the European experience included the importance of controlled distraction, patient selection, prosthesis positioning, and sizing of the implant.

United States Investigative Device Exemption Clinical Trial

In a prospective, randomized, controlled, multicenter FDA-regulated trial, the success rate of the Charité artificial disk was hypothesized to be at least as good as the ALIF BAK cage, thus making the trial a noninferiority study.[1] The FDA set forth six primary end points that the study had to achieve to be a success. These included improvement in the Oswestry Disability Index (ODI) by more than 15 points, a noninferiority margin of 10%, no additional surgery at the treated level, no major complications (vessel or nerve injury), maintenance or improvement of neurologic status, and no device failures. Secondary effectiveness end points included the visual analogue scale (VAS) score, range of motion, duration of hospitalization, and patient satisfaction. Radiolucencies were also observed, and more than 3 mm of displacement of the device was considered significant.

Between March 2000 and December 2001, 375 patients were randomized in a 2:1 ratio of Charité to BAK fusion. The overall success of the Charité, as measured by the above predefined end points, was achieved in 58% of patients compared with 54% of patients receiving the BAK cage fusion. Thus qualifying for approval by the FDA, the Charité implant was released in October 2004. However, the nature of this noninferiority study greatly underestimates the clinical success of the Charité implant. Closer analysis of the data reveals the clinical potential and efficacy of the device when considering patient pain scores, return to work, and patient satisfaction instead of merely considering FDA-defined success of meeting the preset clinical end points.

In summary, the Charité implant provided superior clinical short-term improvement in terms of the ODI, VAS, duration of hospital stay, and patient satisfaction at 2-year follow-up compared with the BAK cage fusion. At 24-month follow-up, 75% of patients responded that they would definitely agree to have the surgery again. Out of the 205 randomized Charité patients, only five patients had clinically significant migration (>3 mm) and all but one remained in place and stable after initial migration. In 2005, McAfee submitted to *Spine* data on all 205 randomized study cases combined with 71 nonrandomized "practice" cases, and 313 continued access cases preformed between the end of the study and the date of FDA approval. Key points of these data are that 92.4% of these patients at 2 years had clinically successful surgery with a mean range of motion of 7 degrees.

At the Spine Arthroplasty Society conference in 2005, Yoon reported on 800 patients treated with 825 disks. His data revealed a mean decrease in VAS for back pain of 5.4 and leg pain of 4.7. Ninety percent of patients returned to work within 2 weeks. He correlated less desirable outcomes with poor implant positioning, violation of the end plate, and patient obesity. The U.S. IDE study specifically analyzed the impact of implant positioning on clinical results. Superior functional outcomes in terms of ODI and VAS were attained with implants within 3 mm of midline on both anterior-posterior and lateral planes **(Fig. 23.2)**.

Analysis of the less than optimal outcomes also provides spinal surgeons with important strategies to avoid potential complications. In reviews of the Charité study cases, the training cases, and the continued access cases, the catastrophic complications of subsidence, anterior migration, and vascular injury range from 0.4 to 1.88%. Again, information from the European experience with Charité and from the now extensive worldwide use of the implant has led to strategies to avoid these and other complications.

In analyzing the economic data from the study, Guyer et al[5] showed that from the hospital prespective. Charité compared well with fusion procedures, being 12.0% less expensive than ALIF with bone graft, 36.5% less expensive than ALIF with infuse and cases, and 36.5% less than instrumented PLIF. When considering the payer's perspective, including the cost of revision surgery, the Charité and ALIF with bone graft were nearly equivalent (only 4.4% difference) and were 16.9% less costly than ALIF with infuse and cages and 27.2% less expensive that instrumented PLIF. Of note, the data were not compared with 360-degree fusions, but this comparison does take into account the cost savings for faster return to work.

■ Surgical Pearls

The success of the IDE Charité study proved Charité total disk arthroplasty to be at least as effective as ALIF BAK fusion for the treatment of degenerative disk disease. In fact, Geisler presented at the Spine Arthroplasty Society meeting of 2006 statistical analysis of the IDE study including the 71 training cases with the randomized study patients showing statistically marked improvement in Charité clinical outcomes versus ALIF with BAK cages. Although some critics may point out that the training cases may be positively skewed because of more stringent adherence to proper indications and patient selection, these critics fail to credit proper patient selection as integral to avoiding complications and achieving an excellent clinical result with the Charité implant.

The success of the study and subsequent cases relies on strict adherence to the inclusion and exclusion criteria. To avoid poor pain response and surgery at inappropriate levels, total disk arthroplasty should be performed only on patients failing conservative (nonoperative) therapy for 6 months or longer and with discogenic pain, which the authors recommend be confirmed by positive diskography. Patient selection is extremely important, not only to rule

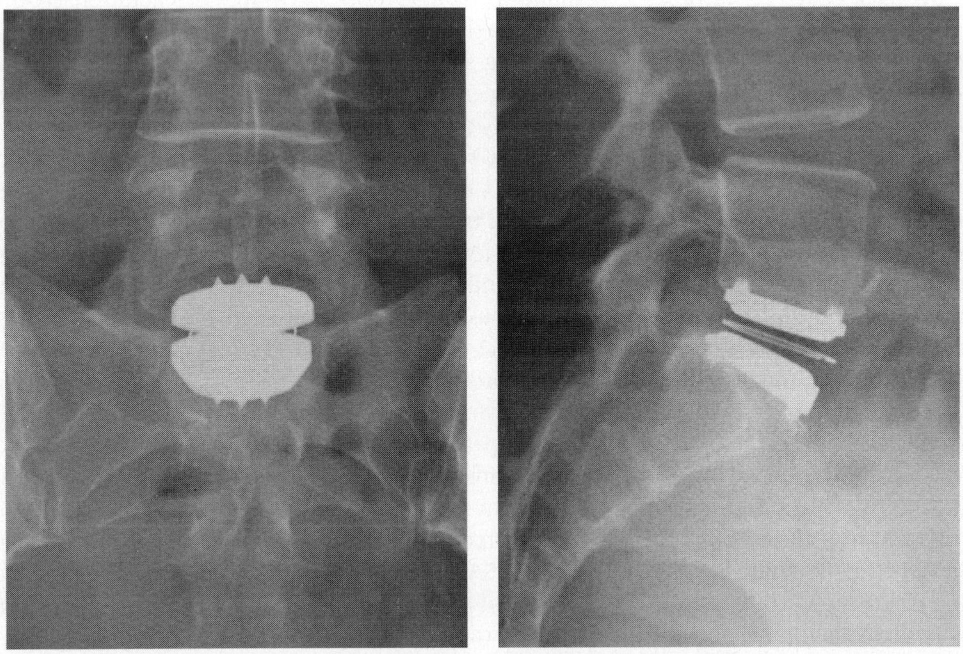

A B

Fig. 23.2 Anteroposterior **(A)** and lateral **(B)** radiographs demonstrating ideal positioning of the Charité implant.

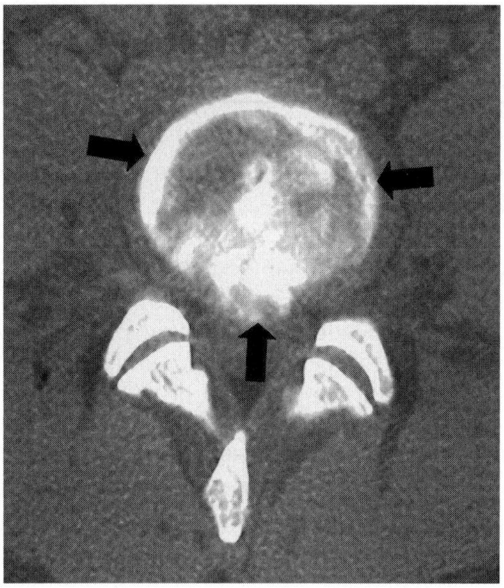

Fig. 23.3 Postdiskogram computed tomography depicting radial and concentric tears/morphology *(arrows)* while demonstrating facet complexes without degenerative changes.

out moderate to severe degenerative facet disease, as well as pars defects, but also to disqualify those patients who have underlying psychological issues **(Fig. 23.3)**.

Despite its apparent use in positively identifying pathologic, painful disk disease, diskography has proven to be a controversial diagnostic tool. First introduced from Europe in the United States by Wise in the 1950s, diskography was scrutinized by several authors who accurately described morphologic disk disruption and who correlated positive results with the presence of low back pain.[24–26] Carragee et al[27] have contributed to the controversy by reporting on patients with a false-positive concordant pain response. However, only eight subjects completed the study, and the methodology did not correlate abnormal disk morphology with a concordant pain response. In a more recent study, Madan et al[28] did not show a statistically significant improvement in surgical outcome in a homogeneous population with low back pain screened with positive diskography compared with another homogeneous group with similar low back pain not undergoing diskography. In contrast to these studies that were unfavorable to the effective use of diskography, Lim et al[29] recently showed a statistical correlation of concordant pain on diskogram with evidence of morphologic degeneration on both magnetic resonance imaging (MRI) and CT scan. Walsh et al[30] developed in 1990 the principles of modern diskography with accurate need placement (i.e., placed into the center of the disk), postdiskography CT evaluation, and less caustic contrast, while simultaneously demonstrating diskography to be a valuable diagnostic tool with false-positive rates between 0 and 10%. From these principles, many authors have furthered the effectiveness of diskography when combining a positively concordant pain response with morphologic disruption visualized both with MRI and postdiskography CT.[31]

Subsidence is a concern that can be largely avoided, again by strict adherence to inclusion/exclusion criteria. The IDE study excluded all patients with a bone density t-score of –1.0 or less as measured by dual-energy x-ray absorptiometry (DEXA) scan or with known metabolic bone disease. In the IDE study itself, this practice contributed to a 0.0% incidence of subsidence and less than 0.2% in continued access cases as well as cases performed after the FDA approval of Charité. The recent release of hybrid end plates with wider diameters without increasing the anterior/posterior dimension has allowed surgeons to better match patients' anatomy, providing more extensive coverage and theoretically preventing subsidence.

The anterior/posterior dimension is also significant not only for matching the native disk's posterior center of rotation, but also for preventing the potentially life-threatening complication of anterior migration. Complete diskectomy with particular attention to removing the posterolateral disk to ensure posterior placement and avoiding the temptation to oversize the implant allows for proper recession of the implant in the prepared disk space. The introduction of porous-coated end plates to allow bony ingrowth also enhances the avoidance of anterior migration. McAfee et al[32] demonstrated the effective bony ingrowth to be approximately 47% by 6 months with no evidence of histopathologic loosening.

The stability and integrity of the implant are also optimized both with patient selection and proper technique. Thoroughly evaluating standing x-rays with flexion and extension views prevents implantation in potentially unstable segments with spondylolysis. In addition, carefully choosing the correct angles of the implants allows the articulating surfaces of the end plates to approach parallel, thereby decreasing the shear forces across the implant and especially through the polyethylene core.

The IDE study was successful in establishing Charité total disk replacement as an effective, safe, and efficient means of treating low back pain caused by DDD at a level that is at least similar to ALIF with BAK cages. As long as the well-founded surgical principles of patient selection and meticulous technique are utilized, the IDE study and continued access as well as subsequent cases since Charité's FDA approval have shown highly favorable clinical outcomes compared with ALIF in the short-term. Now, with the European experience and the wealth of experience from the commencement of the U.S. IDE study in 2000, more long-term results are becoming increasingly evident. In a recent paper presented by Guyer at the Spine Arthroplasty Society (SAS) meeting in 2006, it was shown that the most important issue differentiating a selective group of patients that had the best results from a selective group of patients that had the worst results was the patients' length of time off from work prior to surgery, implicating the importance of psychosocial issues. This was the only variable that was significant among those studied.

The Future of Charité and its Implications for Total Disk Replacement

As the first total disk arthroplasty implant made available in the U.S., the Charité artificial disk has become a benchmark in both implant and study design in the field of motion-preserving reconstructive spinal surgery. In 1990, Marnay introduced a keeled total disk implant that would eventually become the ProDisc.[33] Over 3 years, 93 disks were implanted into 64 patients, achieving clinical success in terms of pain reduction, patient satisfaction, and low rate of reoperation at 8-year follow-up. These data paved the way for the U.S. IDE ProDisc study that was completed in January 2006. Final results from multiple centers involved in the study also are favorable and clinically superior to 360-degree fusion with autologous bone graft, and entail low complication rates and an average range of motion of about 7 degrees in flexion/extension at 1-year follow-up.[34–36]

As long-term data emerges from these populations, valuable information supporting motion-sparing technology will become increasingly apparent.

The revisability and survivability of the Charité disk has been explored by McAfee et al.[37] Comparing the 688 combined Charité cases and ALIF cages, index level reoperation rate was statistically similar at approximately 10%. Twenty-four total disk implants required removal for anterior migration greater than 3 mm. Of these cases, seven were revised to a different Charité of smaller size. The majority of the remaining cases were successfully converted to fusion with placement of intervertebral bone graft. Although only two of 99 patients in the BAK ALIF arm required surgery for adjacent-level disease at 2-year follow-up, the expectation is that long-term data will demonstrate additional cases from the fusion group with adjacent-level disease treated with additional surgery consistent with previously published frequency. The reoperation rate in the arthroplasty group was 4.6% and with adjacent disease was 0.6%, compared with 13% and 5.6%, respectively, in the fusion group. Huang et al[38] in 2005 reported their experience with the ProDisc implant at 8-year follow-up; 24% of 38 patients experienced adjacent-level disease. All of these patients had a range of motion of the total disk implant of less than 5 degrees. In contrast, none of the patients with 5 degrees of implant motion or greater developed adjacent level disease, at least implying that range of motion of 5 degrees is protective to the adjacent levels.

Numerous studies that are currently in press discuss several concepts of total disk arthroplasty, including the determining factors of optimal clinical outcome, return to work comparisons between disk and fusion patients, and the impact of total disk arthroplasty on the index level facet joint complexes as well as the adjacent motion segments. Undoubtedly, the numerous studies including both Charité IDE study and ProDisc IDE study conclusively show in the short term that disk patients perform at least as well as patients receiving the surgical standard of care for DDD. As these first patients progress through life with their disk implants, long-term follow-up will conclusively determine if motion-preserving spinal surgery will ultimately re-create functional physiology protective of the adjacent levels. Thus far, examining the available literature indicates a revision rate or need for reoperation of between 10% and 27% for adjacent-level disease in the presence of lumbar arthrodesis.[8,10–12] Revision rates for adjacent-level disease in the presence of total disk arthroplasty, in contrast, has been reported to range from 2.7 to 12%.[15,20,22,37] At the very least, patients do recover faster and they return to work faster while maintaining motion.

Currently, a multicenter retrospective review of Charité patients versus fusion patients is underway at the highest enrolling IDE study sites, evaluating the time to return to work as well as the return to work rate in these two groups. Comparing the two groups, Banko et al in their preliminary data have demonstrated clinical results similar to the original IDE study. Perhaps more relevant and indicative of the potential of motion-sparing technologies such as total disk replacement, Banko's data submitted to *Spine* in 2006 demonstrate that the Charité patients returned to work faster than the fusion patients by an average of 7 weeks.

■ Conclusion

The era of motion-sparing spinal reconstruction has begun. The Charité IDE study as an unprecedented study model initiated scientific and critical evaluation of motion-sparing technologies in general as well as demonstrated the clinical efficacy and safety of a particular device. As technologies expand and surgical techniques improve, new gold standards of treatment will emerge that serve as comparisons to novel treatments that may further revolutionize spinal surgery. As long-term data continually become available on emerging technologies, the accepted standards of care may shift, thereby increasing the accessibility of motion-sparing technologies to the general public. Research, perfection of technique, and improvement in biomaterials will follow accordingly.

Most importantly, the Charité IDE study has solidified the presence and potential of the first generation of total disk replacement, paving the way for the development of later generations of total disks. Second-generation disks will incorporate all physiologic functions of a native intervertebral disk, including varying degrees of load absorption. Third-generation disks will involve even more minimally invasive implantation and partial disk replacement as well as newer biomaterials.

References

1. Blumenthal S, McAfee PC, Guyer RD, et al. A prospective, randomized, multi-center Food Drug Administration investigational device exemptions study of lumbar total disc replacement with the CHARITE artificial disc versus lumbar fusion: part I: evaluation of clinical outcomes. Spine 2005;30:1565–1575
2. Hochschuler SH, Ohnmeiss DD, Guyer RD, et al. Artificial disc: preliminary results of a prospective study in the United States. Eur Spine J 2002;11(suppl 2):S106–S110
3. Gillet P. The fate of the adjacent motion segments after lumbar fusion. J Spinal Disord Tech 2003;16:338–345
4. Ghiselli G, Wang JC, Hsu WK, Dawson EG. L5–S1 segment survivorship and clinical outcome analysis after L4–L5 isolated fusion. Spine 2003;28:1275–1280
5. Guyer RD, Tromanhauser SG, Regan JJ. An economic model of one-level lumbar arthroplasty vs fusion. Spine J 2007;7:558–562
6. Twomey L, Taylor J. Age changes in lumbar intervertebral discs. Acta Orthop Scand 1985;56:496–499
7. Polly DW, Santos ERG, Mehbod AA. Surgical treatment for the painful motion segment: matching technology with the indications: posterior lumbar fusion. Spine 2005;30(suppl):S44–S51
8. Fritzell P, Hagg O, Wessberg P, Nordwall A. 2001 Volvo Award Winner in Clinical Studies: lumbar fusion versus nonsurgical treatment for chronic low back pain: a multicenter randomized controlled trial from the Swedish Lumbar Spine Study Group. Spine 2001;26:2521–2532
9. Kornblum MB, Fischgrund JS, Herkowitz HN, et al. Degenerative lumbar spondylolisthesis with spinal stenosis: a prospective long-term study comparing fusion and pseudarthrosis. Spine 2004;29:726–733
10. Ghiselli G, Wang JC, Bhatia NN, Hsu WK, Dawson EG. Adjacent segment degeneration in the lumbar spine. J Bone Joint Surg Am 2004;86:1497–1503
11. Burkus JK, Gornet MF, Dickman CA, Zdeblick TA. Anterior lumbar interbody fusion using rhBMP-2 with tapered interbody cages. J Spinal Disord Tech 2002;15:337–349
12. Rillardon L, Guigui P, Veil-Picard A, Slulittel H, Deburge A. [Long-term results of surgical treatment of lumbar spinal stenosis.] Rev Chir Orthop Reparatrice Appar Mot 2003;89:621–631
13. Rao RD, David KS, Wang M. Biomechanical changes at adjacent segments following anterior lumbar interbody fusion using tapered cages. Spine 2005;30:2772–2776
14. Fernström U. Arthroplasty with intercorporal endoprostheses in herniated disc and in painful disc. Acta Chir Scand Suppl 1966;355:154–159
15. McAfee PC, Cunningham B, Holtsapple G, et al. A prospective, randomized, multi-center FDA IDE study of the Charité™ artificial disc: a radiographic outcomes analysis, correlation of surgical technique accuracy with clinical outcomes, and evaluation of the learning curve. Spine 2005;30:1576–1583
16. Cunningham BW, Gordon JD, Dmitriev AE, et al. Biomechanical evaluation of total disc replacement arthroplasty: an in vitro human cadaveric model. Spine 2003;28:S110–S117
17. Buechel FF, Buechel FF, Pappas MJ, et al. Twenty-year evaluation of meniscal bearing and rotating platform knee replacements. Clin Orthop Relat Res 2001;388:41–50
18. Trouillier H, Kern P, Refior HJ, Muller-Gerbl M. A prospective morphological study of facet joint integrity following intervertebral disc replacement with the Charite Artificial Disc. Eur Spine J 2006;15:174–182
19. Liu J, Ebraheim NA, Haman SP, et al. Effect of the increase in the height of lumbar disc space on facet joint articulation area in sagittal plane. Spine 2006;31:E198–E202
20. Lemaire JP, Carrier H, Sariali el-H, Skalli W, Lavaste F. Clinical and radiological outcomes with the Charite artificial disc: a 10-year minimum follow-up. J Spinal Disord Tech 2005;18:353–359
21. David T. Lumbar disc prosthesis: five year follow-up study on 96 patients. Presented at the North American Spine Society, New Orleans, October 25–28, 2000
22. David T. A long-term multi-center retrospective study of 226 patients with the Charite artificial disc: minimum 10-year follow-up. Spine 2006;6:16S–17S
23. van Ooij A, Oner FC, Verbout AJ. Complications of artificial disc replacement: a report of 27 patients with the SB Charite disc. J Spinal Disord Tech 2003;16:369–383
24. Zdeblick TA. A prospective, randomized study of lumbar fusion. Preliminary results. Spine 1993;18:983–991
25. Feinberg SB. The place of discography in radiology as based on 2,320 cases. AJR Am J Roentgenol 1964;92:1275–1281
26. Collis JS, Gardner WJ. Lumbar discography: an analysis of one thousand cases. J Neurosurg 1962;19:452–461
27. Carragee EJ, Tanner CM, Yang B, Brito JL, Truong T. False-positive findings on lumbar discography. Reliability of subjective concordance assessment during provocative disc injection. Spine 1999;24:2542–2547
28. Madan S, Gundanna M, Harley J, et al. Does provocative discography screening of discogenic back pain improve surgical outcome? J Spinal Disord Tech 2002;15:245–251
29. Lim CH, Jee WH, Son BC, et al. Discogenic lumbar pain: association with MR imaging and CT discography. Eur J Radiol 2005;54:431–437
30. Walsh TR, Weinstein J, Spratt K, et al. Lumbar discography in normal subjects: a controlled prospective study. J Bone Joint Surg Am 1990;72:1081–1088
31. Resnick DK, Malone DG, Ryken TC. Guidelines for the use of discography for the diagnosis of painful degenerative lumbar disc disease. Neurosurg Focus 2002;13:E12
32. McAfee PC, Cunningham BW, Orbegoso CM, et al. Analysis of porous ingrowth in intervertebral disc prostheses: a nonhuman primate model. Spine 2003;28:332–340
33. Zigler JE. Clinical results with ProDisc: European experience and U.S. Investigation Device Exemption Study. Spine 2003;28:S163–S166
34. Bertagnoli R, Yue JJ, Shah RV, et al. The treatment of disabling multilevel lumbar discogenic low back pain with total disc arthroplasty utilizing the ProDisc prosthesis: a prospective study with 2-year minimum follow-up. Spine 2005;30:2192–2199
35. Delamarter RB, Fribourg DM, Kanim LE, Bae H. ProDisc artificial total lumbar disc replacement: introduction and early results from the United States clinical trial. Spine 2003;28:S167–S175
36. Zigler JE, Vialle EN, Burd TA, et al. Lumbar spine arthroplasty: early results using the ProDisc II—a prospective randomized trial of arthroplasty versus fusion. J Spinal Disord Tech 2003;16:352–361
37. McAfee PC, Geisler FH, Saiedy SS, et al. Revisability of the Charité artificial disc replacement: analysis of 688 patients enrolled in the U.S. IDE study of the Charité Artificial Disc. Spine 2006;31:1217–1226
38. Huang RC, Girardi FP, Cammisa FP, et al. Correlation between range of motion and outcome after lumbar total disc replacement: 8.6-year follow-up. Spine 2005;30:1407–1411

Index

Note: Page numbers followed by *f* and *t* indicate figures and tables, respectively.

D